1991
YEAR BOOK OF
ANESTHESIA®

The 1991 Year Book® Series

Year Book of Anesthesia®: Drs. Miller, Kirby, Ostheimer, Roizen, and Stoelting

Year Book of Cardiology®: Drs. Schlant, Collins, Engle, Frye, Kaplan, and O'Rourke

Year Book of Critical Care Medicine®: Drs. Rogers and Parrillo

Year Book of Dentistry®: Drs. Meskin, Currier, Kennedy, Leinfelder, Matukas, and Rovin

Year Book of Dermatology®: Drs. Sober and Fitzpatrick

Year Book of Diagnostic Radiology®: Drs. Hendee, Keats, Kirkpatrick, Miller, Osborn, Reed, and Thompson

Year Book of Digestive Diseases®: Drs. Greenberger and Moody

Year Book of Drug Therapy®: Drs. Lasagna and Weintraub

Year Book of Emergency Medicine®: Drs. Wagner, Burdick, Davidson, Roberts, and Spivey

Year Book of Endocrinology®: Drs. Bagdade, Braverman, Halter, Horton, Kannan, Molitch, Morley, Odell, Rogol, Ryan, and Sherwin

Year Book of Family Practice®: Drs. Berg, Bowman, Dietrich, Green, and Scherger

Year Book of Geriatrics and Gerontology®: Drs. Beck, Abrass, Burton, Cummings, Makinodan, and Small

Year Book of Hand Surgery®: Drs. Dobyns, Chase, and Amadio

Year Book of Health Care Management: Drs. Heyssel, King, and Steinberg, Ms. Avakian, and Messrs. Berman, Brock, Kues, and Rosenberg

Year Book of Hematology®: Drs. Spivak, Bell, Ness, Quesenberry, and Wiernik

Year Book of Infectious Diseases®: Drs. Wolff, Barza, Keusch, Klempner, and Snydman

Year Book of Infertility: Drs. Mishell, Paulsen, and Lobo

Year Book of Medicine®: Drs. Rogers, Des Prez, Cline, Braunwald, Greenberger, Utiger, Epstein, and Malawista

Year Book of Neonatal and Perinatal Medicine: Drs. Klaus and Fanaroff

Year Book of Neurology and Neurosurgery®: Drs. Currier and Crowell

Year Book of Nuclear Medicine®: Drs. Hoffer, Gore, Gottschalk, Sostman, Zaret, and Zubal

Year Book of Obstetrics and Gynecology®: Drs. Mishell, Kirschbaum, and Morrow

Year Book of Occupational and Environmental Medicine: Drs. Emmett, Brooks, Harris, and Schenker

Year Book of Oncology: Drs. Young, Longo, Ozols, Simone, Steele, and Weichselbaum

Year Book of Ophthalmology®: Drs. Laibson, Adams, Augsburger, Benson, Cohen, Eagle, Flanagan, Nelson, Reinecke, Sergott, and Wilson

Year Book of Orthopedics®: Drs. Sledge, Poss, Cofield, Frymoyer, Griffin, Hansen, Johnson, Springfield, and Weiland

Year Book of Otolaryngology–Head and Neck Surgery®: Drs. Bailey and Paparella

Year Book of Pathology and Clinical Pathology®: Drs. Brinkhous, Dalldorf, Langdell, and McLendon

Year Book of Pediatrics®: Drs. Oski and Stockman

Year Book of Plastic, Reconstructive, and Aesthetic Surgery: Drs. Miller, Cohen, McKinney, Robson, Ruberg, and Whitaker

Year Book of Podiatric Medicine and Surgery®: Dr. Kominsky

Year Book of Psychiatry and Applied Mental Health®: Drs. Talbott, Frances, Freedman, Meltzer, Perry, Schowalter, and Yudofsky

Year Book of Pulmonary Disease®: Drs. Green, Loughlin, Michael, Mulshine, Peters, Terry, Tockman, and Wise

Year Book of Speech, Language, and Hearing: Drs. Bernthal, Hall, and Tomblin

Year Book of Sports Medicine®: Drs. Shephard, Eichner, Sutton, and Torg, Col. Anderson, and Mr. George

Year Book of Surgery®: Drs. Schwartz, Jonasson, Robson, Shires, Spencer, and Thompson

Year Book of Ultrasound: Drs. Merritt, Mittelstaedt, Carroll, and Nyberg

Year Book of Urology®: Drs. Gillenwater and Howards

Year Book of Vascular Surgery®: Drs. Bergan and Yao

Roundsmanship '91–'92: A Year Book® Guide to Clinical Medicine: Drs. Dan, Feigin, Quilligan, Schrock, Stein, and Talbott

1991

The Year Book of ANESTHESIA®

Editor

Ronald D. Miller, M.D.
Professor and Chairman of Anesthesia and Professor of Pharmacology, Department of Anesthesia, University of California, San Francisco

Associate Editors

Robert R. Kirby, M.D.
Professor of Anesthesiology, University of Florida College of Medicine, Gainesville

Gerard W. Ostheimer, M.D.
Associate Professor of Anaesthesia, Harvard Medical School; Vice Chairman, Department of Anesthesia, Brigham and Women's Hospital, Boston

Michael F. Roizen, M.D.
Professor and Chairman, Department of Anesthesia and Critical Care; Professor of Medicine, University of Chicago

Robert K. Stoelting, M.D.
Professor and Chairman, Department of Anesthesia, Indiana University School of Medicine, Indianapolis

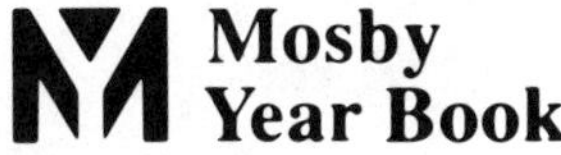

**Mosby
Year Book**

St. Louis   Baltimore   Boston   Chicago   London   Philadelphia   Sydney   Toronto

Editor-in-Chief, Year Book Publishing: Nancy Gorham
Sponsoring Editor: Gretchen C. Templeton
Manager, Medical Information Services: Edith M. Podrazik
Senior Medical Information Specialist: Terri Strorigl
Senior Medical Writer: David A. Cramer, M.D.
Assistant Director, Manuscript Services: Frances M. Perveiler
Associate Managing Editor, Year Book Editing Services: Elizabeth Fitch
Production Coordinator: Max F. Perez
Proofroom Manager: Barbara M. Kelly

Editorial Office:
Mosby-Year Book, Inc.
200 North LaSalle St.
Chicago IL 60601

International Standard Serial Number: 0084-3652
International Standard Book Number: 0-8151-5926-9

Table of Contents

The material in this volume represents literature reviewed through October 1990.

Journals Represented

Mosby—Year Book subscribes to and surveys nearly 850 U.S. and foreign medical and allied health journals. From these journals, the Editors select the articles to be abstracted. Journals represented in this YEAR BOOK are listed below.

Acta Anaesthesiologica Scandinavica
Acta Chirurgica Scandinavica
Acta Paediatrica Scandinavica
American Journal of Cardiology
American Journal of Neuroradiology
American Journal of Obstetrics and Gynecology
American Journal of Physiology
American Journal of Public Health
American Journal of Roentgenology
American Journal of Surgery
American Review of Respiratory Disease
American Surgeon
Anaesthesia
Anesthesia and Analgesia
Anesthesia and Intensive Care
Anesthesiology
Annals Chirurgiae et Gynaecologiae
Annals of Emergency Medicine
Annals of Internal Medicine
Annals of Surgery
Annals of Thoracic Surgery
Annals of Vascular Surgery
Annals of the Royal College of Surgeons of England
Archives of Emergency Medicine
Archives of Internal Medicine
Archives of Surgery
British Journal of Anaesthesia
British Journal of Radiology
British Journal of Surgery
British Journal of Urology
British Medical Journal
Canadian Journal of Anaesthesia
Canadian Journal of Surgery
Chest
Circulation
Clinical Pharmacology and Therapeutics
Critical Care Medicine
Diseases of the Colon and Rectum
European Heart Journal
European Respiratory Journal
Intensive Care Medicine
Israel Journal of Medical Sciences
Journal of Allergy and Clinical Immunology
Journal of Applied Physiology

Journal of Biomedical Engineering
Journal of Bone and Joint Surgery (American Volume)
Journal of Electrocardiology
Journal of Laboratory and Clinical Medicine
Journal of Obstetrics and Gynaecology
Journal of Occupational Medicine
Journal of Parenteral and Enteral Nutrition
Journal of Thoracic and Cardiovascular Surgery
Journal of Trauma
Journal of Vascular Surgery
Journal of the American College of Cardiology
Journal of the American Medical Association
Lancet
Laryngoscope
Nature
New England Journal of Medicine
Obstetrics and Gynecology
Oral Surgery, Oral Medicine, Oral Pathology
Pain
Pediatric Emergency Care
Pediatric Pulmonology
Proceedings of the National Academy of Sciences
Radiology
Regional Anesthesia
S.A.M.J./S.A.M.T.—South African Medical Journal
Scandinavian Journal of Thoracic and Cardiovascular Surgery
Surgery
Surgery, Gynecology and Obstetrics
Therapeutic Drug Monitoring
Thorax

STANDARD ABBREVIATIONS

The following terms are abbreviated in this edition: acquired immunodeficiency syndrome (AIDS), central nervous system (CNS), cerebrospinal fluid (CSF), computed tomography (CT), electrocardiography (ECG), and human immunodeficiency virus (HIV).

Introduction

The 1991 YEAR BOOK OF ANESTHESIA continues to emphasize articles that are of special concern to anesthesia in particular and to society overall. It is increasingly difficult for anesthesiologists to keep themselves well informed because of the exponentially increasing numbers of journals and publications that are available. In his recent address to the International Anesthesia Research Society, the outgoing Editor-in-Chief of *Anesthesia and Analgesia*, Dr. Nicholas Greene, M.D., suggested that one of the adverse effects of the increasing number of publications is to dilute the impact of significant and important contributions to our literature. Putting this concept more bluntly, it is often more difficult to identify the important articles because so many relatively unimportant articles have to be screened initially.

The YEAR BOOK OF ANESTHESIA has more than a 30-year history of attempting to provide a synopsis and screening of the literature. The selections of the Editorial Board undoubtedly reflect some biased views because of our own interests, but we nevertheless have attempted to synthesize all of the literature to provide readers with a more concise approach to selecting that which is "important." Recognizing that most readers will read well-established journals, we have often paid particular attention to those journals that are not widely read by anesthesiologists.

Although many areas are covered in this 1991 YEAR BOOK OF ANESTHESIA, there continues to be an increasing emphasis on operating room environment. This emphasis ranges from the toxicity of anesthetics and the risk of hepatitis and AIDS to operating room personnel, to the effects of the environment on patients themselves, e.g., noise. Furthermore, there are increasing numbers of articles examining the cost and efficiency of utilizing the operating room. These are now starting to appear in the YEAR BOOK OF ANESTHESIA. Undoubtedly, epidemiologically based articles will become increasingly important as society and third-party carriers demand to know how effective health care is. It is distressing to have individuals outside the medical profession intruding into our arena, but the Editorial Board feels that some of their concerns are legitimate and "outcome" studies need to be emphasized.

As before, the Editorial Board of the YEAR BOOK OF ANESTHESIA will continue to seek out those anesthetic-related articles that provide a broad spectrum of clinical and scientific data as they relate to anesthesia.

Ronald D. Miller, M.D.

1 General

Anesthetic Practice

Designing a Practice Policy: Standards, Guidelines, and Options
Eddy DM (Duke Univ)
JAMA 263:3077–3084, 1990   1–1

The process of designing a practice policy is analogous to making a decision for an individual patient except that it is much more complex and of great potential importance. The higher stakes involved magnify the effect of uncertainty. Practitioners must have flexibility to tailor a policy to individual cases. Although standards are intended to be applied rigidly, guidelines are more flexible, although they usually should be followed. Options, in contrast, are neutral with respect to recommending an intervention. Nearly universal agreement is needed to formulate standards, and appreciable agreement is required for writing guidelines. If preferences for a given option are split, practitioners must describe outcomes to their patients.

An example of this approach is colorectal cancer screening, which, because of a lack of information on the desirability of various outcomes to patients, is an option. Few standards actually exist, because information on outcomes and preferences relating to many interventions is lacking. The term standard should not be used unless outcomes and preferences are truly known and the preferences are virtually unanimous. Although it may be difficult and time consuming to discuss outcomes and preferences with patients, such practice accords with a strong tradition of individual decision making. Most practicioners resent being thought of as mere technologists who follow preformed rules. Discussing options with patients is the heart of the physician-patient relationship.

▶ This article is another in the excellent series by David Eddy on clinical decision making that attempts to teach us how to influence the guidelines set by policymakers concerning how practice will be reimbursed and what utilization to expect in the next decade. Dr. Eddy is very good at describing what can and can't be done. He defines standards, guidelines, and options. Practitioners, he states, must be given flexibility to tailor policy to individual cases. Standards are intended to be applied rigidly. They must be followed in virtually all cases. He says that there will be few standards because we lack information on outcomes and patient preferences related to many interventions. He goes on to define guidelines. Guidelines are intended to be more flexible, but they should be followed in most cases. He further states that guidelines can and should be tailored to fit individual needs.

Options are neutral with respect to recommending the use of an intervention. He then details the need to understand outcomes before one can write about whether something should or should not be a policy. The outcome could be death or life, but the probability of the outcome must be known with some degree of certainty. To write a standard for or against the use of something, the main health and economic consequences of the intervention must be known sufficiently well, he states, to permit decisions, and there must be virtual unanimity among patients and physicians about the desired outcome and probability of the outcome.

An indication that outcomes are sufficiently well known, he states, is that policymakers should be able to fill out what he calls a balance sheet, referred to in a previous article (1). This balance sheet article, I think, is important reading for everyone; it states basically that one should be able to look at benefits and risks of both patient outcomes for health and in terms of dollar cost and risks to individual patients. For instance, he says, about the strategy of screening for colorectal cancer in high-risk populations, i.e., those in which a first-degree relative has cancer, to do the fecal occult blood test and sigmoidoscopy — the preferred approach because of its lesser risk and higher benefit than other strategies — would decrease the risk of colon cancer from 10.3% over a 26-year period to 7.3%, and the probability that an individual would die of colon cancer goes down by 2.4%. On the cost side of the balance sheet, 40% of individuals who have false positive test results will undergo more invasive testing than they might otherwise; further, because of this more invasive testing, 3 of every 1,000 persons will have colon perforations and need reparative surgery that would not have been needed had they not been screened.

He further states that with screening there is an increased dollar cost to society based on both the extra cost of the screening and of the treatment. He also states that this is in face even of the strategy of treating the additional individuals in whom colon cancer develops but who were not screened. He goes on to say that, on average, the length of life saved because of fecal occult blood screening is approximately 1 month per person. He states that we don't know the preference for screening, but when he asked various medical groups and health professionals what their preferences were, their wish to undergo this screening ranged from 100% to less than 5%.

Thus he believes that colorectal screening in high-risk groups cannot be a standard or even a guideline but should be presented as an option. He goes on to say that, to write a guideline, at least some of the important outcomes of an intervention must be known, and what is known about the outcomes must be preferred or not preferred by an appreciable, but not necessarily unanimous, majority of people. Such a majority might be said to exist if 60% to 95% agreed on the overall desirability of an intervention. That is why, in the fecal occult blood and sigmoidoscopy screening process for colorectal cancer, this cannot be a guideline but must be an option.

He further states that the classification of practice policies has important implications because (1) we lack information on outcomes and the probability of outcomes, and (2) because it is dangerous to call something a standard unless the outcomes are truly known, the preferences are truly known, and the preferences are truly virtually unanimous.

I think we're lucky as a specialty, because the standards written today (as of for medical care services and would be unable to pay for them. Presently, health care in most provinces consumes more than one third of the total provincial budget, and costs are still rising. A heated debate is ongoing over whether Canada can continue the publicly funded universal health care system. The politicians are restricting access to medical care, and they have blamed physicians for the crisis.

One scenario of where American medicine will be at the end of this century involves increased funding for health care for the poor from a direct tax increase or other form of taxation and coverage for all working Americans by a basic employer-funded program. Costs of care will decline as insurance companies pay health benefits according to scientifically developed guidelines. Health maintenance organizations will be limited to Kaiser-style staff model plans.

Another scenario involves a governmental 1-payer system with unlimited demand for services, as in Canada. Delays in testing and treatment will result, and physicians will be blamed for overusing resources to increase their personal incomes. The overall quality of care will decline as physicians lose their autonomy. The quality of incoming medical students will continue to decrease. The choice will depend on the involvement of physicians in the process.

▶ This article is very important because it describes what can tip the balance between the scenarios of having meaningful free choice in American medicine with good access to care vs. a system in which practice parameters and administrators tell us what we can and can't do. Dr. Bronow comes to the conclusion that what could tip the difference between the 2 scenarios is our own involvement. Will we physicians lead, or will we watch from the sidelines? I recommend this article to you if you don't want to be told how to practice in the future.—M.F. Roizen, M.D.

Theatre Delay for Emergency General Surgical Patients: A Cause for Concern?
Wyatt MG, Houghton PWJ, Brodribb AJM (Derriford Hosp, Plymouth, England)
Ann R Coll Surg Engl 72:236–238, 1990   1–4

With less money now available for staffing and equipping hospital operating theaters, there may be adverse effects on emergency surgical services. The delay in operating on emergency general surgical patients was examined prospectively in a district general hospital serving a catchment population of 450,000. During a 16-week period the data on 204 consecutive general surgical emergency operations were analyzed.

After essential resuscitation the median delay in operating on emergency general surgical patients was 3 hours. A delay of more than 6 hours was experienced by 15% of these patients. Although an operating theater was required after midnight in only 10% of cases, 26% procedures were performed between midnight and 8 AM. Delays were caused by a combination of factors: theater delay was mentioned in 47% of cases, anesthetic delay was mentioned in 30%, and overrunning of routine lists was mentioned in 14%.

The results suggest that unnecessary theater delay results in an unacceptable number of emergency general surgical procedures being performed after midnight. If theater and anesthetic availability was insured in the afternoon and early evening, and if routine afternoon lists were not overrun, the after-midnight workload could be cut from 26% to 10%. This would result in more efficient use of theater capacity, cost effectiveness, and perhaps a safer emergency surgical service.

▶ This study was performed in the United Kingdom; efforts at cost containment in the United States will undoubtedly constrict our ability to respond in an immediate fashion. The data were objectively obtained with regard to what the delays actually were, but one wonders, how objective was the finger pointing?—R.D. Miller, M.D.

Outcome

The Outcomes Movement: Will It Get Us Where We Want to Go?
Epstein AM (Brigham and Women's Hosp, Boston)
N Engl J Med 323:266–270, 1990   1–5

There is increasing activity today directed at assessing outcomes, analyzing efficacy, and assuring quality. Federal funding of these activities has risen rapidly and presently totals more than $30 million. While acknowledging that research on outcomes is able to clarify the efficacy of different interventions, it may be questioned whether this information is sufficient for establishing guidelines for rational decision-making in medical care.

Emphasis on outcome assessment has come from pressures to contain costs, a renewed sense of competition in the health care area, and findings of substantial geographic differences in the use of various medical procedures. Emphasis on the use of large computerized databases continues to increase, offering the opportunity to conduct very large natural experiments. This approach is most useful when data on the severity of illness are available. A wider range of outcomes now is being considered, including functional state, emotional health, social interaction, cognition, and degree of disability.

An attempt was made to determine outcomes as a useful extension of basic clinical research. A focus on outcomes that are meaningful to patients (e.g., dribbling, rather than urine flow, measurements) is welcome. Much more controversial is the attempt to develop guidelines for the use of physicians in providing care and of third-party payers to insure the appropriate use of services. Development of guidelines may be particularly problematic when patients' preferences are an important factor in clinical decision making. There also are potential difficulties with the implementation and monitoring of guidelines. Expectations in this area must be modest if disappointment is to be avoided.

▶ This article details the development of the outcomes movement and shows how it came out of a number of individuals working together, but the person who was instrumental in popularizing the concept of health maintenance organizations (HMOs), Paul Ellwood, has also been important in popularizing this outcomes movement. The outcomes movement is a national program in which clinical standards and guidelines are based systematically on patient outcome. The author states that this movement is now being driven by research dollars, with the National Center for Health Services Research (now called the Agency for Health Care Policy and Research) given 1.9 million to spend in 1988, 5.5 million in 1989, and 30 million allotted in fiscal year 1990.

The outcomes movement is based on 3 factors: First is the need for cost containment and the substantial fear that administrative and payment policies designed to control the increase in medical services would have deleterious effects on the quality of care. The outcomes movement arose from the need to eliminate unnecessary expenditure and is part of the vital monitoring system directed not so much to improving the quality of care as to making sure it doesn't deteriorate. The second factor is a renewed sense of competition, and the fact that HMOs can no longer compete on cost and want to compete on quality; thus the outcomes measures of functional status, not just whether you're alive or dead, are being judged by HMO players. The third factor arises from the key work of John Wennberg and others who found substantial geographic differences in the use of various medical procedures not attributable to disease but to uncertainty by physicians as to what was right.

The Epstein article further shows how this movement not only uses randomized clinical trials, but also uses large computer databases, to look for retrospective outcome advantages of one treatment vis-à-vis another. He cautions us at several points: He says that, so far, there aren't good enough measures of comorbidity in the databases to provide meaningful answers, and also that our expectations must be moderate if we are to avoid disappointment. The danger we face is that we will undermine a healthy evolution and allow revolutionary zeal to lead us to carry a good thing too fast and too far. The result will be that rigid practice procedures will be imposed that don't allow for improvement in practice, or there will be unrealistic expectations on the part of policymakers that aren't met, dooming medicine to disrespect in the future. One can't help but wonder whether one shouldn't use David Eddy's balance sheets to do a balance sheet for all these practice policies. Are the costs of the practice policies worth the benefit? Have the few limitations in our standards led to improvement in quality of care? What has been the cost? Have some of the standards and practice policies and efforts to assure patients' well-being left us being less human in our approach to patients?—M.F. Roizen, M.D.

Death Due to Anesthesia at Groote Schuur Hospital, Cape Town—1956–1987: II. Causes and Changes in Aetiological Pattern of Anaesthetic-Contributory Death
Harrison GG (Univ of Cape Town, South Africa)
S Afr Med J 77:416–421, 1990

1–6

In analyzing anesthesia-related deaths over the period 1956–1987, distinctions were made between failure to control respiratory or circulatory homeostasis, complications of regional anesthesia, and miscellaneous causes (Fig 1–1). Mechanisms involved in the 145 deaths ascribed to anesthesia are outlined in the table. From 20% to 25% of the total were attributed to failures of airway management, pulmonary ventilation management, and blood volume management, and fewer deaths to failure of arrhythmia control.

Failures in airway management were the most common general cause of anesthetic-contributory death in this series. Apart from technical fail-

Causes or Mechanisms of Anaesthetic-Contributory Deaths (ACD)

Causes/mechanisms of ACD			No. of deaths	% ACD
1. Failures in control of respiratory homeostasis			83	57
Failures in airway management			39	27
Vomiting/regurgitation	5	(3%)		
Complications, ET intubation	26	(18%)		
Bronchial obst.	8	(6%)		
Failures in ventilation management			29	20
During operation	7	(5%)		
Postoperative hypoventilation				
Relaxant	20	(14%)		
Narcotic	2	(1%)		
Deficient post-op. nursing			7	5
Tension pneumothorax			3	2
Technical/equipment failure			5	3
2. Failures in control of circulatory homeostasis			51	35
Failures in blood volume management			27	19
Hypovolaemia/hypotension	23	(15%)		
Hypervolaemia/over-transfusion	4	(3%)		
Failures in arrhythmia control			24	17
Drug related	10	(7%)		
Vagal and other	11	(8%)		
Uncertain	3	(2%)		
3. Complications of regional anaesthesia			6	4
4. Miscellaneous			5	3
Total			145	100

(Courtesy of Harrison GG: *S Afr Med J* 77:416–421, 1990.)

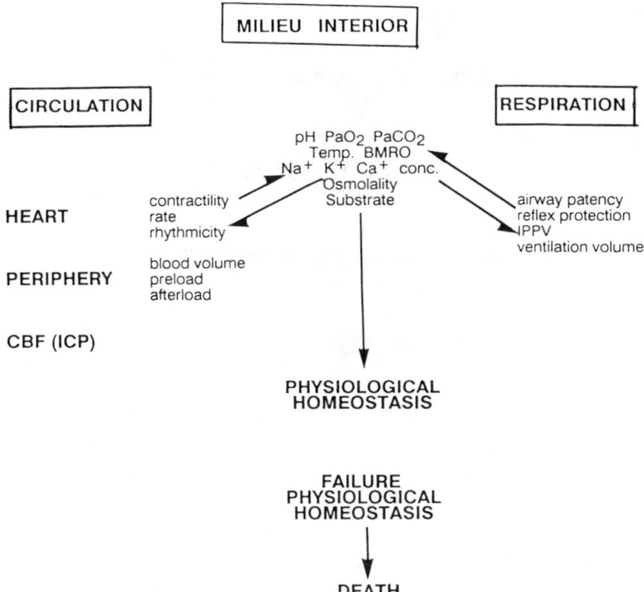

Fig 1–1.—The interrelated system failure of anesthetic-contributory deaths (ACD). (*Abbreviations: CBF*, cerebral blood flow; *ICP*, intracranial pressure; *Temp*, temperature; *BMRO*, basal metabolic rate for oxygen. (Courtesy of Harrison GG: *S Afr Med J* 77:416–421, 1990.)

ures of intubation after administration of a muscle relaxant, there were disconnections and dislodgments of the endotracheal tube and cases of anoxia as a result of failure to clear lower airway obstruction. Most deaths caused by failed pulmonary ventilation management occurred at

CAUSES OF DEATH EXPRESSED AS
% ACD BY DECADE

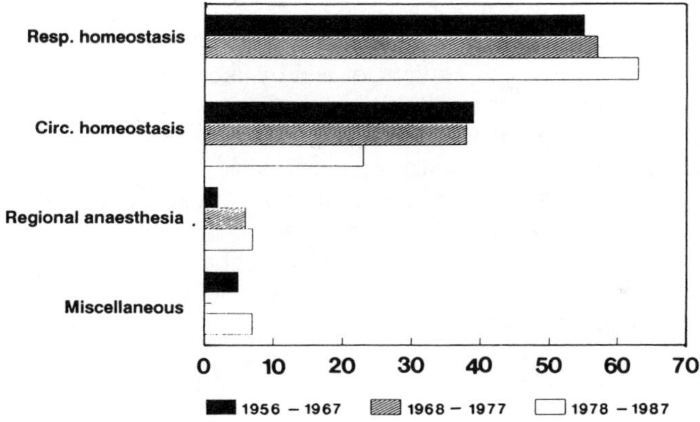

Fig 1–2.—Proportional distribution of causes of anesthetic-contributory deaths (ACD) by decade. (Courtesy of Harrison GG: *S Afr Med J* 77:416–421, 1990.)

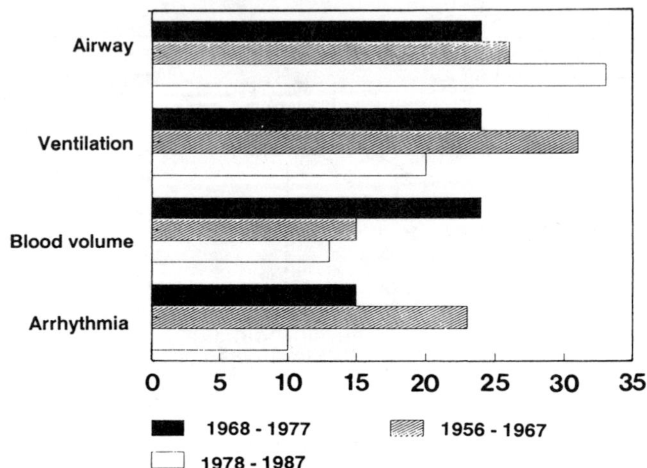

Fig 1–3.—Proportional distribution of the most common clinical management failures responsible for anesthetic-contributory deaths, by decade. (Courtesy of Harrison GG: *S Afr Med J* 77:416–421, 1990.)

the end of anesthesia or shortly afterward. The most frequent fault was the too-extended application of a "wait and see" policy after attempted reversal of neuromuscular blockade. Failure to control respiratory homeostasis has increased over time as failure to control circulatory homeostasis declined in frequency (Fig 1–2). Failures in airway management are responsible for the increase in respiratory deaths (Fig 1–3). Data on anesthetic-contributory deaths ignore the many cases of near-death. More refined identification of hazards is necessary to make anesthesia safer overall.

▶ This article reviews a large number of patients seen in a 30-year period at the Groote Schuur Hospital in Cape Town. It is interesting that no Methods section is presented in this part of the study, and the ways of reaching decisions are not stated. Thus this article, of and by itself, will not stand alone. One needs to read Part I on methods. Nevertheless, the article does imply that, from 1956 to 1987, there have been changes in the cause of death, with respiratory failure increasing and circulatory hemostasis decreasing in frequency. In addition, the overall rate of anesthetic contributory deaths decreased by sixfold, from .43/1,000 to .07/10,000 in this same period.

When one analyzes the deaths on an individual basis, perhaps 18 of the total 145 deaths could have been prevented by end-tidal CO_2 monitoring. More than 22 could have been prevented by appropriate monitoring of muscle relaxant effect, i.e., twitch tension. Thus, were one to design standards of care based on what kills patients and use this hospital as a model, one would institute a standard of muscle relaxant monitoring, especially for reversal, to be done before the institution of end-tidal CO_2 monitoring. Most of the respiratory deaths were related to failure of intubation after administration of a muscle relaxant; i.e., at no time could an endotracheal tube be secured—the surgical team knew it, they didn't need more monitoring to detect it, they just couldn't do it. This again brings up an adage that I was taught a long time ago: demonstrate that you can ventilate for a person before you paralyze him with a muscle relaxant. I recommend this article to anyone who has an interest in quality assurance because it does do an excellent job of reviewing the causes of morbidity and the patient factors that contribute to it.—M.F. Roizen, M.D.

Multicenter Study of General Anesthesia: I. Design and Patient Demography

Forrest JB, Rehder K, Goldsmith CH, Cahalan MK, Levy WJ, Strunin L, Bota W, Boucek CD, Cucchiara RF, Dhamee S, Domino KB, Dudman AJ, Hamilton WK, Kampine J, Kotrly KJ, Maltby JR, Mazloomdoost M, MacKenzie RA, Melnick BM, Motoyama E, Muir JJ, Munshi C (Mayo Clinic and Found, Rochester, Minn; McMaster Univ; Med College of Wisconsin, Milwaukee; Univ of Calgary, Alta; Univ of California, San Francisco; et al.)

Anesthesiology 72:252–261, 1990   1–7

A prospective trial of enflurane, fentanyl, halothane, and isoflurane anesthesia was carried out in 17,201 patients stratified as receiving or not receiving preanesthetic medication. Patients at 15 university-affiliated centers in the United States and Canada participated.

The mean age of the study patients was 43 years; two thirds were females. About 90% were ASA Physical Status 1 or 2. Just over a third of the patients smoked. Patients for whom any of the 4 study agents were considered unsuitable were considered ineligible. Access to data was limited to data management center personnel and members of the policy committee. The most frequent operations were musculoskeletal, gynecologic, and abdominal procedures.

This large randomized trial effectively matched the numbers of patients with each of 4 study agents in each participating center. Because data pooling was valid, the database will be a valuable resource for assessing the relative efficacy and safety of the anesthetics studied.

▶ This article is a model for those who would think of doing large outcome-based research studies. The authors had a policy committee that was different from the investigative group, and they had independent persons to stop or allow the study to continue. They designed their statistical tests appropriately and, after examining approximately 25% of the patients, estimated whether they would meet their goals. They did all these things right, yet they missed finding differences. Why? Was it because differences didn't exist, or because they didn't have a very sick patient population?

Thus, although 10 institutions and 15 hospitals participated in the study, it was basically a study of very healthy individuals; 90.7% were ASA I or II. When the study group is basically healthy, an awful lot of patients are needed to see if the anesthetic makes a difference.

The authors did the study right from a planning standpoint and from a patient enrollment standpoint, and there were no differences between anesthetic agents with regard to the criteria for entry into the study or the randomization. I think it's important to note this, because the study is a major event in anesthesia but a major problem may exist with it. If randomization doesn't work, the study isn't a random study even though it started out to be one. Here, in this study comparing isoflurane, enflurane, halothane, and fentanyl, randomization did work. The study starts out correctly, but are their patients typical of yours?—M.F. Roizen, M.D.

Multicenter Study of General Anesthesia: II. Results

Forrest JB, Cahalan MK, Rehder K, Goldsmith CH, Levy WJ, Strunin L, Bota W, Boucek CD, Cucchiara RF, Dhamee S, Domino KB, Dudman AJ, Hamilton WK, Kampine J, Kotrly KJ, Maltby JR, Mazloomdoost M, MacKenzie RA, Melnick BM, Motoyama E, Muir JJ, Munshi C (Mayo Clinic and Found; McMaster Univ; Med College of Wisconsin, Milwaukee; Univ of Calgary; Univ of California, San Francisco; et al.)

Anesthesiology 72:262–268, 1990 1–8

A 15-center study including 17,201 patients intended to compare the efficacy and safety of 4 commonly used general anesthetics—enflurane, fentanyl, halothane, and isoflurane. Patients were followed for up to a week after anesthesia. The study was successfully completed by 16,023 subjects.

In 7 of 19 deaths the anesthetic may have been a contributing factor. Rates of death, myocardial infarction, and stroke all were less than .15%, with no apparent differences in the various anesthetic groups. Severe ventricular arrhythmia was more frequent with halothane, and severe hypertension and bronchospasm with fentanyl. Severe tachycardia was most frequent in patients anesthetized with isoflurane. Patients given halothane recovered most slowly. Those given fentanyl had less pain in the first hour after surgery than did patients given other anesthetics.

There are few clinically important differences between major anesthetics in the large majority of healthy persons. It remains the case, however, that certain diseases and medications may contraindicate the use of 1 or more of these agents.

▶ In this article, the authors note the fact that before starting the study, the level of α error was set at .01 and the power of the test, i.e., the probability of accepting the null hypothesis when the opposite is true, was set at .95 for comparing outcomes among the 4 study agents. The 66 possible adverse outcomes listed were reviewed independently and without knowledge of the anesthetic used by a committee of 3.

The rates of 16 of 66 types of adverse outcomes were significantly different among the 4 agents, with severe ventricular arrhythmia more common with halothane, severe hypertension and severe bronchospasm more common with fentanyl, and severe tachycardia more common with isoflurane. The overall death rate in these predominatly ASA I and II patients was 11/10,000, with anesthesia contributing to perhaps 4 deaths per 10,000 persons. The rates of death, myocardial infarction, and stroke combined were so low that you would have to study approximately 200,000 patients overall before you would have a 95% chance of finding a difference of 50% between agents if, in fact, such a difference existed.

It is interesting to note that no patient with an ASA Physical Status of I died; 3 of 7,131 patients in AA Physical Status II died (.04%), 9 of 1,519 patients in ASA III died (.59%), and 7 of 88 patients classified as AA Physical Status IV (7.95%) died. Of interest to note is that nausea and vomiting were most frequent in the fentanyl group and shivering lowest in that group—things that one would expect and confirm one's impression about the reliability of the study.

This is a landmark study, and although the results are not very surprising, it is a study showing that, at least in health patients, when minor outcome differences are sought, one can find them. Perhaps a major outcome study is needed. Perhaps there is a difference in serious outcomes based on the agent alone, and not just based on the anesthesiologist. Although I believe that the anesthesiologist is most important to the outcome, I also believe that the differences between anesthetic agents make a difference to outcome in sick patients.—M.F. Roizen, M.D.

Comparing Benefits and Harms: The Balance Sheet
Eddy DM (Duke Univ)
JAMA 263:2493, 2498–2505, 1990   1–9

Medical decisions may be analyzed in terms of the consequences of the intervention under consideration, its benefit, harm, and cost. Take screening for colorectal cancer as an example: Screening may lower the risk that a person will have the disease or die of it. On the other hand, a false positive result leads to an unneeded and costly work-up and measures that themselves entail some risk. The expected costs of work-ups after false positive test results and of treating perforations may be offset by potential savings in initial treatment costs.

Balance sheets can provide the information needed to exercise clinical discretion and good judgment. They also help policymakers and decision makers to organize their thinking. There is, however, a danger that the use of numbers can falsely imply that outcomes are known more precisely than is in fact the case. The inherent uncertainty in the procedure should be described explicitly and the quality of the evidence should be specified. A present lack of adequate information with which to make out a balance sheet is the result of failing to ask the correct questions.

▶ I believe this is a very important article and series for us. David Eddy is essentially writing a series of articles in *JAMA* that appear once or twice a month on clinical decision making and are excellent articles to introduce the practitioner to "practice guidelines" or what the AMA calls "practice parameters." For example, Dr. Eddy presents a balance sheet of risks and benefits of screening for bowel cancer. Screening decreases the risk of an undiagnosed cancer, but there are probabilities of a range of uncertainty and the quality of the evidence that is presented. In addition, if you as a physician find something abnormal on a screening test, you then tend to do something that may increase patient risk, such as a colonoscopy or biopsy or surgery; the benefit of earlier detection must be balanced against the possibly increased risk of the next step that is taken.

David Eddy is very careful to present both the major dangers and major benefits of this type of analysis. The major danger of a balance sheet, he says, is that use of numbers might falsely imply that outcomes are known with greater precision than is in fact the case. He goes on to state that this can be guarded against by stressing the uncertainty, describing it explicitly, and describing the quality of the evidence. He further states that the main barrier to using balance sheets is the poor quality of the evidence. As he says, when looking at benefits and harms from any treatment, the major problem is that we do not have good information to fill out balance sheets today because we did not ask the right questions yesterday.

An important goal for the next 5 years, and one that the government is attempting to achieve by a major effort on the part of the Agency for Health Care Policy and Research, is to develop balance sheets for a thousand of the most important clinical decisions. We are in this era, and I commend you to read this series of articles by David Eddy that regularly appear in *JAMA*. I believe these articles are outstanding; they will educate us as to the limitations of balance sheets and of clinical decision theory so that if you are challenged about what you did, you will be able to speak with conviction and accuracy about why you did it and how you used your art to guide choices among the uncertainties in medical practice.—M.F. Roizen, M.D.

Pediatric Anesthesia Morbidity and Mortality in the Perioperative Period
Cohen MM, Cameron CB, Duncan PG (Univ of Manitoba, Winnipeg; Univ of Saskatchewan, Saskatoon)
Anesth Analg 70:160–167, 1990   1–10

Relatively little is known about the risks of general anesthesia for pediatric patients. Data were reviewed from a pediatric anesthesia follow-up program at Winnipeg Children's Hospital from 1982 through 1987, which included more than 29,000 cases. Most of the children operated on were healthy and 70% had no preoperative medical disorder. Infants younger than age 1 month were more likely to have major cardiac or vascular surgery, and older children had mainly orthopedic and otolaryngologic procedures.

Infants younger than age 1 month had the highest rate of adverse events both during surgery and in the recovery room (Table 1). Respiratory and cardiovascular problems predominated in this group. Postoperative nausea and vomiting were frequent in children older than age 5 years. Overall, adverse events occurred in 35% of children. Perioperative morbidity rates were fairly constant during the review period. Rates were about twice as great for children as for adults (Table 2).

TABLE 1.—Perioperative Events, Summary by Age Group (Percent of Total Anesthetics)

	<1 mo ($n = 361$)	1–12 mo ($n = 2,544$)	1–5 yr ($n = 13,484$)	6–10 yr ($n = 7,184$)	11+ yr ($n = 5,647$)
Any intraoperative event	14.96	7.31	7.10	12.22	9.69
Any recovery-room event	16.61	7.23	12.20	14.88	15.23
Any postoperative					
Minor event*	13.57	10.30	20.32	31.49	32.44
Major event†	23.82	7.51	3.26	3.37	3.33
Any event‡					
Among patients seen	48.89	25.92	37.50	50.52	51.33
Among all patients	41.55	23.47	33.16	45.04	45.78

*Includes problems with nausea and vomiting, sore throat, muscle pain, headache, dentition, position, extremities, eyes, croup, temperature, behavior, thrombophlebitis, arterial line, awareness, and "other."
†Includes "other respiratory" and cardiovascular problems, nerve palsy, hepatic or renal problems, seizures, surgical complications, and death.
‡Percentage of total anesthetics in which there was at least 1 event in intraoperative, recovery room, or later postoperative period.
(Courtesy of Cohen MM, Cameron CB, Duncan PG: *Anesth Analg* 70:160–167, 1990.)

TABLE 2.—Perioperative Events, Summary Over Time (Percent of Total Anesthetics)

	Children (%)			Adults (%)
	1982–83	1984–85	1986–87	1979–83
Any intraoperative	9.52	9.00	8.58	10.6
Any recovery room	12.91	13.24	13.03	5.9
Any postoperative				
Minor*	27.38	26.21	20.86	9.4
Major†	3.82	4.39	3.55	0.5
Any event‡				
Among cases seen	44.58	42.95	40.82	31.6
Among all cases	40.23	38.61	35.35	17.8

*Includes problems with nausea and vomiting, sore throat, muscle pain, headache, dentition, position, extremities, eyes, croup, temperature, behavior, thrombophlebitis, arterial line, awareness, and "other."

†Includes "other respiratory" and cardiovascular problems, nerve palsy, hepatic or renal problems, seizures, surgical complication, and death.

‡Percentage of total anesthetics in which there was at least 1 event in intraoperative, recovery room, or later postoperative period.

(Courtesy of Cohen MM, Cameron CB, Duncan PG: *Anesth Analg* 70:160–167, 1990.)

Neonates tend to have a high rate of perioperative morbidity. Respiratory disorders are an important form of perioperative morbidity in younger children, but gastrointestinal effects are more prominent in older children. The number of deaths in this study was too small to detect time trends.

▶ Large-scale epidemiologic studies such as this are necessary throughout the field of anesthesia to determine problems that can develop during the anesthetic experience.—G.W. Ostheimer, M.D.

AIDS

Recommendations for Control and Prevention of Human Immunodeficiency Virus (HIV) Infection in Intravenous Drug Users
Brickner PW, Torres RA, Barnes M, Newman RG, Des Jarlais DC, Whalen DP, Rogers DE (St Vincent's Hosp and Med Ctr, New York; Columbia Univ School of Law; Beth Israel Med Ctr; New York State Div of Substance Abuse Services; Cornell Univ)
Ann Intern Med 110:833–837, 1989
1–11

In New York City, one third of patients with AIDS are intravenous drug users. There is good evidence that drug users may respond to health education measures, and that they wish to know their HIV status to avoid infecting needle sharers or sex partners. Nevertheless, mandatory reporting has compromised attendance at HIV testing sites. Feedback of test results can lower high-risk behavior if combined with extensive pretest counseling and if confidentiality is assured.

Proposals to distribute free needles and syringes have elicited strong objections. Treatment programs must be made available on demand to reduce HIV infection. There is reason to think that education has discouraged high-risk behavior among sexually active homosexual men. Education must be an ongoing process.

Educational efforts can serve allied goals such as enhancing security, controlling medical costs, and discouraging drug use. Education presently is the only definitive way of controlling the spread of HIV infection among intravenous drug users, their sex contacts, and fetuses.

▶ This article summarizes current knowledge of the science of prevention and what we know about HIV infection. The article is disquieting. The knowledge we have about how to prevent infections, excluding the ability of immunization, is in fact small. We don't know if education works; we don't know what education factors work; we don't know even if giving needles works or has any benefit, or in fact just encourages the rest of society to use drugs. The assumptions the authors make in coming to their conclusions are grossly untested. This article is useful, however, not in its conclusions but more for the data it presents. I've been uncomfortable with our knowledge about transmission of AIDS before, but this article highlights the uncertainty clearly.—M.F. Roizen, M.D.

Farr's Law Applied to AIDS Projections

Bregman DJ, Langmuir AD (Univ of Southern California)
JAMA 263:1522–1525, 1990   1–12

In his Law of Epidemics, promulgated in 1840 and resurrected by Brownlee in the early 1900s, Farr stated that epidemics tend to rise and fall in a nearly symmetric pattern that approximates a bell-shaped curve. This law was applied to the reported annual incidence rates of AIDS in the United States from 1982 through 1987. The incidence data closely fit a normal distribution that crested in late 1988 and then declined to a low point by the mid-1990s. Approximately 200,000 cases are projected in the epidemic. The occurrence of endemic cases is expected to continue but at a low level.

This projection was based only on adult cases and should be increased by at least 12%. In any event, the AIDS epidemic appears to have crested and will probably decline steadily. The number of survivors will increase as medical advances prolong the duration of illness. Further experience will make it possible to confirm or refute the Farr-Brownlee concept.

▶ One can hope that Farr's Law and Bregman and Langmuir's interpretation of it are correct. It would mean that we've seen the worst as far as the rate of increase of the epidemic of AIDs is concerned, and by now, in 1991, it should be well on the way to a downward trend in the total number of new individuals with HIV infections. I think a lot of this depends on the success of safe sex education. Although I hope that the beliefs presented in this abstract prove true, I fear that they won't. Nevertheless, the public policy implications of this study are important and impinge on the money we are spending on AIDS and on what research needs to be done. The importance of this article, I suppose, can be judged by the fact that there was not just one editorial related to it, but several, in that issue of *JAMA* and in subsequent issues.—M.F. Roizen, M.D.

2 Pharmacology

Mechanisms of Anesthesia

Multiple Sites of Action of Volatile Anesthetics in *Caenorhabditis elegans*
Morgan PG, Sedensky M, Meneely PM (Case Western Reserve Univ; Fred Hutchinson Cancer Research Ctr, Seattle)
Proc Natl Acad Sci USA 87:2965–2969, 1990   2–1

The site and mechanism of action of volatile anesthetics remain uncertain, but studies to date suggest that the site has properties similar to the lipid used to determine oil-gas partition coefficients. In addition, all volatile anesthetics appear to act at a single site.

The nematode *Caenorhabditis elegans* is a useful model with which to investigate volatile anesthetics. Two mutants, *unc-79* and *unc-80*, confer large increases in sensitivity to very lipid-soluble agents but little or no increase in sensitivity to other agents. In addition, there are extragenic suppressor mutations that suppress some altered sensitivities but not that to diethyl ether.

Observations of the response to anesthetics in *C. elegans* appear to indicate that volatile anesthetics cause immobility of the nematode by interacting with more than 1 site. A pure lipid-binding model is unlikely.

▶ Although this article is of no clinical value, it does represent the state of the art in research regarding the elusive question as to the mechanisms of anesthesia.—R.D. Miller, M.D.

Mechanism of Age-Related and Nitrous Oxide-Associated Anesthetic Sensitivity: The Role of Brain Catecholamines
Roizen MF, Koblin DD, Johnson BH, Eger EI II, Bainton CR, Lurz FW (Univ of Chicago; Univ of California, San Francisco)
Anesthesiology 69:716–720, 1988   2–2

Brain catecholamine levels were measured in mice selectively bred for resistance (HI) and susceptibility (LO) to nitrous oxide anesthesia. The possibility of a relationship was considered because altered central catecholamine availability significantly influences anesthetic requirements. Drugs that lower CNS levels of norepinephrine or dopamine lead to a dose-related fall in the minimum alveolar concentration of halothane, whereas those elevating central norepinephrine levels have the opposite effect.

Whole brain levels of norepinephrine and dopamine were 26% and 13% higher, respectively, in HI mice than in LO mice. There was no difference in levels of 3,45-dihydroxyphenylacetic acid, a major dopamine metabolite. The norepinephrine content of the medulla, but not of other brain regions, correlated significantly with the N_2O requirement. Differences in both medullary norepinephrine levels and anesthetic requirements declined as the animals aged. Changes in catecholamine content in specific parts of the brain may underlie the difference in anesthetic requirements between HI and LO mice.

▶ It is difficult to comment on one's own work, but this paper is one of the end products of a long line of outstanding research done by Don Koblin and Ted Eger with whom I was lucky enough to participate. It relates to the basic mechanism of anesthesia. The model that was developed by Don Koblin relates to a genetic predisposition to have either large or small anesthetic requirements and the production of that state over 20 generations. At least part of the anesthetic mechanism may be induced by a change in brain catecholamines in small areas of the brain that may induce confirmational changes in other receptor moieties that move toward the creation of the state we now call anesthesia.—M.F. Roizen, M.D.

Nitrous Oxide

Nitrous Oxide Does Not Exacerbate Pulmonary Hypertension or Ventricular Dysfunction in Patients With Mitral Valve Disease
Konstadt SN, Reich DL, Thys DM (Loyola Univ Med Ctr, Maywood, Ill; Mount Sinai Med Ctr, New York)
Can J Anaesth 37:613–617, 1990   2–3

Nitrous oxide is a valuable supplement to opioid anesthesia. Nitrous oxide increases pulmonary vascular resistance in adults, but the clinical implications of this increase are unclear. The effects of nitrous oxide on ventricular function and pulmonary function during high-dose fentanyl anesthesia were assessed in 10 patients with pulmonary hypertension who were undergoing mitral valve replacement or repair.

Patients were premedicated with morphine and scopolamine, and peripheral venous, radial arterial, and rapid-response thermistor pulmonary arterial catheters were placed. Fentanyl anesthesia was induced intravenously and a transesophageal echocardiographic probe was introduced. Then, 70% nitrous oxide/30% oxygen and 70% nitrogen/30% oxygen were administered in random sequence. Measurements were made when stable end-tidal concentrations were reached, after which 100% oxygen was administered and a "return-to-baseline" measurement obtained. Surgery was performed after completion of the study protocol.

Nitrous oxide caused small but significant changes in mean arterial pressure (Fig 2–1), mean pulmonary arterial pressure, and cardiac output compared with baseline values. There were no significant differences in reaction to nitrogen and reaction to nitrous oxide for any variable examined. There were no significant changes from baseline when 100% oxygen was readministered.

Patients with pulmonary hypertension had significant but clinically mi-

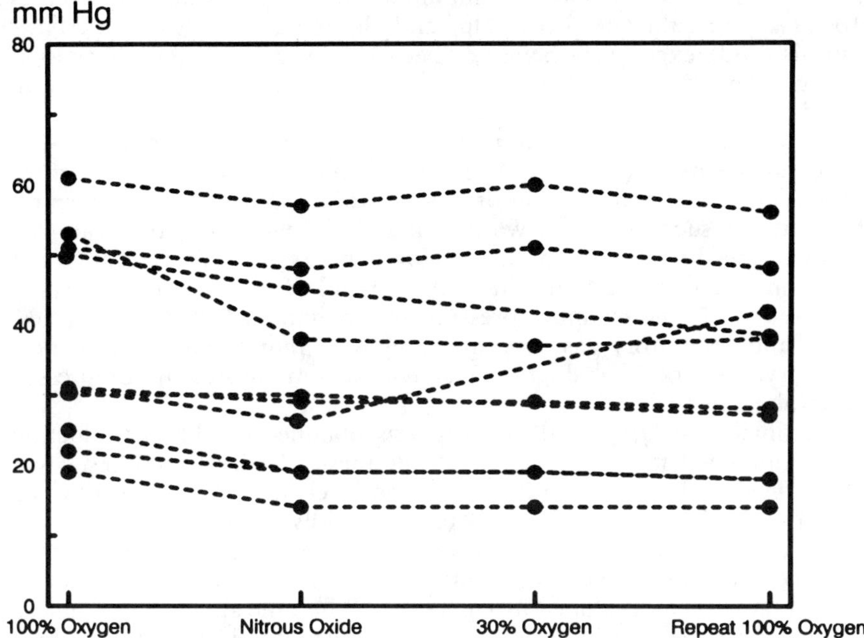

Fig 2–1.—Individual patient responses in mean pulmonary arterial pressure (mm Hg) to nitrous oxide administration. (Courtesy of Konstadt SN, Reich DL, Thys DM: *Can J Anaesth* 37:613–617, 1990.)

nor changes in mean arterial pressure, cardiac output, mean pulmonary arterial pressure, right ventricular end-systolic volume, and pulmonary capillary wedge pressure in response to nitrous oxide in fentanyl anesthesia. Nitrous oxide appears to have no adverse effects on either ventricle or on pulmonary circulation. With appropriate monitoring, it may be used in patients with pulmonary hypertension.

▶ I agree that nitrous oxide seems rarely to have detrimental effects on the pulmonary circulation. Nevertheless, a high index of suspicion should always be maintained, especially in patients with mitral valve disease and preexisting pulmonary hypertension. In this regard, unexplained increases in right heart filling pressures should be recognized as being possibly drug induced.—R.K. Stoelting, M.D.

Hyperbaric Nitrous Oxide as a Sole Anesthetic Agent in Humans
Russell GB, Snider MT, Richard RB, Loomis JL (Pennsylvania State Univ, Hershey)
Anesth Analg 70:289–295, 1990   2–4

Nitrous oxide is commonly used as an adjunctive anesthetic agent, but it cannot be used as the sole anesthetic agent. General anesthesia using nitrous oxide exclusively can be obtained only under hyperbaric conditions, as nitrous oxide has a minimum alveolar concentration (MAC) of 104%. Because the anesthetic value and physiologic effects of hyperbaric nitrous oxide exclusively have not been clearly defined, the physiologic changes that occur with hyperbaric nitrous oxide anesthesia were investigated.

Eight healthy male volunteers aged 20–31 years underwent anesthesia using nitrous oxide only in a hyperbaric chamber at 2 atmospheres absolute (ATA). After stabilization of blood pressure, pulse rate, and respiratory pattern, succinylcholine was administered, followed by tracheal intubation. Anesthesia was maintained for 4 hours in 6 volunteers, for 3 hours in 1, and for 2 hours in 1. At the end of anesthesia, awakening occurred while the chamber pressure was maintained at 2 ATA. Anesthetic and respiratory gas concentrations were monitored by mass spectrometry. Electroencephalographic activity was monitored by compressed spectral array analysis.

Maximal alveolar partial pressure was obtained quickly at induction and maintained for the duration of anesthesia. General anesthesia was maintained with end-tidal nitrous oxygen levels of 836–1,368 mm Hg, or 1.1–1.8 ATA. All 8 volunteers passed rapidly through the excitement phase to deeper anesthesia levels. Increased sympathetic nervous system activity resulted in marked stimulation of the cardiovascular system. Prolonged tachypnea developed in 1 man, and 2 became apneic and required manually assisted ventilation; 4 men had opisthotomic posturing, which subsided and cleared in response to an increase in the inhaled nitrous oxide concentration. Severe nausea and vomiting occurred in 1 man in the postanesthesia period, and 4 others had mild to moderate gastrointestinal tract upset. None of the 8 study participants experienced decompression sickness. There were no prolonged residual effects. Nitrous oxide used as the sole anesthetic agent under hyperbaric conditions is less than ideal because it is associated with hypertension, tachycardia, and tachypnea.

▶ Nitrous oxide is not a useful drug when hyperbaric conditions make it possible to administer partial pressures of the anesthetic (836–1,368 mm Hg) that are anesthetic. This conclusion is supported by the present data and by an earlier report (1).—R.K. Stoelting, M.D.

Reference

1. Hornbein TF, et al: *Anesth Analg* 61:553, 1982.

Recovery of Bowel Motility After High Dose Fentanyl or Morphine Anaesthesia for Cardiac Surgery

Yukioka H, Tanaka M, Fujimori M (Osaka City Univ, Japan)
Anaesthesia 45:353–356, 1990

2–5

High-dose fentanyl or morphine anesthesia is used commonly for cardiac surgery. Because little is known about the recovery of bowel func-

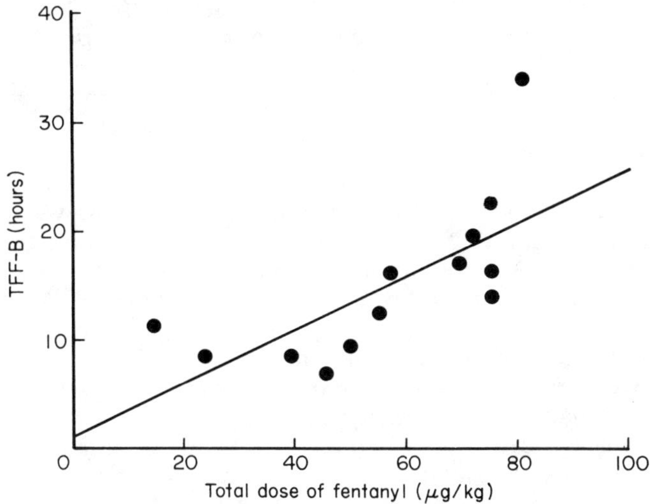

Fig 2–2.—Relationship between total dose of fentanyl and time from the patient's arrival in the intensive care unit to passage of the first flatus *(TFF-B)*. $y = .25 + 1.12$; $n = 13$; $r = .709$; $P < .01$. (Courtesy of Yukioka H, Tanaka M, Fujimori M: *Anaesthesia* 45:353–356, 1990.)

tion after high-dose opioid anesthesia, studies were made in 22 adults undergoing elective cardiac surgery during high-dose fentanyl or morphine anesthesia. Time to first passage of flatus (TFF) was measured, using a carbon dioxide analyzer, as an indication of the return of coordinated bowel motility.

The total dose of fentanyl was 56.3 μg/kg and of morphine, 1.3 mg/kg. The time from the patient's arrival in the intensive care unit to TFF was significantly longer in the group given fentanyl than in the group given morphine, although the time from administration of the opioid to TFF did not differ. There was a good correlation between TFF and total dose of fentanyl, but not for morphine (Fig 2–2). These findings suggest that high-dose fentanyl anesthesia delays recovery of bowel motility in a dose-dependent manner in patients undergoing cardiac surgery. However, there may be other factors that could have influenced these results, including the use of diazepam and morphine as premedication, increased sympathetic activity after surgery or catecholamine administration, and hypothermia; these factors are known to depress gastrointestinal tract motility.

▶ The article preceding this report describes the presumed effect on bowel motility of 70% nitrous oxide in the presence of a modest dose of fentanyl (3 μg/kg⁻¹/h⁻¹). This study describes the presumed effect on bowel motility of fentanyl (56 ± 21 μg/kg⁻¹) in the presence of a modest dose of nitrous oxide (50% to 60%). It is intriguing to speculate about the likely time to first flatus in a study that combined high doses of both fentanyl and nitrous oxide.—R.K. Stoelting, M.D.

Peroperative Nitrous Oxide Delays Bowel Function After Colonic Surgery
Scheinin B, Lindgren L, Scheinin TM (Central Univ Hosp, Helsinki)
Br J Anaesth 64:154–158, 1990   2–6

Nitrous oxide diffuses into air-containing closed body cavities more rapidly than nitrogen diffuses out. In dogs, gas volume in the intestinal lumen increased by up to 200% with nitrous oxide administration. Because distended bowel may influence the recovery of bowel function, a randomized, prospective study was conducted to determine the effect of peroperative nitrous oxide on bowel function in 40 patients undergoing colonic surgery; 20 patients were given nitrous oxide (N_2O) and 20 patients were given air during surgery. Anesthetic management included isoflurane, vecuronium by infusion, and fentanyl.

There were no significant differences between groups with regard to preoperative management, surgery, parenteral therapy, and postoperative analgesics. The mean inspired concentration of isoflurane in the group given air was twice that in the N_2O group. The duration of surgery, blood loss, need for postoperative analgesia, and postoperative nausea did not differ.

The group given air had significantly less gas in the small and large bowel than the N_2O group had. After surgery, the former group had significantly faster recovery of bowel function in terms of earlier passage of flatus and feces, resulting in fewer days of parenteral nutrition and a shorter hospital stay. These data indicate that the peroperative administration of N_2O delays bowel function after colonic surgery.

▶ I have always been a skeptic regarding the undesirable effects of N_2O when administered to patients undergoing bowel surgery, especially in the absence of intestinal obstruction. The above data cast doubt on the "benign" effect of N_2O in these patients. Nevertheless, this is likely to be a dose-related effect: The present study administered 70% N_2O for an average duration of 282 minutes.—R.K. Stoelting, M.D.

Differential Effects of Nitrous Oxide on Baroreflex Control of Heart Rate and Peripheral Sympathetic Nerve Activity in Humans
Ebert TJ (Med College of Wisconsin, Milwaukee)
Anesthesiology 72:16–22, 1990   2–7

Acute regulation of blood pressure in human beings is mediated by the arterial baroreflex regulation of heart rate, cardiac contractility, and peripheral sympathetic outflow. Most studies have only examined heart rate responses to increasing blood pressure, and little is known regarding reflex regulation of sympathetic outflow in human beings.

To determine the effects of nitrous oxide (N_2O) on baroreceptor-mediated increases in heart rate and efferent muscle sympathetic nerve activity to skeletal muscle blood vessels (MSNA), studies were made using an epoxy-coated tungsten needle placed into the peroneal nerve. Data were obtained from 6 healthy volunteers before and during brief reductions of blood pressure with intravenously administered sodium nitroprusside while they breathed 40% N_2/60% O_2 (control), during administration of N_2O (40% N_2O/60% O_2), and during recovery (40% N_2/60% O_2). Another 5 individuals acted as time controls breathing 40% N_2 in O_2 throughout the protocol.

Inhalation of N_2O resulted in a significant 59% increase in MSNA from baseline, compared with a 17% nonsignificant reduction in MSNA from baseline in the controls. Reductions in blood pressure produced linear increases in MSNA and decreases in R-R interval. Exposure to N_2O produced a 39% reduction in the slope of the R-R interval response but no significant change in the MSNA slopes.

Brief exposure to 40% N_2O in human beings stimulates sympathetic nerve activity directed to the vascular smooth muscle in skeletal muscles and reduces baroreceptor-mediated tachycardia. However, baroreflex-mediated augmentation in muscle sympathetic outflow is well maintained during N_2O inhalation, which may partially explain the relatively stable cardiovascular effects when N_2O is administered in combination with other inhalational agents.

► Baroreceptor-mediated control of the heart rate seems to be vulnerable to influence by nearly every drug studied, ranging from volatile anesthetics to vasodilating drugs. It is now acceptable to add N_2O to the list. Nevertheless, I doubt that clinicians will find much solace in the ever-growing length of this list.—R.K. Stoelting, M.D.

Halothane, Desflurane, and Xenon

Respiratory and Hemodynamic Effects of Halothane in Status Asthmaticus
Saulnier FF, Durocher AV, Deturck RA, Lefèbvre MC, Wattel FE (Hôp Albert Calmette, Lille, France)
Intensive Care Med 16:104–107, 1990   2–8

Inhalational anesthetics such as halothane are often used for anesthesia in patients with asthma. The effects of halothane were studied in 12 patients with status asthmaticus who required mechanical ventilation. A flow-generated ventilator was used to administer 1% halothane for 30 minutes.

Peak inspiratory pressure fell significantly after halothane administration. The dead space-tidal volume ratio decreased significantly. The $PaCO_2$ was decreased by 10 mm Hg within 30 minutes after halothane administration and the arterial pH rose significantly. Intravascular pressures decreased after halothane administration, whereas cardiac index, vascular resistances, and the left ventricular stroke work index remained normal. Mean systemic blood pressure decreased but remained at acceptable levels. Arrhythmias did not develop during halothane exposure.

Halothane rapidly controls bronchospasm in patients with status asthmaticus and improves respiratory efficiency. Adverse hemodynamics are not observed. Administration of 1% halothane appears to be effective.

▶ There is no question that halothane is a useful drug in patients with acute increases in airway resistance described as status asthmaticus. There is some question as to the advantages of halothane over isoflurane in such patients, especially if sympathomimetic drugs are being administered simultaneously.—R.K. Stoelting, M.D.

General Anesthesia Does Not Alter the Viscoelastic or Transport Properties of Human Respiratory Mucus
Rubin BK, Finegan B, Ramirez O, King M (Univ of Alberta, Edmonton)
Chest 98:101–104, 1990   2–9

Mucus transport rates are depressed in anesthetized animals and humans. This observation has led to speculation that general anesthesia depresses ciliary activity or adversely changes the physical properties of the respiratory mucus (RM). The possibility that anesthesia changes the physical properties of RM in such a way as to depress ciliary transport was investigated.

Thirty-three samples of RM were collected from the endotracheal tubes of 25 patients aged 1–79 years. All were undergoing elective surgery and had no clinical evidence of lung disease. The rigidity, viscoelasticity, spinnability, and percentage of solid composition of the specimens were measured. The transport of the collected RM across the mucus-depleted frog palate also was assessed. There was no significant difference between these properties and those of RM collected from awake volunteers using the bronchoscopy brush collection method. Differences in spinnability, transportability, and solid content of paired mucus samples from the inside and outside of the endotracheal tubes suggested altered RM hydration.

General anesthesia does not alter the physical properties of RM in healthy persons. The observed decrease in mucus transport rates is probably caused by ciliary depression as a direct effect of anesthetic gases, or the effect of anesthesia on mucus transport rates occurs only in some individuals.

▶ Whether this information is clinically useful is difficult to judge. It is unlikely to change how we administer anesthetics, but it is of interest nevertheless. Will it cause us to rethink the necessity of providing humidification for short cases?—R.R. Kirby, M.D.

Effects of Halothane on the Conduction System of the Heart in Humans
Scheffer GJ, Jonges R, Holley HS, Grimbergen CA, Ros HH, Peper A, Booij LHDJ (Free Univ Hosp, Amsterdam; Univ of Amsterdam)
Anesth Analg 69:721–726, 1989   2–10

Invasive His bundle ECG studies in dogs have indicated that halothane impairs conduction in the specialized conducting system of the heart. However, because of the considerable risk involved, similar invasive assessments cannot be performed in humans. The electrical activity of the His-Purkinje system (HPS) during halothane anesthesia was measured noninvasively, using a real-time recording system to detect surface His-Purkinje potentials. A signal averaging technique was used to increase the signal-to-noise ratio to recover the signals of the HPS.

Twenty-three patients (mean age, 22 years) who were undergoing a variety of minor elective surgical procedures were studied. The first HPS recordings were obtained with the patients breathing oxygen for approximately 4 minutes. Anesthesia was then induced with the patients breathing halothane in oxygen via a facemask until the exhaled halothane concentration corresponded with a minimum alveolar concentration (MAC) of 2, at which point the second recording was made. Conduction time intervals and heart rates were measured with the help of the computer system.

Atrial (P-H) and His-Purkinje conduction times could be measured in 18 of the 23 patients. Because of excessive noise or P-wave overlap, HPS activity could not be detected in the other 5 patients. There was a slight but significant decrease in the P-H conduction time, from 115.8 ms before halothane inhalation to 110.8 ms thereafter. During halothane inhalation, the P-H interval decreased in 13 patients, remained the same in 2 patients, and increased in 3 patients. His-Purkinje conduction times did not change significantly. Heart rates decreased significantly from 87.6 beats per minute before to 74.8 beats per minute after halothane inhalation. Systolic blood pressures decreased from 118.9 mm Hg before anesthesia to 103.6 mm Hg after halothane inhalation, and diastolic blood pressures decreased from 75.8 mm Hg to 64.7 mm Hg.

Measurements obtained with noninvasive signal averaging techniques during anesthesia induction with 2 MAC halothane did not show a significant effect of halothane on His-Purkinje conduction times, but it yielded an unexpected decrease in P-H conduction times, in combination with a decreased heart rate.

▶ As the authors conclude, these changes are consistent with the occurrence of atrial dysrhythmias that may manifest during the inhalation of halothane. The importance of these data is related to establishing the mechanism of halothane-induced effects on heart rate and cardiac impulse conduction. The clinical significance of small changes in atrial conduction times produced by 2 MAC halothane is questionable.—R.K. Stoelting, M.D.

Kinetics and Potency of Desflurane (I-653) in Volunteers
Jones RM, Cashman JN, Eger EI II, Damask MC, Johnson BH (Guy's Hosp, London; Univ of California, San Francisco)
Anesth Analg 70:3–7, 1990   2–11

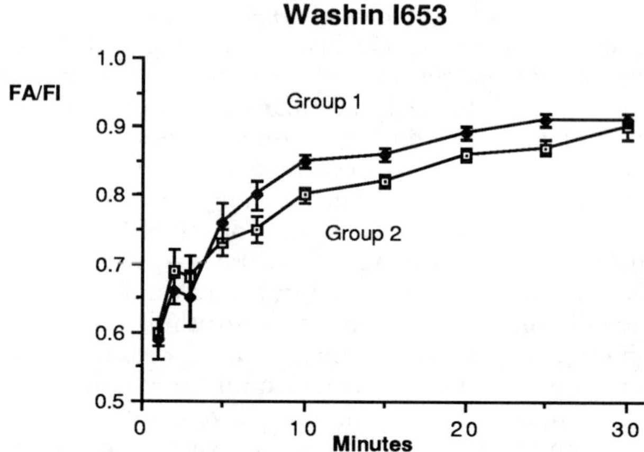

Fig 2–3.—Ratio of alveolar to inspired concentration (F_A/F_I) for desflurane given to 10 volunteers increased rapidly whether inspired concentration was 1.8% or 5.4%. In both groups respiration was spontaneous and normal as defined by end-tidal CO_2 levels of 5% to 6.5%. (Courtesy of Jones RM, Cashman JN, Eger EI II, et al: *Anesth Analg* 70:3–7, 1990.)

The inhalation anesthetic desflurane (I-653) is a methyl ethyl ether that is halogenated wholly with fluorine. It differs from isoflurane only in the substitution of fluorine for chlorine on the α-ethyl carbon. Desflurane has low blood-gas and oil-gas partition coefficients compared with currently used potent inhalation anesthetics. Thus desflurane will undergo rapid wash-in and wash-out and have a MAC value of about 5%. The kinetics and potency of desflurane were investigated in 10 healthy young male volunteers in ASA physical status I.

After a 10-minute exposure to desflurane, the ratio of alveolar to inspired concentration was .82. Wash-out was also rapid. Ten minutes after administration of desflurane was discontinued, the alveolar concentration, compared with the last concentration during administration of anesthetic, was .11. These values are comparable to those for nitrous oxide. The volunteers responded to commands at an average of 2.7 minutes after discontinuation of anesthetic administration. The values for MAC-awake and MAC were 2.42% and 4.58%, respectively. The ratio of the former to the latter was .53 (Fig 2–3).

Desflurane has a rapid uptake and wash-out, and it is potent. The low blood-gas partition coefficient may be especially advantageous because it allows for rapid induction of and recovery from anesthesia and should permit rapid adjustments of the depth of anesthesia.

▶ The hope for a rapid-onset, short-acting nondepolarizing muscle relaxant to replace succinylcholine and a potent volatile anesthetic with solubility characteristics similar to those of nitrous oxide is on the "wish list" of many anesthesiologists. Desflurane may well become the long-sought replacement for nitrous oxide.—R.K. Stoelting, M.D.

Biotransformation and Hepato-Renal Function in Volunteers After Exposure to Desflurane (I-653)
Jones RM, Koblin DD, Cashman JN, Eger EI II, Johnson BH, Damask MC (United Med and Dental Schools, London; Guy's Hosp, London; Univ of California, San Francisco; Anaquest, Milburn, NJ)
Br J Anaesth 64:482–487, 1990 2–12

The molecular structure of desflurane, a new inhalational anesthetic, differs from isoflurane only in the substitution of fluorine for chlorine at the α-ethyl carbon. Its physical stability equals or exceeds that of other potent inhaled agents that are used clinically. Results of animal studies have shown that desflurane undergoes minimal biotransformation and does not have hepatic or renal toxicity.

Hepatic and renal functions, and standard hematologic and biochemical indices, were investigated in 10 healthy unpremedicated male volunteers before and after exposure to desflurane in oxygen. Two sensitive tests of renal integrity were also performed: measurement of urinary retinol-binding protein and β-N-acetyl-D-glucosaminidase. Serum and urinary concentrations of inorganic fluoride and total urinary organic fluoride were measured to define the degree of biotransformation of desflurane.

All persons were exposed to desflurane for 89 minutes at an average inspired concentration of 3.6%. Results of standard hematologic and biochemical tests did not change significantly after exposure to desflurane, except for a significant increase in white blood cell counts. Similarly, renal function and liver function were unchanged by exposure to desflurane. Neither serum or urinary inorganic fluoride nor urinary nonvolatile organic fluoride concentrations changed after exposure to desflurane.

These findings confirm those of animal studies, showing that desflurane undergoes minimal biotransformation and is free of hepatic and renal toxicity. Further studies are warranted to define the safety of desflurane in higher concentrations and in other patient populations.

▶ This is certainly a promising new inhaled anesthetic. It appears to have many of the positive attributes of isoflurane, and also allows patients to recover more rapidly from anesthesia.—R.D. Miller, M.D.

Safety and Efficacy of Xenon in Routine Use as an Inhalational Anaesthetic
Lachmann B, Armbruster S, Schairer W, Landstra M, Trouwborst A, Van Daal G-J, Kusuma A, Erdmann W (Univ Hosp Dijkzigt; Erasmus Univ, Rotterdam)
Lancet 335:1413–1415, 1990 2–13

Xenon offers many advantages over routinely used inhalational anesthetic gases. It is nonexplosive, probably does not undergo transformation, is nontoxic, and offers rapid induction of and recovery from anesthesia. Its main drawback is the nonavailability of anesthesia machines in which to use the gas. The anesthetic efficacy and safety of a mixture of 70% xenon/30% oxygen and 70% nitrous oxide/30% oxygen were compared in a randomized, double-blind study of 40 patients aged 21–59 years undergoing routine surgery of similar duration. In accordance with the balanced anesthesia method, the patients received fentanyl, .1 mg, for each increase in blood pressure of more than 20% of the preanesthetic level. The total amount of fentanyl required per patient was used as an index of anesthetic potency of the 2 gases.

The average amount of fentanyl required was about 5 times greater in the nitrous oxide group than in the xenon group (.24 mg of fentanyl vs. .05 mg of fentanyl, per kg). Furthermore, fentanyl was required in 95% of the nitrous oxide group but in only 35% of the xenon group. Changes in blood pressure were significantly higher in the nitrous oxide group. Oxygen saturation did not differ between groups at the end of the operation, but oxygen saturation decreased to less than 92% in 8 patients in the nitrous oxide group during the first 20 minutes after induction. Thorax-lung compliance was significantly lower in the group given nitrous oxide. Recovery time from anesthesia was similar in both groups. The anesthetic and postoperative courses were uneventful in both groups. Xenon, at a concentration of 70%, is a potent and effective anesthetic that can be used safely under routine conditions. It is a very promising anesthetic agent for routine use.

▶ Xenon has been used, mainly for research, for more than 25 years. It was also very expensive. Overall, most of the anesthetic qualities have already been demonstrated. Is it reasonable to reconsider a reexamination of xenon?—R.D. Miller, M.D.

Toxicity of Inhaled Anesthetics

Anaesthetic Agents and the Ozone Layer
Westhorpe R, Blutstein H (Royal Children's Hosp, Melbourne; Environment Protection Authority, East Melbourne, Vic, Australia)
Anaesth Intens Care 18:102–104, 1990   2–14

A hole, found in the ozone layer over Antarctica in 1985, forms in September and dissipates in about 8 weeks for climatic reasons. A marked short-term movement of ozone-depleted air was observed over southern Australia when the hole filled in, leading to ultraviolet levels normally incurred later in midsummer. A decline in the ozone layer could lead to increases in nonmelanomatous skin cancers as well as certain types of malignant melanoma. In addition, ultraviolet radiation may suppress immune functions.

Several halogenated hydrocarbons now are used in anesthesia. Halogenated hydrocarbon and chlorofluorocarbons have varying ozone-depletion potential, depending on the stability of a given molecule, its lifetime in the stratosphere, and its breakdown products. Catalytic destruction of ozone depends on the halide breakdown products, bromide being the most potent.

Whereas the anesthetic use of halothane and nitrous oxide does not constitute a major threat to the ozone layer, ozone-depleting chemicals such as chlorofluorocarbon aerosol propellants should not be used unnecessarily. Care is in order when using halothane with high-flow open or semi-open circuits.

▶ This article goes on to tell us what has happened to the ozone layer and its relationship to anesthetic agents. In essence, it says that the ozone layer is a protective layer comprised of ozone molecules in the stratosphere 10–15 km above the earth's surface. These scattered particles absorb a large portion of the sun's radiation, especially ultraviolet, in particular, the harmful ultraviolet-B. Further, the amount of ozone decreased by approximately 2.5% from October 1978 to October 1985, and the predictions are that this current decrease, especially as it appears that there are holes forming in the ozone layer in specific areas, could mean increases in the number of squamous cell and basal cell carcinomas and malignant melanomas that develop. The authors further state that, for each 1% depletion of the total column ozone, the increase in carcinogenically effective ultraviolet rays is approximately 1.5%. Thus, for the 2.5% depletion, there is approximately a 4% increase in the effective dose of ultraviolet B, which translates into an increase in malignant melanomas of approximately 2% per year. In addition, there is an increase in the number of cataracts and depression of immune function, of which we do not understand the mechanism.

Should we as anesthesiologists feel guilty because of using the chlorofluorocarbons and halogenated hydrogenased hydrocarbons, which have ozone-depleting potential? The current contribution of anesthetics to ozone depletion is less than .001%, that is, less than $\frac{1}{1,000}$ of the depletion is attributable to the use of anesthetic agents cumulatively over all the years that anesthetic agents have been administered.

The authors also explain the effect of nitrous oxide in causing a warming effect. They state that the medical use of nitrous oxide probably contributes less than 1% of the total of nitrous oxide flux but, by virtue of its ability to absorb thermal infrared radiation, nitrous oxide contributes to maintenance of the warm surface temperature and the "greenhouse effect," which is the warming effect of the earth. Nitrous oxide contributes approximately 14% of the total effect compared to that of carbon dioxide, and the nitrous oxide used medically thus contributes .14%. Of all the things for anesthesiologists to worry about, one of them does not appear to be the effect of anesthetics in changing the atmosphere. Obviously, if you are concerned about that, you can go to low-flow and closed systems and have even less guilt.—M.F. Roizen, M.D.

Tropospheric Lifetimes of Halogenated Anaesthetics
Brown AC, Canosa-Mas CE, Parr AD, Pierce JMT, Wayne RP (Univ of Oxford; Southampton Gen Hosp, England)
Nature 341:635–637, 1989   2–15

The halogenated anesthetics halothane, enflurane, and isoflurane have the potential for contributing to stratospheric ozone destruction and global warming. Almost all administered doses of these popular inhalation anesthetics will end up in the atmosphere, but the damage they may cause depends on their atmospheric lifetime.

The absolute rates of reaction with hydroxyl (OH) radicals were chosen as a measurement because such reactions are likely to be the main homogeneous sink for halogenated species in the troposphere. A uniform OH radical concentration of 7.7×10^5 molecule cm^{-3} and a tropospheric temperature of 300 K were assumed. Comparison with a 1-dimensional model indicates that, with respect to this reaction, the lifetimes of halothane, enflurane, and isoflurane are 2, 6, and 5 years, respectively.

To evaluate the greenhouse warming potential of each anesthetic, the infrared spectra were measured and their integrated absorption cross sections in the range of $800-1,200$ cm^{-1} from the area under the peaks in the spectra were estimated. The potential of these anesthetics for ozone depletion and greenhouse warming is much smaller than for chlorofluorocarbons 11 and 12, the most important ozone-depleting molecules. At most, halothane, enflurane, and isoflurane contribute a fraction of about 5×10^{-4} to the total atmospheric content of chlorine-containing species.

▶ This is not a clinical article, but it is intriguing to speculate that halogenated anesthetics contribute to global warming. That this article was published in a very prestigious journal adds some validity to this questionable concept.—R.D. Miller, M.D.

Variation of Tumour Radiosensitivity With Time After Anaesthetic

Nias AHW, Perry PM (St Thomas' Hosp, London)
Br J Radiol 62:932–935, 1989

2–16

Anesthesia has been known to change the radiosensitivity of malignant tissues. To investigate further, the radiosensitivity of the C_3H mouse mammary adenocarcinoma was studied at various time intervals after the start of anesthesia in mice breathing oxygen or air at 1 atm. Diazepam and ketamine anesthesia was used. The radiation response to single doses of 25 Gy was determined based on the time taken to reach 3.5 times the treatment volume. The radiation response was also measured in animals that were not anesthetized but were irradiated.

At all times after the administration of anesthesia, there was more growth delay in tumors irradiated in pure oxygen than in air. At 10 minutes after the administration of anesthesia, the radiation response in both air and oxygen showed a reduction below the level for nonanesthetized control mice. After 25 minutes the response in air had returned to the control level, but the group exposed to oxygen had a highly significant increase in response. After 40 minutes the group given air showed slight sensitization, whereas the oxygen-exposed group still showed significant sensitization by the anesthetic. In contrast, radiation response did not vary significantly at all time intervals in nonanesthetized control mice.

There is considerable variation in the radiosensitivity of C_3H mouse mammary tumors depending on the time interval after induction of anesthesia. Effective radiosensitization of tumors may be achieved in mice breathing normobaric oxygen.

▶ This article is published in a journal that anesthesiologists are highly unlikely to read. Furthermore, the clinical implications with respect to anesthetic practice are limited at best. The reason this article was selected is because it does relate to anesthesia and therefore, might be of interest to the clinician.—R.D. Miller, M.D.

Antibody Assays for the Detection of Patients Sensitized to Halothane
Martin JL, Kenna JG, Pohl LR (Natl Heart, Lung, and Blood Inst, Bethesda, Md; Johns Hopkins Med Insts)
Anesth Analg 70:154–159, 1990   2–17

Halothane hepatitis is a rare and severe complication that appears to be an immune-mediated toxicity. An enzyme-linked immunosorbent assay (ELISA) that uses the trifluoroacetyl (TFA) hapten as the test antigen reportedly is useful in detecting serum antibodies. A more complete evaluation of this method was done in a larger population of patients with halothane hepatitis and controls.

Serum samples were obtained from both groups. In the ELISA procedures, TFA-rabbit serum albumin, liver microsomes, and purified TFA-proteins were used as antigens. Gel electrophoresis and immunoblotting also were done.

Of the 44 serum samples from halothane hepatitis patients, the TFA-rabbit serum albumin ELISA was positive in 26 (59%). Of the 126 serum samples from controls, 15 tested positive by this method but not by the others. Reaction with the carrier protein rabbit serum albumin occurred in 27% of the halothane hepatitis patients and 29% of controls. The TFA-rabbit serum albumin ELISA was then compared with assays using either liver microsomes or purified TFA proteins from halothane-treated rats as test antigens. With this method, 67% of 24 halothane hepatitis patients tested had a positive result. When the purified TFA-57 kDa, TFA-76 kDA, and TFA-100 kDa proteins were used as test antigens, this value rose to 79%. In all, 63% of patients reacted with each purified TFA neoantigen and 3 patients tested negative by each procedure.

The TFA-rabbit serum albumin ELISA appears to have only limited ability to detect patients sensitized to halothane. Use of the purified TFA-microsomal proteins as test antigens appears to increase significantly the specificity and sensitivity of these methods. Sensitivity will be improved when all of the TFA neoantigens are included as test antigens.

▶ Currently, halothane hepatitis is a diagnosis of exclusion. A reliable and specific antibody assay would be helpful in taking some of the guesswork out of this diagnosis.—R.K. Stoelting, M.D.

Hepatic Blood Flow in Humans During Isoflurane-N$_2$O and Halothane-N$_2$O Anesthesia

Goldfarb G, Debaene B, Ang ET, Roulot D, Jolis P, Lebrec D (Hôp Beaujon; Univ Paris; Hôp Beaujon, Clichy, France)
Anesth Analg 71:349–353, 1990

2–18

Halothane reportedly reduces hepatic blood flow and oxygen supply in experimental animals. Isoflurane has a lesser effect on these parameters. The effects of anesthesia induction with intravenous agents and of maintenance of anesthesia with halothane plus nitrous oxide and isoflurane plus nitrous oxide in humans were examined.

Anesthesia was induced with thiopental, fentanyl, and nitrous oxide in 11 patients. Five received halothane and 6, isoflurane. Hepatic blood flow (HBF), cardiac index, and hepatic venous oxygen saturation were measured before and after induction of anesthesia and again during halothane or isoflurane anesthesia before surgery. Hepatic blood flow was assessed by plasma clearance and hepatic extraction of indocyanine green.

The induction of anesthesia reduced HBF and the cardiac index. Before volatile anesthetics were administered, HBF, the cardiac index, and hepatic venous oxygen saturation were similar in both treatment groups. The cardiac index remained stable in both groups during anesthesia, but HBF rose significantly only with isoflurane. Hepatic venous oxygen saturation was also significantly higher during isoflurane compared with halothane anesthesia (Fig 2–4).

Hepatic blood flow decreases after induction of anesthesia in humans. Isoflurane appears to increase HBF in anesthetized patients and is accom-

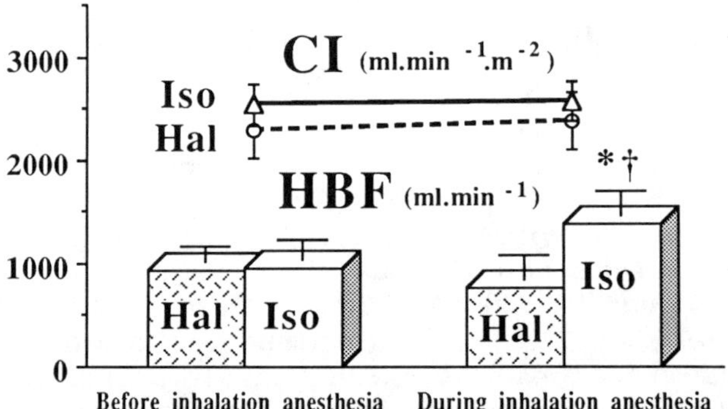

Fig 2–4.—Cardiac index *(CI)* and hepatic blood flow *(HBF)* before and after 30 minutes of stable end-tidal concentration of halothane *(Hal,* no. = 5) or isoflurane *(Iso,* no. = 6), plus nitrous oxide. Results are expressed as mean ± 1 SEM. *Dotted line* represents variation of CI in anesthetized patients given halothane (1 MAC). *Solid line* represents variation of CI in anesthetized patients given isoflurane (1 MAC). *Shaded bars* represent values of HBF in anesthetized patients before and during halothane anesthesia. *Open bars* represent values of HBF in anesthetized patients before and during isoflurane anesthesia. *Different from value measured before administration of isoflurane ($P < .05$). †Different from value measured in patients given halothane ($P < .05$). (Courtesy of Goldfarb G, Debaene B, Ang ET, et al: *Anesth Analg* 71:349–353, 1990.)

panied by a greater hepatic venous oxygen saturation when compared with halothane. The effects of halogenated agents are not related to cardiac output changes but to direct effects on splanchnic circulation.

► These data support findings previously reported when halothane or isoflurane was administered in the absence of adjuvant drugs (1). It is tempting to speculate that the greater incidence of liver damage observed after halothane, compared with isoflurane, is related to such findings. Proof, however, is still lacking.—R.K. Stoelting, M.D.

Reference

1. Gelman S, et al: *Anesthesiology* 61:726, 1984.

Immunological Basis of Anesthetic-Induced Hepatotoxicity
Hubbard AK, Gandolfi AJ, Brown BR Jr (Univ of Connecticut, Storrs; Univ of Arizona, Tucson)
Anesthesiology 69:814–817, 1988   2–19

Halothane-induced hepatotoxicity is seen both in a mild form occurring shortly after anesthesia and in a delayed, severe, and often lethal form, which may reflect an allergic response. Christ et al. suggested the potential for metabolic hepatotoxic reactions to enflurane anesthesia. Such reactions presumably are produced by covalently bound liver antigens that are recognized by antibodies generated by patients with halothane hepatitis.

The finding that metabolites can bind covalently to liver tissue indicated that they may act as haptens to evoke an immune response. Animals oxidatively biotransform halothane to a trifluoroacetyl halide moiety during anesthesia, and this in turn acetylates endogenous liver protein, making it immunogenic. The antibodies produced against this nonself protein create the immune response. Five liver proteins have been induced in rabbits and guinea pigs exposed on multiple occasions to halothane inhalation.

Any fluorohalocarbon volatile anesthetic has the potential to acetylate a liver protein and thereby evoke an immune response. It appears that such responses are relatively unique to the fluorocarbon acetylated intermediates produced from the volatile halogenated anesthetics.

► The debate about the mechanism of anesthetic-induced hepatotoxicity and whether there is a specific immunologic basis continues to exist. The epidemiologic facts are that there is a higher incidence after repeat exposures to halothane. This article and editorial summarize the evidence for this immunologic basis and show the oxidative biotransformation of halothane to a trifluoroacetyl halide moiety, which then acetylates endogenous liver protein. This endogenous liver protein is, in effect, changed from self to non-self, thus becoming immunogenic. Antibodies are elicited against this non–self-protein, creating an immunologic response. Why some individuals have this immunologic response and others do not remains a mystery, however. It does point up the fact that an enzyme-linked immunosorbent assay for halothane hepatotoxicity, and perhaps enflurane hepatotoxicity, is possible.—M.F. Roizen, M.D.

Narcotics

Differences in Magnitude and Duration of Opioid-Induced Respiratory Depression and Analgesia With Fentanyl and Sufentanil
Bailey PL, Streisand JB, East KA, East TD, Isern S, Hansen TW, Posthuma EFM, Rozendaal FW, Pace NL, Stanley TH (Univ of Utah)
Anesth Analg 70:8–15, 1990   2–20

Fentanyl and sufentanil are potent opioids that are commonly used in anesthesia. Although both analgesics are classified as pure μ agonists, sufentanil-nitrous oxide produces less respiratory depression and greater analgesia in the immediate postoperative period than does fentanyl-nitrous oxide. A double-blind, randomized study was done to evaluate the magnitude and duration of analgesia and respiratory depression induced by fentanyl and sufentanil.

The study group included 30 healthy nonsmoking volunteers aged 18–35 years who were divided into 3 groups of 10. Each group received 1 intravenous dose of sufentanil on 1 study day and the corresponding equipotent dose of fentanyl on another day. The study days were separated by at least 48 hours. The 3 sufentanil doses evaluated were .1, .2, and .4 μg/kg, and the 3 fentanyl doses were 1, 2, and 4 μg/kg. End-tidal carbon dioxide (CO_2) and ventilatory and occlusion pressure responses to CO_2 rebreathing were used to measure drug-induced respiratory effects. Analgesic efficacy was assessed by changes in pain threshold to electric shock applied to the forearm. Plasma sufentanil and fentanyl levels were measured by radioimmunoassay. Sampling was performed at baseline and at regular intervals up to 360 minutes after drug administration.

Sufentanil caused significantly less depression of the ventilatory and occlusion pressure response than did fentanyl, regardless of the dose (Fig 2–5). After sufentanil administration, ventilatory and occlusion pressure responses both returned to control values by 30 minutes. In contrast, ventilatory pressure responses did not return to baseline until 240 minutes after fentanyl administration, and the occlusion pressure response took 120 minutes to return to control values. Pain thresholds returned to control values within 180 minutes after sufentanil administration, but after only 90 minutes with fentanyl administration.

Sufentanil produces less depression of ventilatory drive and greater and

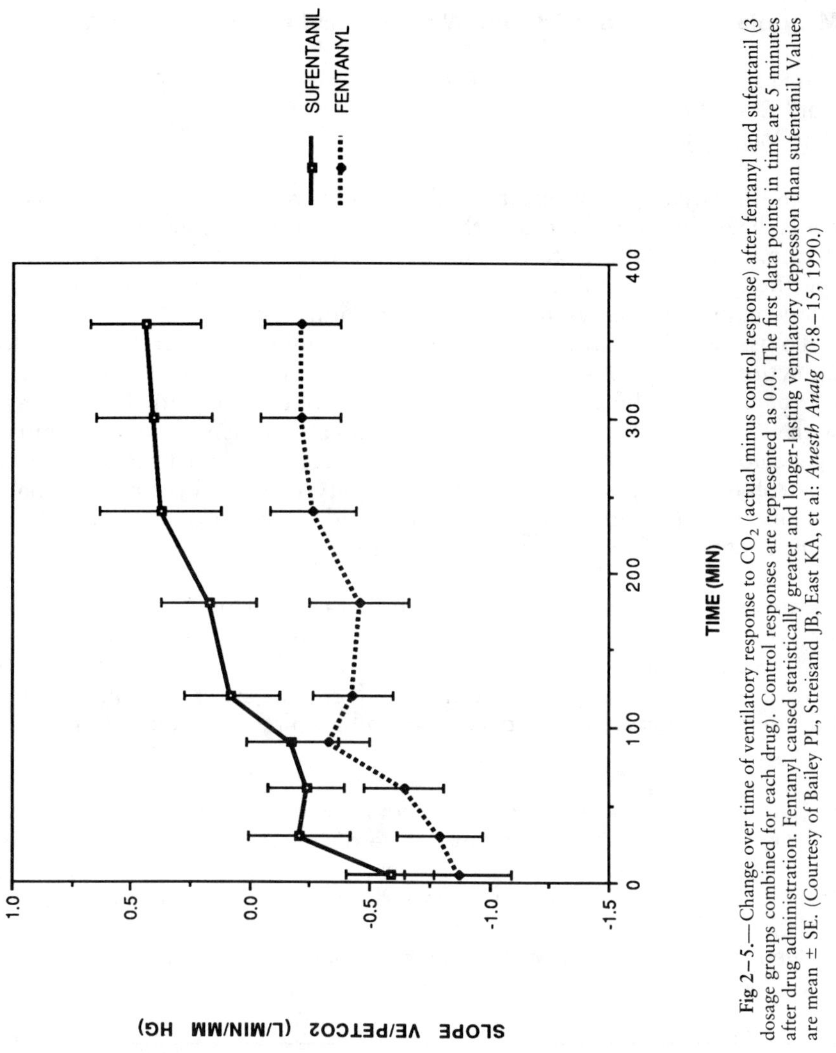

Fig 2–5.—Change over time of ventilatory response to CO_2 (actual minus control response) after fentanyl and sufentanil (3 dosage groups combined for each drug). Control responses are represented as 0.0. The first data points in time are 5 minutes after drug administration. Fentanyl caused statistically greater and longer-lasting ventilatory depression than sufentanil. Values are mean ± SE. (Courtesy of Bailey PL, Streisand JB, East KA, et al: *Anesth Analg* 70:8–15, 1990.)

longer-lasting analgesia than fentanyl. Sufentanil may thus provide better patient comfort with less respiratory depression than fentanyl.

▶ Fentanyl and sufentanil have both been useful additions to the anesthesiologist's menu of drugs designed to produce predictable and desirable responses in the perioperative period. There are those who argue that sufentanil is simply a more potent fentanyl. To those who disagree with this comparison, the above data are reassuring but are not likely to cause those who favor fentanyl to change opioids.—R.K. Stoelting, M.D.

Midazolam Acts Synergistically With Fentanyl for Induction of Anaesthesia

Ben-Shlomo I, Abd-El-Khalim H, Ezry J, Zohar S, Tverskoy M (The 'Rebecca Sieff' Govt Hosp, Safed, Israel)
Br J Anaesth 64:45–47, 1990
2–21

Life-threatening complications have occurred with combinations of benzodiazepines and opioids, which are used to induce anesthesia and sedation. Several studies have reported mutual potentiation of effects by specific drugs from these 2 groups, but there has been no attempt to define whether this represents synergism or additivity.

To assess the specific interaction between midazolam and fentanyl for induction of anesthesia, the induction dose-response of midazolam was compared with the dose-response of its combination with fentanyl and with that of fentanyl alone in 3 groups of 60 women undergoing minor gynecologic surgery. All of the women were unpremedicated, with an ASA physical status of I or II. The inability to open eyes on command was used as the end point of anesthesia induction. Dose-response curves were determined for each group with a probit procedure and compared with an isobolographic analysis.

Midazolam acted in synergism with fentanyl for induction of anesthesia. Twenty-five percent of the median effective dose (ED_{50}) of fentanyl was needed in combination with 23% of the ED_{50} for midazolam to attain the ED_{50} of the combination. The degree of synergism may explain the mutual potentiation between benzodiazepines and opioids reported previously.

▶ These data are consistent with a common clinical observation: The previous intravenous administration of a small dose of fentanyl (50–150 μg) or sufentanil (10–30 μg) greatly facilitates the rapidity of onset of unconsciousness after the subsequent injection of midazolam. This is a useful drug interaction during the induction of anesthesia, but exaggerated and undesirable responses may occur when this combination is used during monitored anesthetic care.— R.K. Stoelting, M.D.

Inhaled Fentanyl as a Method of Analgesia

Worsley MH, MacLeod AD, Brodie MJ, Asbury AJ, Clark C (Royal Infirmary, Edinburgh; Victoria Infirmary, Glasgow; Western Infirmary, Glasgow)
Anaesthesia 45:449–451, 1990
2–22

Fentanyl is effective for postoperative analgesia because it has a rapid onset of action, is potent, and has a short duration of action. To determine whether nebulized fentanyl would be suitable for postoperative analgesia, 30 patients aged 18–65 years who had a variety of elective surgical procedures were studied. While in the recovery room, patients with significant pain were randomly assigned to receive either nebulized placebo, nebulized fentanyl at a dose of 100 μg, or nebulized fentanyl at a dose of 300 µg. Pain was assessed on a linear visual analogue (LVA) scale at 5, 15, 30, 60, 120, and 180 minutes after completion of nebulization. Escape analgesia was available if pain relief was inadequate. Venous blood samples for the determination of serum levels of fentanyl were taken before and at regular intervals after inhalation of fentanyl.

Ten patients were excluded from the study because they did not complain of any significant pain while in the recovery room. Seven patients received placebo, 6 received the 100-µg dose of fentanyl, and 7 received 300 µg. There was significant improvement in postoperative pain as assessed by the LVA scale in patients treated with the 300-µg dose of nebulized fentanyl. With either dose of fentanyl the mean time to escape analgesia was significantly longer than that for placebo.

After inhalation of fentanyl 300 µg a peak of about .4 ng/mL was reached and serum levels plateaued at 15 minutes at about .1 ng/mL. No peak was detected after inhalation of 100 µg and serum levels plateaued at 15 minutes at about .04 ng/mL. No respiratory depression, bronchospasm, nausea, or drowsiness occurred with either dose of inhaled fentanyl. Inhaled fentanyl appears to provide effective analgesia during the immediate postoperative period despite its low serum levels.

▶ In the absence of data to confirm that inhalation of fentanyl is better than continuous infusion of fentanyl, I would prefer the latter. Keep in mind that transdermal administration is also effective and lacks the possible misconceptions generated by "sniffing" a drug for therapeutic purposes.— R.K. Stoelting, M.D.

Morphine and Metabolite Behavior After Different Routes of Morphine Administration: Demonstration of the Importance of the Active Metabolite Morphine-6-Glucuronide

Osborne R, Joel S, Trew D, Slevin M (St Bartholomew's Hosp, London; Homerton Hosp, London)
Clin Pharmacol Ther 47:12–19, 1990   2–23

The presence of significant quantities of morphine-6-glucuronide, a morphine metabolite, after morphine administration has been demonstrated. This morphine metabolite has analgesic activity. The pharmacokinetics of morphine, morphine-6-glucuronide, and morphine-3-glucuronide were evaluated after single-dose morphine administration by 5 different routes.

The study was done in 10 normal volunteers aged 25–44 years who were qualified medical practitioners. The 5 forms of morphine therapy used in this study included a 5-mg intravenous bolus injection, an 11.7-mg oral tablet, an 11.7-mg sublingual tablet, an 11.7-mg buccal tablet, and a 14.2-mg sustained-release buccal tablet. Blood samples were collected at baseline and at predetermined intervals thereafter, up to 12 hours after morphine therapy. Urine was collected for 24 hours after each morphine dose. All plasma and urine samples were assayed for mor-

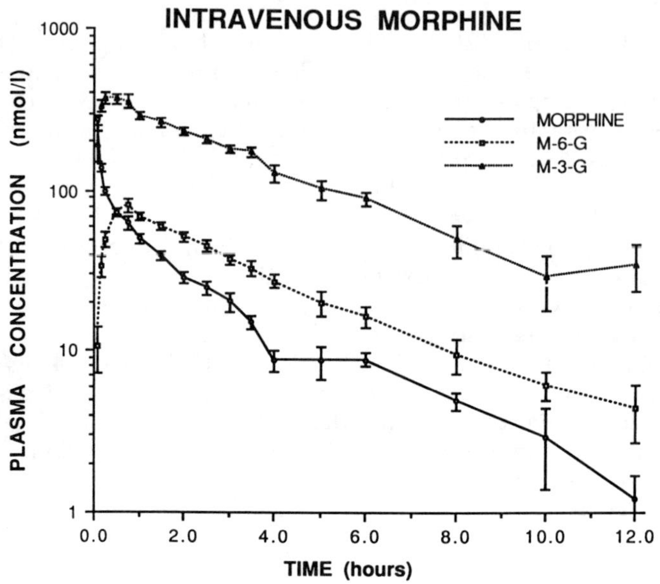

Fig 2–6.—Mean plasma concentrations (± SEM) of morphine, morphine-6-glucuronide (M-6-G), and morphine-3-glucuronide (M-3-G) after intravenous administration of morphine. (Courtesy of Osborne R, Joel S, Trew D, et al: *Clin Pharmacol Ther* 47:12–19, 1990.)

phine, morphine-6-glucuronide, and morphine-3-glucuronide, using high-performance liquid chromatography.

After intravenous morphine therapy, morphine was present in measurable quantities for 4–6 hours (Fig 2–6). Metabolism of morphine to morphine glucuronides proceeded extremely fast, as detectable quantities of morphine-6-glucuronide and morphine-3-glucuronide were found in plasma samples as early as 5 minutes after morphine administration. The mean plasma levels of morphine-3-glucuronide exceeded those of morphine within 6 minutes after dosing. The mean plasma levels of morphine-6-glucuronide exceeded those of morphine at 30 minutes after dosing. Very low plasma morphine levels were observed after the oral administration of morphine, with morphine-6-glucuronide plasma levels exceeding those of morphine by a factor of 9:1. Administration of sublingual, buccal, and sustained-release buccal morphine tablets resulted in delayed absorption with attenuation and delay of peak morphine and metabolite levels.

The findings confirm the quantitative importance of morphine-6-glucuronide after parenteral morphine administration. Recognition of the potential contribution of this morphine metabolite to analgesia has profound clinical implications. Studies of morphine pharmacokinetics should therefore always include the measurement of glucuronides to be clinically relevant.

► Recognition that the morphine-6-glucuronide metabolite of morphine has analgesic and ventilatory depressant effects has important implications. For example, elimination of this active metabolite may be impaired in patients with renal failure. Indeed, depression of ventilation lasting for up to 7 days has been observed in patients in renal failure after the administration of small doses of morphine.—R.K. Stoelting, M.D.

Reference

1. *Anesthesiology* 42:745, 1975.

Absorption Characteristics of Transdermally Administered Fentanyl
Varvel JR, Shafer SL, Hwang SS, Coen PA, Stanski DR (Stanford Univ; Alza Corp, Palo Alto)
Anesthesiology 70:928–934, 1989   2–24

A transdermal fentanyl delivery system was developed for the management of moderate to severe pain. The absorption characteristics and systemic bioavailability of the transdermal fentanyl delivery system, with a predicted nominal delivery rate of 100 μg/hr, were evaluated. Fentanyl was administered as an intravenous infusion, 150 μg/min for 5 to 6.5 minutes, to 8 surgical patients, and transdermally on the first postoperative day (24 hours after the intravenous dose). The transdermal fentanyl system was left in place for 24 hours.

Serum fentanyl concentrations reached a plateau (mean, 1.8 ng/mL) within about 14 hours after placement of the transdermal system and remained relatively constant until removal of the system at 24 hours. The mean terminal half-life after removal of the system was 17 hours. The rate of fentanyl absorption was relatively constant until removal of the system (mean, 91.9 μg/hr). The mean terminal half-life of the rate of absorption after removal was 16.6 hours. At time of removal of the system, 1.07 mg of the drug remained in the cutaneous depot at the site of placement. Systemic fentanyl bioavailability was .92, indicating that transdermally administered fentanyl was neither significantly degraded by the skin's bacterial flora nor susceptible to significant first-pass cutaneous metabolism.

The transdermal administration of fentanyl produces relatively constant serum fentanyl concentrations for prolonged periods of time in the postsurgical patient. The prolonged terminal half-life of fentanyl results from continued absorption of fentanyl from a peripheral depot of drug. Because of the initial time lag of 10–14 hours in obtaining analgesic serum fentanyl concentrations, either the transdermal system should be placed before surgery, or parenterally administered opioids should be used for the first few hours postoperatively.

▶ Although there are some very interesting calculations in this article, perhaps most important to note is that there is an initial time lag of 10–14 hours in obtaining analgesic serum fentanyl concentrations after placement of the system, suggesting that you either need to place it preoperatively, or that you use other forms of opioids for analgesia for the first few hours. Transdermal administration obviously is convenient, but it should be noted that, after the patch is removed, there is a depot in the skin that continues to provide increased absorption for at least 12 and perhaps as long as 24 hours. This depot appears to be in the subcutaneous skin. In addition, not all of the transdermally administered fentanyl is absorbed, as at least a milligram on average is left in these patches. The net result may be that the wastebaskets of patients who have transdermal fentanyl administered may be highly sought after by drug addicts.—M.F. Roizen, M.D.

Non-Narcotic Intravenous Anesthetics

Pregnanolone Emulsion: A Preliminary Pharmacokinetic and Pharmacodynamic Study of a New Intravenous Anaesthetic Agent
Carl P, Høgskilde S, Nielsen JW, Sørensen MB, Lindholm M, Karlen B, Bäckstrøm T (Municipal Hosp of Copenhagen; Hvidovre Hosp, Denmark; Karolinska Inst, Stockholm; Univ of Umeå, Sweden)
Anaesthesia 45:189–197, 1990   2–25

Pregnanolone is a naturally occurring metabolite of progesterone that lacks notable endocrine action and is anesthetically active in several animal species. However, its lack of water solubility has prevented its development for clinical practice. Pregnanolone is available in a stable emulsion for use in a clinical setting. A preliminary pharmacokinetic and pharmacodynamic study was carried out in 6 healthy male volunteers with no history of anesthetic complications or drug allergy.

All 6 were given 2 bolus doses of pregnanolone emulsion (PE) with at least 2 weeks between doses. The initial dose was .05 mg/kg. Increasing doses were given in consecutive men until anesthesia was induced for about 10 minutes, until a maximum dose of 1.6 mg/kg was reached, or until unacceptable side effects were observed. Plasma concentrations of pregnanolone were measured in arterial blood before injection of PE and at regular intervals thereafter.

The minimum dose of PE required to induce sleep was .4 mg/kg. However, only 1 of 2 men given this dose and 1 of 2 men given a dose of .5 mg/kg fell asleep; both men given a dose of .6 mg/kg fell asleep. The time to loss of eyelash reflex varied from 75 to 90 seconds, and the time to stop counting varied from 20 to 39 seconds. The men opened their eyes on command 5 minutes after the .4 mg/kg dose, 7.3 minutes after the .5 mg/kg dose, and 7.4–15.2 minutes after the .6 mg/kg dose. Thus PE caused rapid induction of anesthesia of short duration.

The plasma concentration-time curves of pregnanolone fit a 2-compartment model. Elimination half-life ranged from .9 to 1.4 hours, volume of central compartment ranged from .95 to 2.10 L/kg, volume of distribution ranged from 3.75 to 5.58 L/kg, and total body clearance ranged from 1.80 to 3.07 L/hour/kg. Urinary excretion of unchanged pregnanolone was less than .1%. Injection of PE only slightly affected hemodynamics. Minor side effects after injection of PE were slight respiratory depression of short duration, excitation in 1 volunteer, and involuntary muscle movement in another. There were no venous sequelae. No clear conclusions of clinical efficacy could be drawn from this small sample trial, but PE appears to be a safe short-acting anesthetic that merits further clinical investigation.

▶ At first glance, this drug does not seem to exhibit attributes that would challenge the historic role of thiopental and the emerging place of propofol for the induction of anesthesia. Allergic reactions may be unlikely considering the naturally occurring origin of the active drug. Nevertheless, the contents of the emulsion may introduce this risk. Indeed, the authors suggest that the anesthetic and anticonvulsive properties of pregnanolone are very similar to another steroidal anesthetic, Althesin, a drug that found disfavor because of an unacceptable incidence of associated allergic reactions.—R.K. Stoelting, M.D.

Pain on Injection of Propofol: Methods of Alleviation
Johnson RA, Harper NJN, Chadwick S, Vohra A (Manchester Royal Infirmary, Manchester, England)
Anaesthesia 45:439–442, 1990   2–26

The intravenous anesthetic agent propofol is increasingly being used because it provides high-quality anesthesia and rapid recovery. A disadvantage of propofol is that injection into small veins is often painful. To determine whether injecting lidocaine before injecting propofol or adding lidocaine to the propofol induction solution would alleviate the pain and discomfort, 103 adults undergoing elective procedures under general propofol anesthesia were studied in a controlled, double-blind, randomized trial. All patients received 10 mg of diazepam 1 hour before operation. A 23-gauge intravenous cannula was inserted on the dorsum of the hand.

Twenty-two of the 103 patients were pretreated with 2 mL of saline solution, followed by induction of anesthesia with propofol with 2 mL of saline solution added; 21 were pretreated with 2 mL of a solution containing 20 mg of lidocaine, followed by induction with propofol plus saline; 20 were pretreated with 40 mg of lidocaine, followed by induction with propofol plus saline; 18 were pretreated with saline, followed by induction with propofol to which 20 mg of lidocaine had been added; and 22 were pretreated with saline, followed by induction with propofol with 40 mg of lidocaine added.

Three of the 22 control patients who received propofol only felt discomfort and 13 had pain during injection of propofol. In contrast, 4 patients had pain and 1 had discomfort after injection of propofol when pretreated with 20 mg of lidocaine; only 1 patient had pain after pretreatment with 40 mg of lidocaine. Two patients felt discomfort and 1 had pain after injection of propofol with 20 mg of lidocaine added; none of the patients who received propofol with 40 mg of lidocaine added had any pain or discomfort. Sixty-eight percent of the patients who experienced pain or discomfort during injection of propofol recalled the sensation, suggesting that administration of propofol does not insure amnesia of noxious events that occur during induction of anesthesia.

The incidence of pain or discomfort after the injection of propofol for induction of anesthesia is common. Lidocaine, 20 mg or 40 mg, administered as a pretreatment dose or as part of the induction mixture significantly reduces the incidence of pain and discomfort associated with the injection of propofol.

▶ Many drugs used for the induction of anesthesia cause discomfort during their intravenous injection and propofol is no exception. Often alerting the patient to this possibility before initiating injection is sufficient, especially when a small vein is utilized. Adding lidocaine for this purpose to an induction characterized by polypharmacy must be a carefully weighed decision.—R.K. Stoelting, M.D.

Randomized Comparison of Outcome After Propofol-Nitrous Oxide or Enflurane-Nitrous Oxide Anaesthesia in Operations of Long Duration
Korttila K, Östman PL, Faure E, Apfelbaum JL, Ekdawi M, Roizen MF (Univ of Chicago)
Can J Anaesth 36:651–657, 1989   2–27

Propofol compares favorably with other intravenously or inhalationally administered anesthesia in surgical procedures of short duration. In a randomized, prospective study, the safety, efficacy, and speed and quality of recovery from propofol or thiopental-enflurane anesthesia were compared in 60 patients undergoing mainly gynecologic laparotomies. Propofol, 2 mg/kg, was administered to 30 patients for induction followed by propofol infusion; the other 30 patients received thiopental, 4 mg/kg, for induction followed by enflurane, .5% to 2%. All patients received fentanyl, 1.5 μg/kg, before induction and nitrous oxide (66%) in oxygen 1 minute after tracheal intubation. The mean duration of anesthesia was 152 minutes in the propofol group and 162 minutes in the thiopental-enflurane group.

Hemodynamic responses to induction and maintenance of anesthesia with propofol or thiopental-enflurane were comparable and satisfactory except after tracheal intubation, when the mean arterial pressure was significantly lower in the propofol-treated group. The speed of recovery or discharge time from the recovery room did not differ between groups. However, propofol-nitrous oxide anesthesia was associated with significantly less postoperative nausea and vomiting (Fig 2–7). In addition, the propofol-treated group experienced less dizziness, depression/sadness, and hunger than the thiopental-enflurane group.

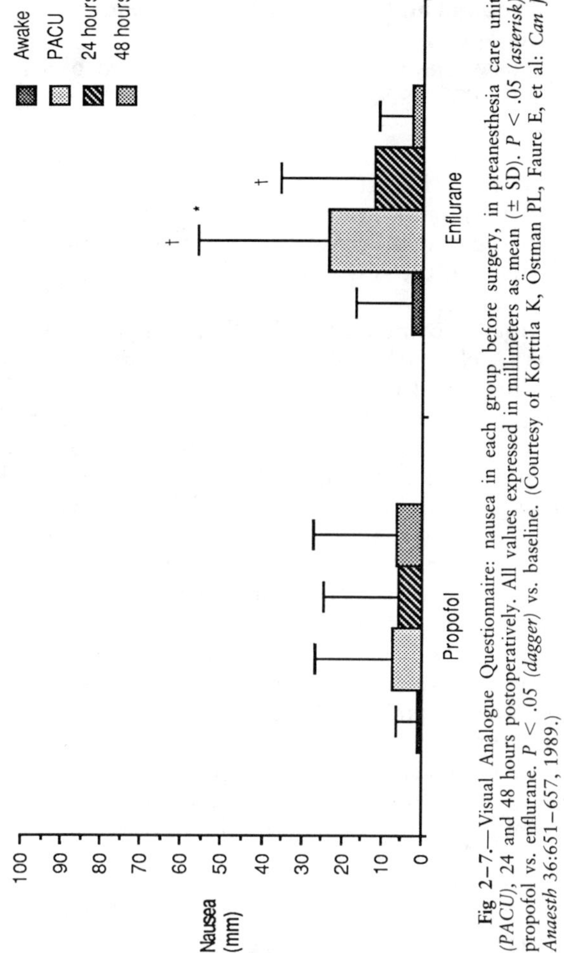

Fig 2–7.—Visual Analogue Questionnaire: nausea in each group before surgery, in preanesthesia care unit (PACU), 24 and 48 hours postoperatively. All values expressed in millimeters as mean (± SD). *P* < .05 (*asterisk*) propofol vs. enflurane. *P* < .05 (*dagger*) vs. baseline. (Courtesy of Korttila K, Östman PL, Faure E, et al: *Can J Anaesth* 36:651–657, 1989.)

These data show that propofol-nitrous oxide anesthesia is as effective as thiopental-enflurane anesthesia during long intra-abdominal operations. However, propofol is associated with less dizziness and emesis than enflurane anesthesia.

▶ An antiemetic effect of propofol has been attributed to its lipid emulsion. nevertheless, this effect for the lipid emulsion has not been documented (1).— R.K. Stoelting, M.D.

Reference

1. Ostman PL, et al: *Anesth Analg* 71:536, 1990.

Comparison of Propofol and Thiopentone as Anaesthetic Agents for Electroconvulsive Therapy

Boey WK, Lai FO (Natl Univ of Singapore; Toa Payoh Hosp, Singapore)
Anaesthesia 45:623–628, 1990   2–28

Electroconvulsive therapy (ECT) requires an anesthetic agent that provides smooth and rapid induction, fast recovery, attenuation of the physiologic effects of ECT, and minimal antagonistic effects on seizure activity. In a repeated measure, crossover study, thiopental, the anesthetic agent routinely used in the researchers' hospital for ECT, was compared with propofol.

Thirty-one patients completed 4 ECT treatments. Twenty-seven patients were in ASA class I and 4 were in ASA class 2. In most patients, ECT was given for failed medical treatment. The mean induction doses were 1.33 mg/kg for propofol and 2.27 mg/kg for thiopental.

Patients receiving propofol had significantly better tonus for the second treatment and the first and second treatments combined and better clonus for the first and second treatments combined. The increase in systolic and diastolic arterial pressures and heart rate after treatment were significantly higher with thiopental. Seizure times were shorter with propofol, but there was significant drug-time interaction. Apnea time was significantly longer with propofol, and propofol caused significantly more discomfort on injection. The quality of walking at 20 minutes after anesthesia was significantly better with propofol for the first, second, and first and second treatments combined (Fig 2–8).

Although the time from induction until electric shock was significantly longer (20 seconds) in the propofol-treated group, this time difference should not affect the conduct of the treatment significantly. Overall, propofol is an effective anesthetic for ECT and causes few side effects.

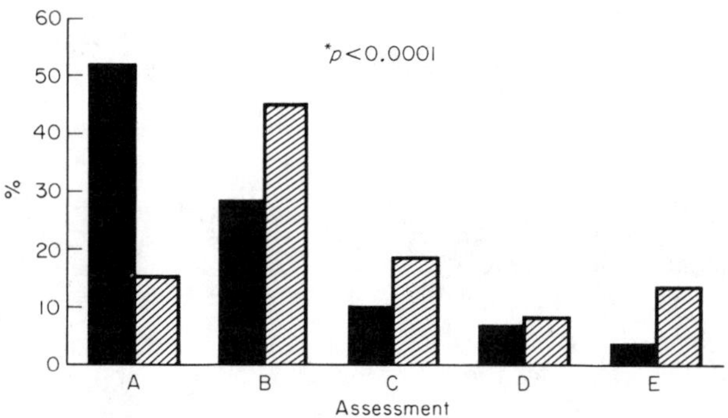

Fig 2–8.—Assessment of patients walking 10 m 20 minutes after induction of anesthesia graded as *(A)* no impairment, *(B)* slight impairment, *(C)* moderate impairment, *(D)* severe impairment, and *(E)* unable to stand. First and second treatment results are combined (no. = 60). Wilcoxon signed rank test was used to compare both groups. *Filled bars,* propofol; *striped bars,* thiopental. *Statistically significant. (Courtesy of Boey WK, Lai FO: *Anaesthesia* 45:623–628, 1990.)

▶ These data support the conclusion that propofol is an acceptable induction drug for ECT, as is thiopental. Many would select methohexital in preference to propofol or thiopental for this procedure.—R.K. Stoelting, M.D.

Flumazenil Reverses Sedation After Midazolam-Induced General Anesthesia in Ambulatory Surgery Patients

Philip BK, Simpson TH, Hauch MA, Mallampati SR (Brigham and Women's Hosp, Boston; Harvard Med School)
Anesth Analg 71:371–376, 1990

2–29

Midazolam is used to induce general anesthesia in day surgery patients, but it can cause prolonged postoperative somnolence. The value of flumazenil, a competitive benzodiazepine antagonist, in reversing sedation was assessed in a double-blind trial in 31 women in ASA physical status I or II who were scheduled for ambulatory gynecologic surgery lasting less than 90 minutes. Those taking any type of sedative were excluded. A mean of 12.4 mg of midazolam was given, followed by nitrous oxide in oxygen, fentanyl, and succinylcholine. Postoperatively, patients received either flumazenil solution or placebo intravenously at 1-minute intervals up to 10 mL, or until they were awake and calm.

The mean dose of flumazenil was .8 mg. Patients given this drug scored significantly better on psychodiagnostic tests than did placebo recipients 5–60 minutes after surgery. No significant difference was noted 2–3 hours after surgery. Estimates of oxygen saturation and end-expired carbon dioxide tension showed improvement 15 minutes after flumazenil injection.

Flumazenil can reverse postoperative sedation in patients given midazolam for induction of general anesthesia. Titrating the dose of flumazenil can maintain a state of wakefulness and calmness. Reversal is not, however apparent after 2 hours, so that caution is needed to avoid premature discharge of day surgery patients.

▶ The effective induction dose of midazolam in the presence of an opioid is usually less than 12.4 ± 2.4 mg as administered in this study.—R.K. Stoelting, M.D.

Effect of Flumazenil on Midazolam-Induced Amnesia

McKay AC, McKinney MS, Clarke RSJ (Belfast City Hosp; Queen's Univ of Belfast, Northern Ireland)
Br J Anaesth 65:190–196, 1990

2–30

Flumazenil is a benzodiazepine antagonist with little agonist activity that blocks the actions of both benzodiazepines and inverse agonists, e.g., β-carbolines. The effects of intravenously administered flumazenil on the amnesic and sedative effects of midazolam were examined in 6 healthy subjects who received midazolam in doses of 2 mg and 5 mg on different days. The dose of flumazenil was .01 mg/kg.

Midazolam produced dose-dependent central neural depression, as determined by estimates of critical flicker fusion frequency. Dose-dependent amnesia for word cards also was observed. Both fusion frequency and memory were restored to baseline levels after flumazenil administration. Flumazenil alone did not influence memory function.

Flumazenil, used to antagonize midazolam-induced sedation, also restores memory for events occurring during the period of antagonism. This is advantageous for dentistry or endoscopy but not when benzodiazepine sedation is used for neurologic assessment.

▶ Flumazenil will be a welcome addition to the anesthesiologist's menu of drugs. Its ultimate application, and even disadvantages, await its widespread usage, much like the naloxone story.—R.K. Stoelting, M.D.

Use of Low-Dose Ketamine Hydrochloride in Outpatient Oral Surgery
Kryshtalskyj B, Direnfeld VN, Johnson TWG (Univ of Toronto; Queensway Gen Hosp; St Michael's Hosp, Toronto)
Oral Surg Oral Med Oral Pathol 69:413–419, 1990   2–31

The quality of anesthesia with low-dose ketamine (LDK) was compared with an already acceptable alternative regimen, methohexital sodium, in a double-blind study of 40 outpatient adults undergoing minor oral surgery. After administration of nitrous oxide, all patients received diazepam and meperidine plus placebo (saline) (group 1), or methohexital sodium when necessary (group 2), LDK (group 3), and LDK and methohexital sodium as necessary (group 4). The anesthetic techniques were evaluated in terms of patients' subjective evaluation of the anesthesia, level of response to local anesthesia, psychomotor ability after surgery, recovery times, and frequency of side effects.

Patients had no preference with regard to the anesthetic technique used. Although there were no significant differences between groups in their response to local anesthesia, there was a less variable response in group 3 than in group 2. There was no significant difference in psychomotor impairment after surgery (Fig 2–9), or in the emergence of adverse reactions. Recovery time was 43.5 minutes in group 2 and 44.5 minutes in group 3.

These data indicate that LDK should be considered as an alternative to light general anesthesia with methohexital sodium in outpatient oral surgery. When used with diazepam, meperidine, and nitrous oxide, LDK is a safe and effective supplement. This technique involves polypharmacy to maximize the desirable effects of each drug through additive-synergistic interactions while minimizing the possible adverse reaction.

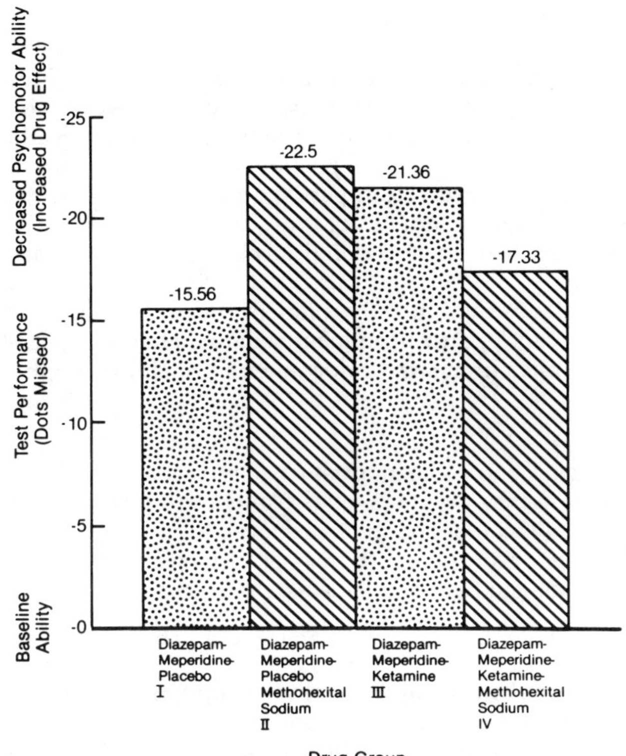

Fig 2−9.—Measure of impairment of psychomotor functions (measured at end of surgery or emergence from anesthesia). (Courtesy of Kryshtalskyj B, Direnfeld VN, Johnson TWG: *Oral Surg Oral Med Oral Pathol* 69:413−419, 1990.)

▶ The authors propose that polypharmacy maximizes the desirable effects of each drug while minimizing the possibility for adverse reactions. However, adverse additive-synergistic interactions are a constant risk, and I find little attraction to a technique that combines diazepam, meperidine, methohexital, and ketamine.—R.K. Stoelting, M.D.

Time-Dependent Pharmacodynamic Effects of Phenobarbital in Humans

Barzaghi N, Gatti G, Manni R, Galimberti CA, Zucca C, Tartara A, Perucca E (Univ of Pavia, Italy)

Ther Drug Monit 11:661−666, 1989

2−32

Most clinical studies of barbiturate tolerance have used subjective assessment criteria in chronically treated patients. Serum phenobarbital levels and pharmacodynamic data were determined in 8 normal men given single oral doses of phenobarbital, 100 mg, or placebo in a double-blind, randomized, crossover study design. Multiple sleep latency tests were carried out.

Visual analogue scales and critical flicker fusion tests indicated CNS depressant effects from phenobarbital. The drug did not, however, alter choice reaction times or the results of tapping and digit symbol substitution tests. The serum level of phenobarbital remained at a plateau through most of the observation period and was not associated with test alterations, which were noted for only up to 9 hours after drug administration. Elevated phenobarbital levels were seen for as long as 72 hours.

A single oral dose of phenobarbital producing subtherapeutic serum concentrations can lead to prominent sedative effects. Multiple sleep latency tests are a useful means of documenting such psychopharmacologic effects.

▶ What this study implies to me, rather than just a pharmacodynamic end point, is that there may well be a difference between the concentration of an active drug at the receptor and the blood level. But maybe there is a pharmacokinetic difference as well as the pharmacodynamic difference. I can't separate the 2 from the studies done to date.—M.F. Roizen, M.D.

A Method for Implementing Programmed Infusion of Thiopentone and Methohexitone With a Simple Infusion Pump

Crankshaw DP, Karasawa F (Royal Melbourne Hosp, Vic, Australia)
Anaesth Intensive Care 17:496–499, 1989   2–33

Infusion rates based on averaged patient data can provide fine control of intravenously administered anesthetics in a manner similar to use of a calibrated vaporizer to deliver volatile anesthetics. In the absence of a programmable infusion pump, it is relatively easy to convert published infusion profiles, derived from either a conventional pharmacokinetic model or from plasma drug efflux profiles, into a series of steps.

Lean body mass (LBM) is used in scaling the infusion to patient size. The size of each patient is estimated using height (in centimeters), total body weight (TBW, in kilograms), and sex according to the following equations:

$$\text{LBM (males)} = 1.10 \times \text{TBW} - 128 \times (\text{TBW/Ht})^2$$

$$\text{LBM (females)} = 1.07 \times \text{TBW} - 148 \times (\text{TBW/Ht})^2$$

Delivery rates needed to maintain a desired thiopental concentration at 10 mg/L are given in Table 1. Rates for maintaining an arterial methohexital level of 5 mg/L are given in Table 2. These tables should prove useful for instituting infusion using standard syringe infusion pumps.

TABLE 1.—Infusion Rates (mL/hr) for Thiopental for a Desired Arterial Concentration of 10 mg/L When a Syringe Concentration of 25 mg/mL Is Used

LBM (kg)	35.0	40.0	45.0	50.0	55.0	60.0	65.0	70.0	75.0
Bolus (ml)	2.8	3.2	3.6	4.0	4.4	4.8	5.2	5.6	6.0
0-5 (min)	26.5	30.2	34.0	37.8	41.6	45.3	49.1	52.9	56.7
5-10	18.5	21.1	23.7	26.4	29.0	31.6	34.3	36.9	39.5
10-20	13.3	15.2	17.1	19.0	20.9	22.8	24.7	26.6	28.5
20-30	10.8	12.4	13.9	15.5	17.0	18.6	20.1	21.7	23.2
30-60	9.6	10.9	12.3	13.7	15.0	16.4	17.8	19.1	20.5
60-90	8.7	10.0	11.2	12.5	13.7	15.0	16.2	17.5	18.7
90-120	8.3	9.4	10.6	11.8	13.0	14.2	15.3	16.5	17.7
120-150	7.9	9.1	10.2	11.4	12.5	13.6	14.8	15.9	17.0
150-180	7.7	8.9	10.0	11.1	12.2	13.3	14.4	15.5	16.6

(Courtesy of Crankshaw DP, Karasawa F: *Anaesth Intensive Care* 17:496–499, 1989.)

▶ These tables are useful and have been reprinted here for that reason. It's pretty close to what I learned as a rule of thumb back during my training—after the initial sleep dose of thiopental, the current level can be maintained by giving 1 mL/min of a 2.5% solution to a 70-kg person for the first 5 minutes, then 1 mL/2 min to a 70-kg person for the next 15 minutes. Another point of importance that I take from this article is that the lean body weight of the patient is

TABLE 2.—Infusion Rates (mL/hr) for Methohexitone for a Desired Arterial Concentration of 5 mg/L When a Syringe Concentration of 10 mg/mL Is Used

LBM (kg)	35.0	40.0	45.0	50.0	55.0	60.0	65.0	70.0	75.0
Bolus (ml)	3.5	4.0	4.5	5.0	5.5	6.0	6.5	7.0	7.5
0-5 (min)	39.6	45.3	50.9	56.6	62.3	67.9	73.6	79.2	84.9
5-10	32.4	37.1	41.7	46.3	51.0	55.6	60.2	64.9	69.5
10-20	26.3	30.0	33.8	37.5	41.3	45.1	48.8	52.6	56.3
20-30	22.1	25.3	28.4	31.6	34.8	37.9	41.1	44.2	47.4
30-60	19.4	22.1	24.9	27.7	30.4	33.2	36.0	38.7	41.5
60-90	18.0	20.5	23.1	25.6	28.2	30.8	33.3	35.9	38.5
90-120	17.3	19.7	22.2	24.7	27.1	29.6	32.1	34.5	37.0
120-150	16.8	19.2	21.6	24.0	26.4	28.8	31.2	33.6	36.0
150-180	16.5	18.8	21.2	23.5	25.9	28.3	30.6	33.0	35.3

(Courtesy of Crankshaw DP, Karasawa F: *Anaesth Intensive Care* 17:496–499, 1989.)

most appropriate to use for calculating the best estimate of dosage for pain therapy requirements. Remember, a patient's requirements for thiopental decrease by 5% per decade because of a smaller distribution to the "pharmaco-kinetic peripheral compartment." (See comment after Abstract 8–8.)—M.F. Roizen, M.D.

Neuromuscular Blocking Drugs

Anticonvulsant Therapy Increases Fentanyl Requirements During Anaesthesia for Craniotomy

Tempelhoff R, Modica PA, Spitznagel EL Jr (Washington Univ)
Can J Anaesth 37:327–332, 1990   2–34

Anesthesiologists often encounter patients who are taking 1 or more anticonvulsant medications, usually in treatment of seizure disorders. To determine whether patients taking chronic anticonvulsant therapy have an altered requirement for fentanyl during anesthesia, 61 patients undergoing craniotomy were studied. Twenty patients had never received anticonvulsants and served as the control group. The remaining 41 patients were epileptics in whom therapeutic plasma concentrations of 1, 2, or 3 different anticonvulsants were recorded.

During anesthesia with 60% to 70% nitrous oxide in oxygen and .2% isoflurane, a maintenance dose of fentanyl was given by using a continuous variable-rate intravenous infusion. This was supplemented by intermittent intravenous boluses of 50 μg. To define the minimal dosage of fentanyl required by each patient, the maintenance dose was titrated according to increases or decreases in the heart rate or mean arterial pressure exceeding 15% of baseline ward values. Epileptic patients required a

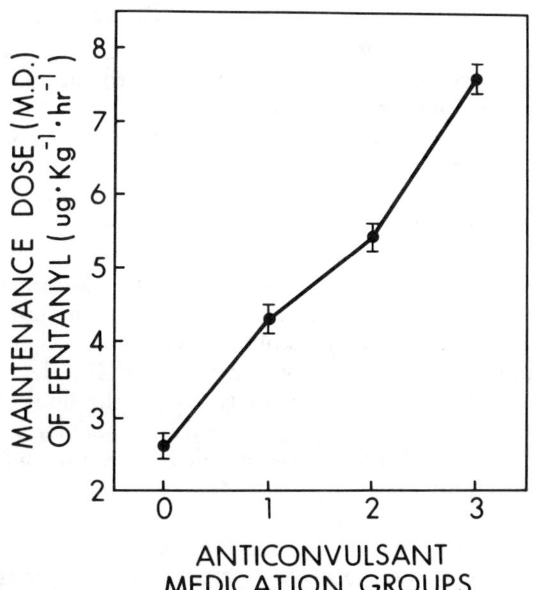

Fig 2–10.—Linear dose-effect relationship between number of anticonvulsants received in each medication (MED) group and maintenance dose (MD) of fentanyl required. Plasma level of each anticonvulsant was in therapeutic range before surgery. Values are expressed as least square means ± standard error. (Courtesy of Tempelhoff R, Modica PA, Spitznagel EL Jr: *Can J Anaesth* 37:327–332, 1990.)

progressively higher fentanyl maintenance dose, compared with controls (Fig 2–10).

Epileptic patients treated chronically with 1 or more anticonvulsant agents have higher requirements of fentanyl for maintenance of anesthesia. Furthermore, there appears to be a dose-effect relationship between the number of anticonvulsants taken and the maintenance dose of fentanyl needed during balanced anesthesia.

► A similar increased drug requirement for long-acting and intermediate-acting nondepolarizing muscle relaxants has been documented (1). In the presence of chronic anticonvulsant drug therapy, the anesthesiologist must consider the possibility that "usual" doses of drugs may be inadequate in these patients.— R.K. Stoelting, M.D.

Reference

1. Tempelhoff R, et al: *Anesth Analg* 71:665, 1990.

Contribution of Prostacyclin to D-Tubocurarine-Induced Hypotension in Humans
Hatano Y, Arai T, Noda J, Komatsu K, Shinkura R, Nakajima Y, Sawada M, Mori K (Kyoto Univ Hosp, Japan; Ono Pharmaceutical Co)
Anesthesiology 72:28–32, 1990   2–35

Histamine release is believed to be the major factor in d-tubocurarine (dTc)-induced hypotension. Histamine releases prostacyclin, a potent vasodilator, which is converted to 6-keto-prostaglandin-(PG)$F_{1\alpha}$. The role of prostacyclin in dTc-induced hypotension was examined through changes in arterial blood pressure and the plasma 6-keto-$PGF_{1\alpha}$ level after administration of dTc to 21 patients, with or without the previous administration of aspirin and histamine H_1 antagonist.

A bolus injection of dTc caused a significant decrease in mean arterial pressure that was associated with a significant increase in plasma 6-keto-$PGF_{1\alpha}$. Pretreatment with aspirin or an H_1 antagonist significantly attenuated these effects. There was a significant correlation between the arterial pressure changes and the changes in 6-keto-$PGF_{1\alpha}$ levels.

Although histamine has been considered to be the final chemical mediator of dTc-induced hypotension, prostacyclin appears to be the actual final mediator. Prostacyclin is released by histamine through H_1 receptors on vascular epithelium.

► For 25 years we have been locked into the concept that if a neuromuscular blocking drug causes hypotension, it is probably related to the release of histamine. There has been indirect evidence that this simplistic approach has been incorrect, especially with atracurium. This study confirms the concept that d-tubocurarine-induced hypotension may be related to factors in addition to histamine release.—R.D. Miller, M.D.

Clinical Observations on the Neuromuscular Blocking Action of Org 9426, a New Steroidal Non-Depolarizing Agent

Wierda JMKH, De Wit APM, Kuizenga K, Agoston S (Univ of Groningen, The Netherlands)
Br J Anaesth 64:521–523, 1990

2–36

Org 9426, the 2-morpholino, 16-allyl-pyrrolidino derivative of the 3-desacetoxy analogue of vecuronium, has a faster onset of neuromuscular blocking action and equal or shorter duration and recovery time than vecuronium, as shown in animal studies. The neuromuscular blocking effects of Org 9426, at doses of 250 µg/kg and 500 µg/kg, were investigated in 22 patients anesthetized with thiopental-fentanyl-65% nitrous

Degree of Block and Onset Characteristics of Org 9426 Compared With Vecuronium in Patients Anesthetized With an Intravenous Anesthetic Technique and 65% Nitrous Oxide in Oxygen

| | | | | | Onset time to | |
| | | | | | | |
Agent	Dose (µg kg^{-1})	n	Max. block (%)	Lag time (s)	75% block (s)	Max. block (s)
Org 9426	250	11	69 (22)	34 (11) †	94 (51)*	231 (59)
Org 9426	500	11	98 (03)	36 (14) †	68 (30)†	204 (72)
Vecuronium	85	8	100 (00)	71 (34)	155 (78)	216 (96)

Note: Values are means ± (1 SD).
*Only 6 patients reached 75% block.
† Significant difference from vecuronium ($P < .05$, Wilcoxons rank sum test).
(Courtesy of Wierda JMKH, De Wit APM, Kuizenga K, et al: *Br J Anaesth* 64:521–523, 1990.)

oxide in oxygen. The doses of Org 9426 were estimated as the ED_{90} and $2 \times ED_{90}$, respectively. The magnitude of the block, onset characteristics, and time course of action were studied with the standard ulnar nerve-adductor pollicis muscle technique.

Comparison with data for vecuronium from an identical study indicated that Org 9426 had approximately 15% of the potency of the vecuronium and offered faster onset of neuromuscular block, with good to excellent intubating conditions 1 minute after administration of 500 μg/kg (table). The duration of action and recovery index of Org 9426 appeared to be similar to those of vecuronium. Cardiovascular and other side effects were not noted. This steroidal nondepolarizing agent offers several advantages over existing nondepolarizing agents in terms of rate of development of good intubating conditions and stability in aqueous solutions.

▶ This new neuromuscular blocking drug is very similar to vecuronium. An intriguing aspect of it is that it may have an onset time more rapid than any other nondepolarizing muscle relaxant.—R.D. Miller, M.D.

Investigation of the Effects of Paralysis by Pancuronium on Heart Rate Variability, Blood Pressure, and Fluid Balance

Greenough A, Gamsu HR, Greenall F (King's College Hosp, London)
Acta Paediatr Scand 78:829–834, 1989   2–37

Paralysis of preterm neonates during mechanical ventilation may reduce the variability of cerebral blood flow, but its effect on intraventricular hemorrhage is inconsistent. The effects of pancuronium bromide in infants who were actively expiring against positive-pressure inflation were examined, and the findings were compared with those in infants of comparable gestational age who were ventilated but received no paralyzing agent. Eighteen of 29 infants in the study were paralyzed to suppress spontaneous respiratory movement.

Heart rate variability declined or disappeared after paralysis. Mean daily blood pressures were similar in the 2 groups, as was pressure variability in the first week of life. Episodes of hypotension and hypertension were similarly frequent in the 2 groups. No infant had renal failure or required marked fluid restriction. No infant in the study had pneumothorax.

Selective treatment of neonates with pancuronium appears to be safe, but close attention to the fluid balance is necessary. The study infants did not have renal failure, but they did gain weight and have persistent edema.

▶ The authors are to be congratulated for trying to obtain objective data in a difficult clinical setting, but the pancuronium group is not comparable with the control group. The readers should review the original article to detect the differences between the 2 groups.—R.D. Miller, M.D.

Concentrations of Atracurium and Laudanosine in Cerebrospinal Fluid and Plasma During Intracranial Surgery
Eddleston JM, Harper NJN, Pollard BJ, Edwards D, Gwinnutt CL (Manchester Royal Infirmary, Manchester, England)
Br J Anaesth 63:525–530, 1989   2–38

Atracurium is a suitable neuromuscular blocking agent during neurosurgical procedures, but concern has been expressed about the accumulation of laudanosine, its major breakdown product, during prolonged infusions of atracurium in intensive care. Because the concentration of laudanosine in the CNS determines toxicity, concentrations of atracurium and laudanosine in the CSF and plasma were determined during infusions of atracurium for neuromuscular block in 9 patients undergoing surgery for intracranial aneurysm.

The mean total dose of atracurium was 1.98 mg/kg (range, 1.57–2.60 mg/kg), and the mean duration of infusion was 166 minutes (range, 111–251 minutes). During infusion, plasma concentrations of laudanosine gradually increased in all patients, reaching a mean concentration of 1,449 ng/mL (range, 560–2,720 ng/mL) after 125–140 minutes of infusion (Fig 2–11). Concentrations of laudanosine in the CSF increased in 8 of 9 patients, reaching a mean concentration of 203 ng/mL (range, 50–570 ng/mL) within 125–140 minutes after infusion. The highest recorded concentration of laudanosine in CSF of 570 ng/mL was found in 1 of only 2 samples of CSF that contained atracurium and blood (Fig 2–12). Two patients had epileptiform seizures in the postoperative period, but none could be attributed to laudanosine.

Laudanosine accumulates in both plasma and CSF during infusion of atracurium. The high concentration in 1 CSF sample that contained atra-

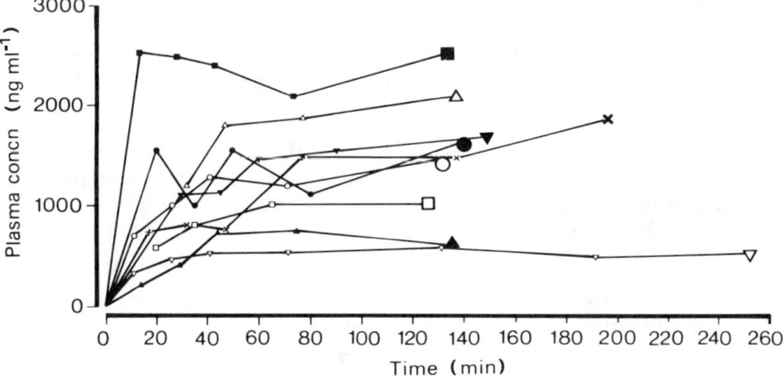

Fig 2–11.—Plasma concentrations of laudanosine for each of 9 patients during infusion of atracurium. (Courtesy of Eddleston JM, Harper NJN, Pollard BJ, et al: *Br J Anaesth* 63:525–530, 1989.)

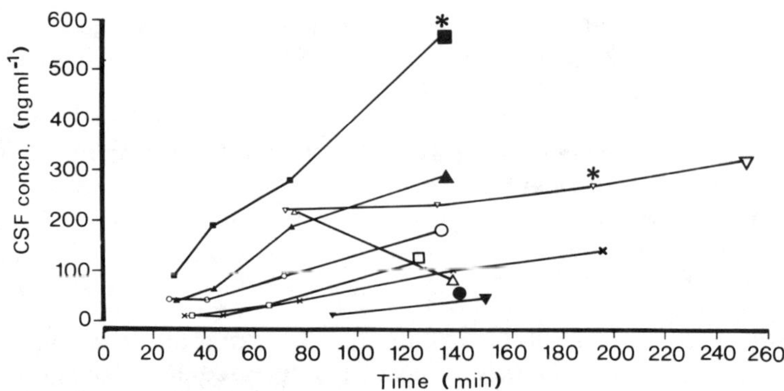

Fig 2–12.—Concentrations of laudanosine in CSF for each of 9 patients during infusion of atracurium. Samples found to contain atracurium. (Courtesy of Eddleston JM, Harper NJN, Pollard BJ, et al: *Br J Anaesth* 63:525–530, 1989.)

curium and blood probably resulted from a breakdown of atracurium from blood contamination from the operative site, loss of blood-brain barrier, and reduced production of CSF.

▶ This is another in the many studies that have attempted to determine whether laudanosine and its seizure activity is of clinical concern. Two of the 9 patients had epileptiform seizures, which the authors stated were thought not to be related to laudanosine. How did they come to this conclusion?—R.D. Miller, M.D.

Reversal of Intense Neuromuscular Blockade Following Infusion of Atracurium

Engbœk J, Østergaard D, Skovgaard LT, Viby-Mogensen J (Herlev Hosp, Rigshospitalet; Univ of Copenhagen)
Anesthesiology 72:803–806, 1990   2–39

It has been claimed that reversal from more intense levels of atracurium-induced block can be conducted safely. Introduction of the posttetanic count (PTC) method has allowed an intense level of blockade to be quantitated. To evaluate reversal time from different levels of very intense neuromuscular blockade induced by continuous infusion of atracurium, 30 patients who were anesthetized with nitrous oxide, fentanyl, and thiopental was studied. The time course of neostigmine-induced reversal from different levels of intense atracurium-induced neuromuscular blockade was evaluated using the PTC and train-of-four (TOF).

Reversal time, defined as the time from administration of neostigmine at the different PTC of a TOF ratio of .7, depended on the degree of blockade at the time of reversal. Reversal time was prolonged with more intense levels of blockade and varied between 19 and 41 minutes. There was wide individual variation in reversal time. Spontaneous recovery time, defined as the time from PTC level of 1–2 when atracurium infusion was stopped to a PTC level at which antagonism was induced, and

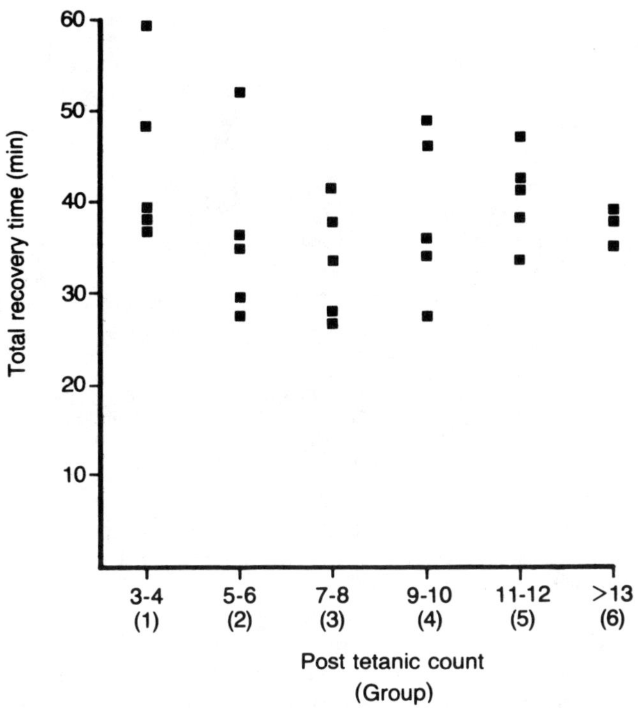

Fig 2–13.—Total recovery time (spontaneous recovery time plus reversal time) in relation to the different PTC levels from which reversal was attempted. Each patient is represented by 1 reading *(square)*. (Courtesy of Engbœk J, Østergaard D, Skovgaard LT, et al: *Anesthesiology* 72:803–806, 1990.)

reversal time were related to the square root of PTC. Total recovery time, which was the sum of spontaneous recovery time and reversal time, was inversely related to the level of blockade at the time of attempted antagonism (Fig 2–13). Neostigmine administration during intense neuromuscular blockade after infusion of atracurium does not shorten total recovery time and offers no clinical advantage.

▶ This study emphasizes that the administration of neostigmine when no twitch or very little twitch is present offers no clinical advantages and probably should not be utilized.—R.D. Miller, M.D.

Can Early Administration of Neostigmine, in Single or Repeated Doses, Alter the Course of Neuromuscular Recovery From a Vecuronium-Induced Neuromuscular Blockade?
Magorian TT, Lynam DP, Caldwell JE, Miller RD (Univ of California, San Francisco)
Anesthesiology 73:410–414, 1990   2–40

It may be necessary to antagonize neuromuscular blockade when there is no muscle response to ulnar nerve stimulation. It is not clear whether

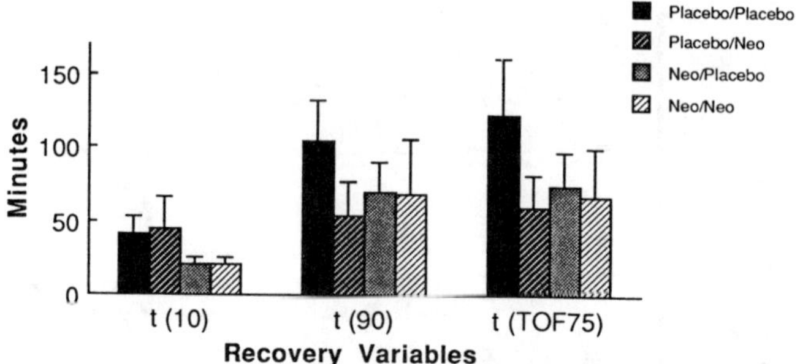

Fig 2–14.—Group comparison: times to recovery. Recovery from neuromuscular blockade as a function of time from administration of vecuronium by treatment group. All results are mean (± SD) times to recovery as a percentage of control muscle twitch t(10) is the time from vecuronium administration to 10% recovery of control twitch tension; t(90) is the time from administration of vecuronium to 90% recovery of control twitch tension; and t(TOF75) is the time from administration of vecuronium to achieving a ratio of 75% of the last twitch to the first twitch in the train-of-four. (Courtesy of Magorian TT, Lynam DP, Caldwell JE, et al: *Anesthesiology* 73:410–414, 1990.)

an antagonist, given before there is any evidence of recovery, alters the time of recovery. Neostigmine was administered to antagonize profound vecuronium-induced blockade in 40 patients scheduled for elective surgery. The dose of neostigmine was 70 µg/kg.

Neostigmine consistently shortened the time to recovery compared with placebo recipients. Initial recovery was most rapid in patients given neostigmine initially, whether or not placebo or neostigmine was given when T1 (train-of-four) had recovered to 10% of control (Fig 2–14). Later recovery was most rapid in patients given placebo and then neostigmine. There is no apparent advantage of giving neostigmine before spontaneous recovery begins. In addition, repeated doses are not indicated in the presence of profound vecuronium-induced neuromuscular blockade.

▶ This study also emphasizes that the administration of neostigmine, when no response to peripheral nerve stimulation is present, produces neither adverse nor desirable outcomes. Therefore, it probably should not be done.—R.D. Miller, M.D.

Cardiovascular

Bolus Doses of Esmolol for the Prevention of Perioperative Hypertension and Tachycardia

Oxorn D, Knox JWD, Hill J (Dalhousie Univ, Halifax, Nova Scotia)
Can J Anaesth 37:206–209, 1990   2–41

Esmolol is an intravenously administered short-acting cardioselective β-blocker with an elimination half-life of only 9.2 minutes. Previous studies have reported that esmolol infusion effectively prevented the hemodynamic alterations produced by tracheal intubation. However, few studies have examined the effectiveness of esmolol administered as bolus doses in the same setting. To determine whether bolus doses of esmolol would prevent postintubation hypertension and tachycardia, 48 women undergoing vaginal or abdominal hysterectomy were studied.

Of the women, 16 were randomly allocated to an intravenous bolus of saline solution, 20 mL; 16 were given a 20-mL bolus containing esmolol, 100 mg; and 16 received 20 mL of a solution containing esmolol, 200 mg. All bolus doses were administered over 15 seconds immediately before anesthesia induction with thiopental and succinylcholine. Tracheal intubation was carried out 90 seconds after administration of the study drug. Anesthesia was maintained with 50% nitrous oxide and enflurane 1% to 3%. Monitoring of the heart rate, systolic, diastolic, and mean blood pressures (BP), and ECG morphology was continued for at least 15 minutes after administration of the study drug.

After anesthesia induction, the heart rate in patients treated with esmolol, 200 mg, was significantly less than that in placebo-treated patients. Following intubation, the heart rate in esmolol-treated patients in both dosage groups was significantly lower than that in placebo-treated patients. However, at 2½ minutes after intubation, no further significant differences among the 3 groups were observed. After anesthesia induction the systolic BP in patients treated with esmolol, 200 mg, was significantly less than that in the esmolol, 100 mg, group or in the placebo group. However, there were no significant differences in systolic, diastolic, or mean BP among the 3 study groups at any time after intubation. The incidence of ventricular arrhythmias after intubation was also lower in esmolol-treated patients than in placebo-treated patients. None of the patients experienced episodes of myocardial ischemia.

Bolus doses of esmolol, 100 mg and 200 mg, were equally effective in ameliorating the tachycardic response to tracheal intubation. Esmolol also decreased the incidence of postintubation ventricular arrhythmias. However, neither dose prevented the hypertensive response to intubation. No side effects attributable to esmolol were observed.

▶ There is no question that bolus doses of esmolol are more practical than a continuous infusion to provide either rapid protection against predictable stimuli or treatment of abrupt increases in heart rate. In fact, my experience in anesthetized adult patients is that a bolus dose of esmolol, 10–30 mg, is often effective in the slowing heart rate to acceptable levels.—R.K. Stoelting, M.D.

Esmolol Reduces Autonomic Hypersensitivity and Length of Seizures Induced by Electroconvulsive Therapy
Howie MB, Black HA, Zvara D, McSweeney TD, Martin DJ, Coffman JA (Ohio State Univ Hosps)
Anesth Analg 71:384–388, 1990   2–42

Electroconvulsive therapy (ECT), used primarily to treat major affective psychiatric disorders, relies on electrically induced grand mal seizure for therapeutic effect. The physiologic changes accompanying ECT can produce cardiovascular stress in patients with heart disease. Several investigators have proposed that the hypertension and arrhythmia induced by ECT be controlled by β-adrenergic receptor blocking drugs. The clinical efficacy of esmolol, an ultra-short-acting, β_1-adrenergic receptor blocking drug, in controlling the sinus tachycardia and increased arterial blood pressures induced by ECT was investigated.

Twenty patients were included in the double-blind, randomized study involving 4 matched-pair trials during ECT. The patients were ASA physical status I to III. Each served as his or her own control. Each received a 4-minute infusion of either placebo or esmolol at 600 μg/kg/min. Anesthesia was induced with methohexital and succinylcholine. After electrical stimulation, the infusion was reduced to a rate of 300 μg/kg/min for 3 more minutes and then discontinued.

Patients given esmolol had significant decreases in mean heart rate from minute 2 until minute 15 and in maximum heart rate (Fig 2–15).

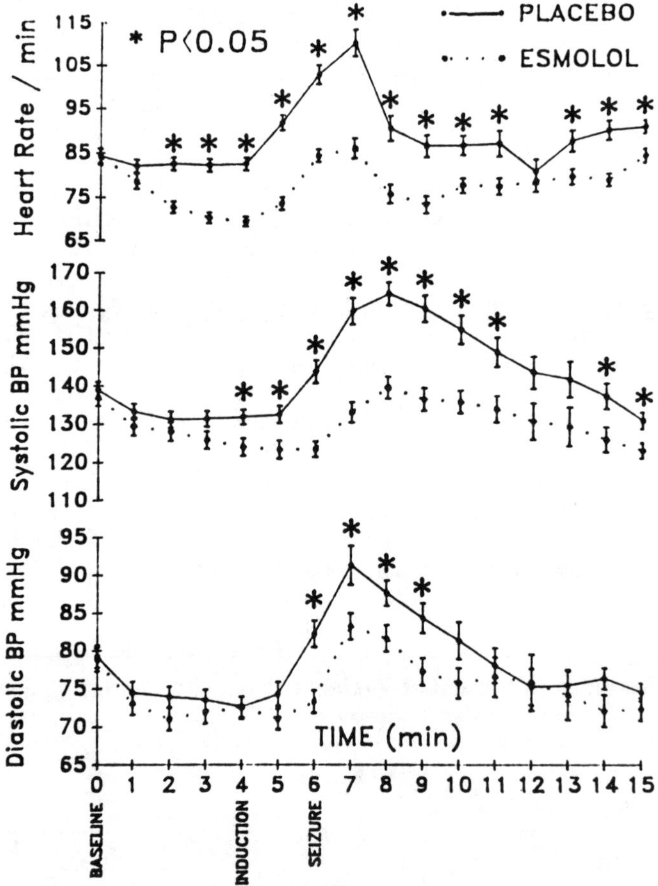

Fig 2–15.—Mean values ± 1 SE for heart rate and systolic and diastolic arterial blood pressures for all 20 patients given either esmolol or placebo during ECT. (Courtesy of Howie MB, Black HA, Zvara D, et al: *Anesth Analg* 71:384–388, 1990.)

Arterial blood pressure was also reduced during and just after infusion. The length of seizures also decreased. The drug effectively attenuates the tachycardic and hypertensive response to ECT. Its use decreases both the clinically documented and electroencephalographically measured seizure length.

► It is unclear why esmolol would influence the duration of an electrically induced seizure. Assuming that shortened seizure activity does not alter efficacy, I find the use of esmolol in selected patients undergoing ECT an attractive addition to the therapeutic menu. My guess is that single or repeated intermittent doses would be equally effective and more practical than a continuous intravenous infusion in these very brief procedures.—R.K. Stoelting, M.D.

Anesthesia and Angiotensin-Converting Enzyme Inhibitors: The Effect of Enalapril on Peri-Operative Cardiovascular Stability

Yates AP, Hunter DN (Univ College Hosp, London)
Anaesthesia 43:935–938, 1988   2–43

The properties of angiotensin-converting enzyme (ACE) inhibitors may prove advantageous during anesthesia and surgery to control hemodynamic responses to stress. The effects of enalapril, used as premedication, on cardiovascular responses to laryngoscopy and on subsequent stability were examined in 22 women undergoing elective gynecologic operations. Either 5 mg of enalapril or placebo was given orally in a double-blind manner 4 hours before surgery.

Patients given enalapril and those given placebo had comparable falls in mean arterial pressure and rises in heart rate after induction of anesthesia. After the induction, those given enalapril had significantly lower arterial pressures, and this effect lasted for 6 minutes after intubation. Postincisional arterial pressure also was lower in patients given enalapril than in the placebo recipients.

Use of an ACE inhibitor before general anesthesia may promote perioperative cardiovascular stability. Hemodynamic stability and control of sympathetic stimulation are especially important in patients who are at risk of complications from hypertension and tachycardia.

► The angiotensin-converting inhibitors, although more expensive, lead to a better quality of life for the patient who must be treated with antihypertensives. This article stresses the importance of these drugs in maintaining normal blood pressure and normal hemodynamic responses during anesthesia and surgery. Although some of these responses are definitely unwanted, others are desired. The perioperative cardiovascular stability thus engendered by the ACE inhibitors in the perioperative milieu is a double-edged sword. But it's a double-edged sword we need to learn to live with, as we'll be seeing more and more patients given these medications, should the data on quality of life in antihypertensives be borne out with repeated study.—M.F. Roizen, M.D.

Local Anesthetic

A New Local Anesthetic, Ropivacaine: Its Epidural Effects in Humans

Concepcion M, Arthur GR, Steele SM, Bader AM, Covino BG (Brigham and Women's Hosp, Boston; Harvard Med School)

Anesth Analg 70:80–85, 1990

2–44

Ropivacaine is an amide local anesthetic that is similar in structure to both bupivacaine and mepivacaine. Experimental studies have shown that ropivacaine has an anesthetic profile similar to that of bupivacaine. To determine the epidural anesthetic properties of ropivacaine, 3 different concentrations were evaluated in 12 men and 3 women, ASA physical status I and II, aged 22–60 years, who were undergoing orthopedic procedures on the lower limbs.

Patients were premedicated orally with diazepam or intravenously with midazolam. A 3-mL ropivacaine test dose was injected when the epidural space was identified. The first 5 patients were given .5% ropivacaine solution, the next 5 patients were given .75% ropivacaine, and the last 5 patients were given the 1% dosage. An additional 17 mL of the designated ropivacaine solution was given after the test dose.

As the concentration of ropivacaine increased from .5% to 1%, the time to onset of sensory anesthesia decreased. Onset of sensory anesthesia to the T_{12} dermatomal level occurred within 6.6 minutes when the .5% ropivacaine solution was used, within 6.4 minutes with the .75% solution, and within 2.4 minutes with the 1% solution. The difference in onset time to T_{12} between the .5% and the .75% solutions was not statistically significant. The degree of motor blockade varied with the concentration used. There was no significant difference in duration of motor blockade between the .75% and the 1% solutions. The time to regression of anesthesia to T_{12} increased from 255 minutes with the .5% ropivacaine solution to 356 minutes with the 1% solution. In only 1 patient was the quality of anesthesia judged unsatisfactory for the surgical procedure performed, as significant amounts of opioids were necessary to provide adequate surgical anesthesia. None of the patients experienced adverse effects from the use of epidurally administered ropivacaine.

These preliminary clinical data indicate that ropivacaine administered at the concentrations used for this study provides satisfactory anesthesia with minimal motor blockade at a concentration of .5%. Increasing the concentration results in more profound motor blockade.

Comparison of 0.5% Ropivacaine and 0.5% Bupivacaine for Epidural Anesthesia in Patients Undergoing Lower-Extremity Surgery

Brown DL, Carpenter RL, Thompson GE (Virginia Mason Med Ctr, Seattle)

Anesthesiology 72:633–636, 1990

2–45

Animal studies of a new amide local anesthetic, ropivacaine, have shown that it is less cardiotoxic than bupivacaine. The clinical effectiveness of ropivacaine and bupivacaine was compared in 45 patients aged 18–70 years undergoing lower-extremity orthopedic operations.

The patients were randomly assigned to receive either .5% ropivacaine, 20 mL, or .5% bupivacaine, 20 mL for local anesthesia. Intermittent sensory and motor measurements were monitored as long as the block was in effect. All patients were premedicated 30–90 minutes before epidural blockade with diazepam, 5–10 mg, administered orally. Midazolam and fentanyl were given for additional sedation immediately before epidural blockade. One patient was subsequently excluded from data analysis as the needle was not in the epidural space when the drug was administered.

The intensity of the sensory and motor blockade obtained with ropivacaine was clinically indistinguishable from that with bupivacaine, except that the duration of motor blockade was slightly longer after bupivacaine. If it is confirmed in future clinical trials that ropivacaine is less cardiotoxic than bupivacaine in humans, ropivacaine may have a better margin of safety for epidural anesthesia.

▶ Ropivacaine will probably be the most studied local anesthetic in history by the time it is approved for clinical use. At present, it appears that ropivacaine has the same properties as bupivacaine but with less cardiovascular toxicity. Initial clinical impressions are that there is less motor blockade with ropivacaine than is seen with bupivacaine at equivalent concentrations. This one aspect may prove to be beneficial in obstetric anesthesia where anesthesia with minimal motor block is desirable. It will be interesting to see if the higher concentrations of ropivacaine give adequate muscle relaxation for major abdominal and orthopedic procedures.—G.W. Ostheimer, M.D.

Reducing the Pain of Intradermal Lignocaine Injection by pH Buffering

McGlone R, Bodenham A (Pinderfields Hosp, Wakefield; St James' Hosp, Leeds, England)
Arch Emerg Med 7:65–68, 1990   2–46

Lidocaine, like other local anesthetics, causes pain when injected, and this pain may be lessened by increasing its pH. Lidocaine is a weak organic base consisting of charged and uncharged fractions, each of which is pH dependent. The value of raising the pH of 1% lidocaine was examined in 20 healthy adults who received 1% lidocaine (Phoenix, pH 5), 1% lidocaine (Astra, pH 6.7), 1% lidocaine (Phoenix, adjusted to pH 7.35), or physiologic saline.

Pain scores were higher with lidocaine at a lower pH and least with a solution at pH 7.35. There was no trend toward increased interstitial spread with a higher pH solution when lidocaine was injected intradermally into the flexor forearm surface.

Pain from injection of local anesthetic appears to depend more on the rate of injection than on the pH of the anesthetic solution. Slower injections will be less painful.

▶ We are indebted to the authors for emphasizing the fact that pain from injection of local anesthetic appears to depend more on the rate of injection rather than the pH of the anesthetic solution.—G.W. Ostheimer, M.D.

pH Adjustment of Local Anesthetic Solutions With Sodium Bicarbonate: Laboratory Evaluation of Alkalinization and Precipitation

Peterfreund RA, Datta S, Ostheimer GW (Massachusetts Gen Hosp; Brigham and Women's Hosp, Boston)
Reg Anesth 14:265–270, 1989

2–47

Results of previous studies on the effect of pH adjustment of commonly used anesthetics have shown that alkalinization with sodium bicarbonate speeds the onset and prolongs the duration of major nerve

Suggested Alkalinization Doses and pH Achieved

Local anesthetic		HCO_3-, ml/20 ml Anesthetic ‡	HCO_3- mEq/20 ml Anesthetic	pH after HCO_3-
2-chloroprocaine	2%	4.0	1.92	7.51
	3%	4.0	1.92	7.43
Mepivacaine	1%	4.0	1.92	7.26
	1.5%	2.0	0.96	7.00
Etidocaine	1%	0.015	0.007	5.90
	1% + epi	0.100	0.048	5.73
	1% + epi †	0.015	0.007	5.85
	1.5% + epi	0.100	0.048	5.76
Bupivacaine	0.25%	0.10	0.048	6.97
	0.5%	0.05	0.024	6.62
	0.5% + epi*	0.30	0.144	6.37
	0.5% + epi †	0.05	0.024	6.78
	0.75%	0.05	0.024	6.56
	0.75% + epi*	0.30	0.144	6.32
	0.75% + epi †	0.05	0.024	6.58
Lidocaine	1%	4.0	1.92	7.43
	1% + epi*	4.0	1.92	7.21
	1% + epi †	4.0	1.92	7.37
	1.5%	4.0	1.92	7.31
	1.5% + epi*	4.0	1.92	7.16
	1.5% + epi †	4.0	1.92	7.35
	2%	4.0	1.92	7.24
	2% + epi*	4.0	1.92	7.08
	2% + epi †	4.0	1.92	7.26

Note: No precipitation before 1 hour with sodium bicarbonate at these doses.
*Commercially added epinephrine 1:200,000.
†Freshly added epinephrine, 1:200,000
‡Data compiled for sodium bicarbonate, 4% (weight/volume), 0.48 mEq/mL.
(Courtesy of Peterfreund RA, Datta S, Ostheimer GW: *Reg Anesth* 14:265–270, 1989.)

blocks. However, a systematic study of alkalinization of commonly local anesthetic solutions in different concentrations is not yet available. Several local anesthetic solutions of different concentrations were pH adjusted, using commercially available bicarbonate solutions. The quantity of bicarbonate required to achieve a physiologic solution pH was quantitated and the onset of precipitation in the alkalinized solutions was recorded.

The anesthetics studied were 2-chloroprocaine, mepivacaine, etidocaine, bupivacaine, and lidocaine solutions in several concentrations, with or without epinephrine 1:200,000 added. Either an 8.4% or a 4% sodium bicarbonate solution was used for alkalinization. Bicarbonate solution was added to 2-mL aliquots of local anesthetic solution. Both solutions were kept at room temperature. In some experiments, test solutions were warmed in a water bath to 37° or 38° C.

Lidocaine and 2-chloroprocaine solutions readily alkalinized to near physiologic pH without precipitation. Mepivacaine solutions showed a tendency for delayed precipitation when adjusted above neutral pH. Bupivacaine and etidocaine solutions precipitated after the addition of only small amounts of sodium bicarbonate and could not be alkalinized to physiologic pH. The addition of epinephrine to plain bupivacaine and etidocaine solutions slightly reduce the pH, but both were still subject to precipitation with small quantities of sodium bicarbonate. Warming the solutions to body temperature caused only small variable differences in pH compared with solutions kept at room temperature. Similar results were obtained after alkalinization with either 4% or 8.4% bicarbonate preparations. The suggested alkalinization doses and the pH achieved in volumes that do not produce precipitation before 1 hour of incubation at room temperature are shown in the table. These data may be useful in a clinical setting whenever rapid onset of major nerve blocks is desirable.

▶ We did this study to supply the clinician with the information necessary to allow alkalinization of local anesthetics in a safe manner. Although we investigated all of the local anesthetics, the reader is cautioned that mepivacaine, bupivacaine, and etidocaine may precipitate with very small amounts of sodium bicarbonate added to the solution. I find that alkalinization is clinically useful only with lidocaine and chloroprocaine. However, because of the incidence of back pain with large volumes of chloroprocaine, I primarily use pH-adjusted lidocaine for the rapid onset of epidural anesthesia when indicated. The onset of chloroprocaine is hastened by 30 seconds with its alkalinization. Quite frankly, I do not find this clinically significant, even in cases of fetal distress when the use of chloroprocaine has been suggested on the theoretical basis that ion trapping of lidocaine could occur in the acidotic fetus. I pH adjust lidocaine for more rapid onset of epidural block to provide pain relief during labor or anesthesia for cesarean delivery.

One must remember that the more rapid onset of the epidural block in this manner is also causally related to the more rapid onset of sympathetic blockade and possible subsequent hypotension in the parturient if there is inadequate intravascular volume expansion with a crystalloid solution. One must always balance the benefits gained versus the problems created when one manipulates the local anesthetics.—G.W. Ostheimer, M.D.

Evaluation of a New Cutaneous Topical Anesthesia Preparation

Maddi R, Horrow JC, Mark JB, Concepcion M, Murray E (Harvard Med School; Brigham and Women's Hosp, Boston)
Reg Anesth 15:109–112, 1990
2–48

Topical anesthetics applied to intact skin are usually ineffective. A new topical anesthetic formulation, EMLA, reportedly provides effective cutaneous anesthesia. The oil in water emulsion contains an equal mixture of 5% lidocaine and 5% prilocaine. Both local anesthetics are contained only in the oil phase of the emulsion. This preparation must be used with an occlusive bandage and remain in contact with the skin for a certain period of time to be effective. To determine whether EMLA can prevent or alleviate the pain associated with percutaneous placement of a large intravenous catheter, and to define the contact time required for optimal topical anesthesia of intact skin, studies were made in 75 patients undergoing orthopedic or cardiac operations.

The anesthetic or placebo was applied to the dorsum of both hands under double-blind randomized conditions. The trial anesthetic was left in contact with the skin for 30 minutes before intravenous cannulation in 30 patients, for 45 minutes in 20 patients, and for 60 minutes in 25 patients. A 16-gauge catheter was inserted through each application area. Patients were then asked to rate pain severity on a 10-cm visual analogue

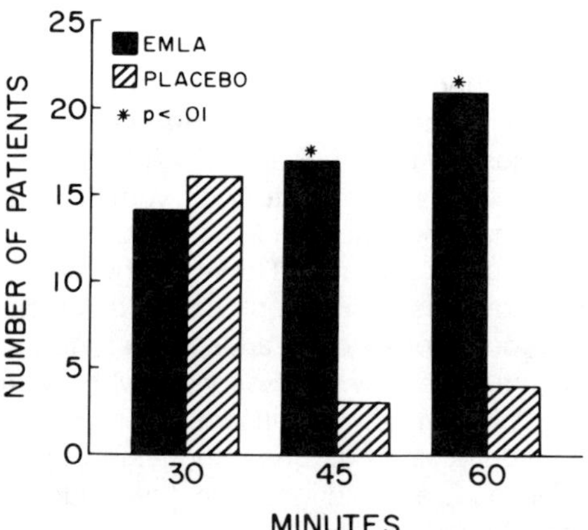

Fig 2–16.—Number of patients who preferred intravenous placement on EMLA side *(filled bar)* and placebo side *(striped bar)* after 30, 45, and 60 minutes of application ($p < .01$ by confidence limits for binomial distribution). (Courtesy of Maddi R, Horrow JC, Mark JB, et al: *Reg Anesth* 15:109–112, 1990.)

scale at each puncture site and to indicate their preference for catheter insertion as the right or the left side.

There was no difference in pain severity between the EMLA-treated and the placebo-treated side with the 30-minute application time. Although contact with the skin for 45 minutes resulted in less reported pain on the EMLA-treated side, the difference was statistically not significant. However, a highly significant difference in pain scores existed in favor of the EMLA-treated side after the 60-minute application. When asked to indicate a preference for placement of the intravenous cannula, a statistically significant preference for the EMLA-treated side was recorded with application times of 45 minutes and longer (Fig 2–16). Thus a minimum application time of approximately 40 minutes is required before EMLA achieves an acceptable degree of analgesia.

▶ I understand the need for a topical preparation that would produce sensory anesthesia for placement of intravenous catheters and the like. It would appear that this topical preparation must be applied for at least 45 minutes to have any significant anesthetic effect. The obvious question: Is the application of EMLA worth the trouble? One can only guess that additional studies in larger numbers of patients will give us a more definitive answer.

The one area in which EMLA may prove to be very effective and important is in the neonate and pediatric patient. One would hope to see appropriate studies in this area in the near future. EMLA or a similar preparation may be the answer to providing pain relief for circumcision. If one is concerned about dorsal penile nerve block or local circumferential infiltration, administration of a metered amount of EMLA or other local anesthetic preparation by means of an occlusive dressing may provide the answer to this vexing problem. Look for further commentary on this interesting problem in future YEAR BOOKS.—G.W. Ostheimer, M.D.

Adrenergic Function

Catecholamines: Study of Interspecies Variation
Hart BB, Stanford GG, Ziegler MG, Lake CR, Chernow B (Uniform Services Univ of the Health Sciences, Bethesda, Md; Massachusetts Gen Hosp, Boston; Univ of California, San Diego)
Crit Care Med 17:1203–1222, 1989   2–49

Catecholamines play an important role in the response to acute illness and injury. Although many studies on catecholamines have been published, no summary article has analyzed species variations in concentrations of circulating catecholamines. Data on the basal plasma catecholamine levels and responses to various commonly used stresses derived from more than 200 publications involving 31 animal groups were reviewed.

Primitive cartilaginous fish have the highest reported basal plasma cate-

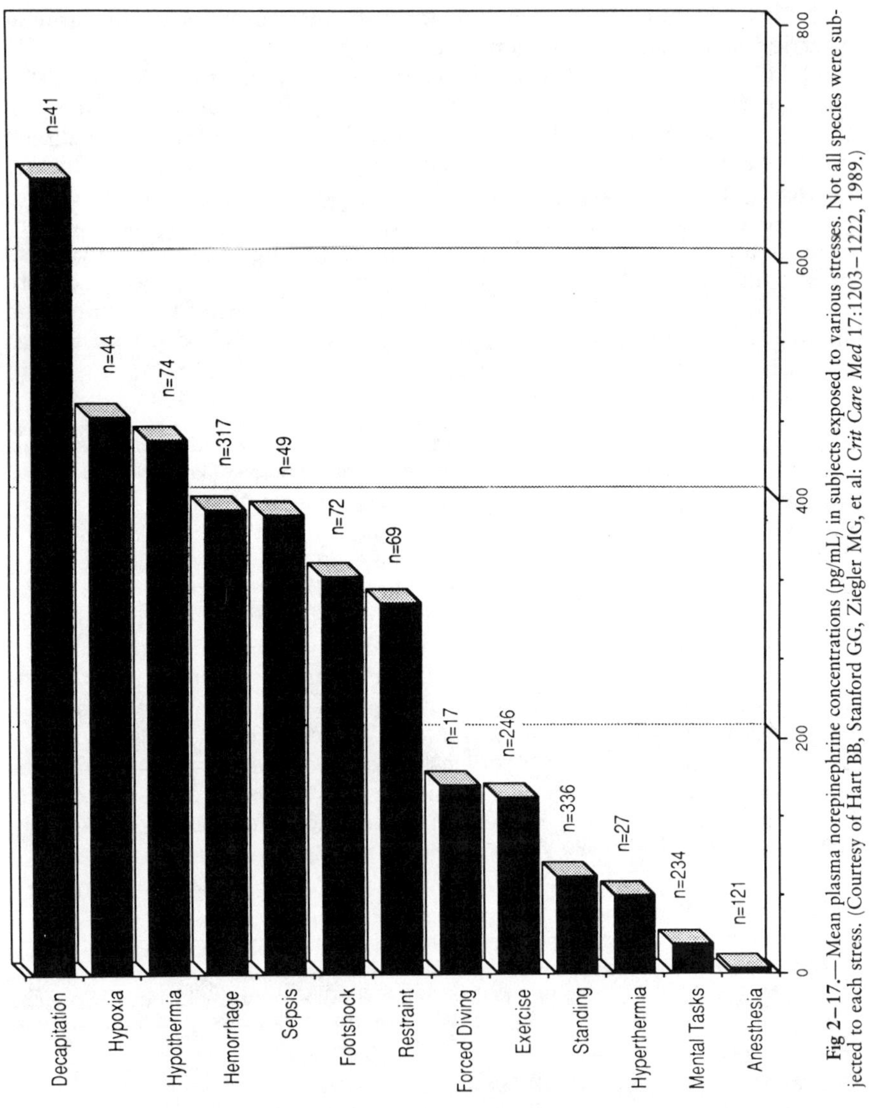

Fig 2–17.—Mean plasma norepinephrine concentrations (pg/mL) in subjects exposed to various stresses. Not all species were subjected to each stress. (Courtesy of Hart BB, Stanford GG, Ziegler MG, et al: *Crit Care Med* 17:1203–1222, 1989.)

cholamine levels, whereas birds, mammals, and teleost fish have lower basal levels. The lower levels of circulating catecholamines in these species parallel anatomical changes in the development of the adrenal medulla and nervous system. The greatest stress-induced changes reported in catecholamine concentrations are associated with decapitation, hypoxia, hemorrhage, and hypothermia (Figs 2–17 and 2–18).

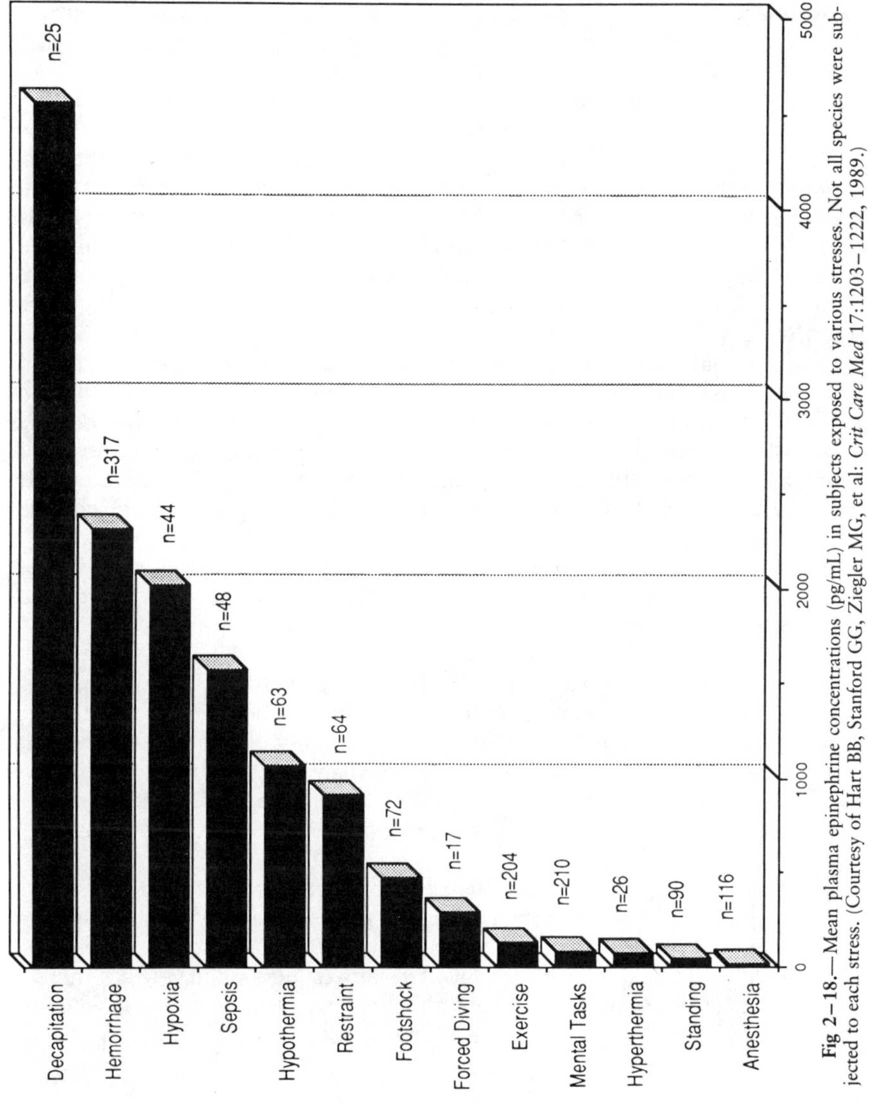

Fig 2–18.—Mean plasma epinephrine concentrations (pg/mL) in subjects exposed to various stresses. Not all species were subjected to each stress. (Courtesy of Hart BB, Stanford GG, Ziegler MG, et al: *Crit Care Med* 17:1203–1222, 1989.)

▶ This article is very useful as a reference in discussions concerning stress in newborns as opposed to adults. It clearly states that anesthesia is not very stressful compared with hemorrhage, trauma (including decapitation), hypoxia, and hypothermia, which are much more stressful in most species. I recommend these tables as useful references for anyone reading another article about catecholamine pharmacology and the stress response.—M.F. Roizen, M.D.

β-Adrenergic Receptor Function Is Acutely Altered in Surgical Patients

Marty J, Nimier M, Rocchiccioli C, Mantz J, Luscombe F, Henzel D, Loiseau A, Desmonts J-M (Hôp Bichat; Univ of Paris)

Anesth Analg 71:1–8, 1990   2–50

Perioperative adrenergic activation from surgical stress is thought to be a major factor in cardiovascular complications of surgery, particularly in patients with heart disease. Changes in lymphocyte β-adrenergic receptor density and affinity were related to changes in plasma catecholamines in 19 generally healthy surgical patients aged 18–60 years. The patients, all ASA physical status I, underwent mild elective procedures under general anesthesia.

Thirteen patients had a rise in mean plasma catecholamines during operation, which was not transient. These patients were older than the others and had higher preoperative heart rates. β-Receptor density was significantly increased in the patients with elevated catecholamine levels, whereas receptor affinity was reduced. No such changes occurred in the other patients. β-Receptor binding did not relate to heart rate changes during surgery.

β-Adrenergic receptor function may be changed acutely during and after nonmajor surgery. Altered receptor affinity could account for the adrenergic hyporesponsiveness seen in some patients.

▶ This is an important study. Jonathan Moss and I tried to prove this in 1975, and I know that Mervyn Maze also tried to determine this. We thought that the β-adrenergic receptor function alterations, both upregulation and downregulation, could account for other than the hemodynamic and dysrhythmic changes we saw perioperatively. We didn't segregate patients the way Marty et al. have done, and perhaps that is why they were able to find changes when we were not.

I think there is more and more evidence to support the fact that stress is an important variable that can affect outcome after surgery, and this is another study supporting that hypothesis. It may be that those patients who already are experiencing stress and have high levels of stress intraoperatively are more at risk of complications postoperatively if they do not also receive supplemental catecholamines in those periods, whereas those who don't normally experience stress will be endangered by intraoperative stress.—M.F. Roizen, M.D.

3 Preoperative Evaluation

General

Preoperative Anxiety: Is It a Predictable Entity?

Domar AD, Everett LL, Keller MG (Beth Israel Hosp–New England Deaconess Hosp, Boston)
Anesth Analg 69:763–767, 1989   3–1

Patients anticipating identical invasive medical or surgical procedures exhibit different levels of preoperative anxiety. Because the predictability of preoperative anxiety has not been well studied, patient characteristics that may serve to warn health care professionals about the potential for increased preoperative anxiety were sought in 523 patients (mean age, 39.7 years) undergoing elective surgery. Each participant completed a Spielberger State-Trait Anxiety Inventory while awaiting registration. The patient's blood pressure and pulse also were measured and recorded. Fourteen different characteristics were recorded for each patient, including demographics, possibility of cancer, presence of a support person, previous surgical experience, and extent of surgery; 81% of the patients were women.

Women had significantly higher anxiety scores than men. The mean blood pressure and pulse immediately before operation were lower than expected. Patients who were accompanied by a support person were more anxious than those who came alone. All other factors were noncontributory to preoperative anxiety.

It has generally been assumed by surgical and anesthesia personnel that the level of a patient's preoperative anxiety is directly related to the type of operation. For instance, cancer patients would have higher anxiety levels than noncancer patients, and patients having major surgery are expected to be more anxious than those having minor surgical procedures. However, this study found that the level of preoperative anxiety reflected the patients' personality and coping style, rather than their actual concerns about the risk of operation or anxiety about anesthesia.

▶ Preoperative anxiety is a predictable and normal reaction that is influenced by a complex array of tangible and intangible characteristics. The present data confirm the importance of the patient's personality and coping style, which are unlikely to be amenable to psychological or pharmacologic manipulation in the few hours preceding elective operations.—R.K. Stoelting, M.D.

Aerobic Exercise Reduces Levels of Cardiovascular and Sympathoadrenal Responses to Mental Stress in Subjects Without Prior Evidence of Myocardial Ischemia

Blumenthal JA, Fredrikson M, Kuhn CM, Ulmer RL, Walsh-Riddle M, Appelbaum M (Duke Univ; Karolinska Inst, Stockholm; Vanderbilt Univ)
Am J Cardiol 65:93–98, 1990   3–2

Aerobic exercise training reduces the standard risk factors of coronary artery disease (CAD). Excessive activation of the sympathetic nervous system has been implicated as a potential risk factor for CAD, but previous studies could not confirm the role of exercise training in reducing stress responses. A randomized clinical study was conducted to assess the cardiovascular and sympathoadrenal responses to a mental stressor in healthy men. Individuals with type A behavior patterns were selected for study because they are considered to be at increased risk for CAD from mental stress.

A total of 37 men aged 30–52 years without previous evidence of CAD were randomly assigned to either an aerobic exercise training program or a strength and flexibility training program. All study participants underwent comprehensive physiologic and behavior assessments before the start of the 12-week program and were re-evaluated at completion of the program. Assessment included graded exercise treadmill testing with direct measurement of oxygen consumption, and measurement of the cardiovascular and neuroendocrine responses to mental arithmetic.

The 12-week program was completed by 35 men. Participants in the aerobic program achieved significant reductions in heart rate at rest and at 5 METs, and increased their treadmill time by almost 2 minutes. Participants in the strength training program almost tripled their leg strength and doubled their arm strength, but made only small gains in aerobic fitness. At the end of the program, the men in the aerobic training group tended to exhibit less cardiovascular reactivity to mental stress compared with those in the strength training group, as evidenced by slightly decreased epinephrine secretion and faster recovery. Aerobic exercise reduces levels of cardiovascular and sympathoadrenal responses during and after mental stress. However, aerobic exercise is more likely to reduce the overall levels of the cardiovascular response to stress, rather than the magnitude of absolute change of responses from rest to mental stress.

▶ This article's abstract is more impressive than are the absolute data presented. I wonder: Should we all participate in aerobic exercise so that we have less stress during the rest of our lives? This article accentuates the fact that much of what anesthesiologists do, much of the capacity to change outcomes, may be attributable to our ability to better manage patients preoperatively. Should every patient we see preoperatively be given aerobic conditioning for 2 or 3 months to achieve the optimal condition for surgery? What would happen to the number of orthopedic cases we saw if such was the case? Some of this is said tongue in cheek, but the essential hypothesis remains true: If we all had a sympathectomy at birth, we might have less myocardial damage, or, failing that, we need to be in optimal condition to allow our hearts to undergo regular sympathetic stress so we can withstand the sympathetic stress that postoperative pain engenders.—M.F. Roizen, M.D.

Cardiopulmonary Complications in High-Risk Surgical Patients: The Value of Preoperative Radionuclide Cardiography

Pedersen T, Kelbaek H, Munck O (Univ of Copenhagen)
Acta Anaesthesiol Scand 34:183–189, 1990   3–3

Can the nuclide estimation of left ventricular function predict cardiopulmonary complications in high-risk patients? In a series of 7,306 patients having noncardiac surgery in 1986–1987, 95 patients with chronic cardiopulmonary insufficiency underwent nuclide cardiography. These patients had predominantly left-sided, chronic cardiac insufficiency or chronic pulmonary insufficiency with symptoms of right-side heart failure.

The risk of cardiovascular complications in high-risk patients having a left ventricular ejection fraction below 50% or above 70% was 58%. In contrast, those with a normal ejection fraction had a cardiovascular complication rate of 12%. High-risk patients with a left ventricular end-diastolic volume above 140 mL had a 37% risk of cardiovascular complications (table).

It seems appropriate to measure the left ventricular ejection fraction in patients with heart failure or severe ischemic heart disease who are ad-

Preoperative Clinical Cardiac Status, LVEF, and LVEDV in
Relation to Cardiovascular Complications, Sensitivity,
Specificity, and Odds Ratios

	No.	Cardiovascular complications	Sensitivity	Specificity	Odds ratio
IHD†	42	29% (12)	31%	56%	0.5
MI†	34	35% (12)	29%	69%	1.0
CHF†	33	42% (14)	42%	72%	1.3
LVEF					
<50% or >70%	36	58% (21)*	75%	78%	8.2
50–70%	59	12% (7)			
LVEDV††					
>140 ml	54	37% (20)	77%	44%	2.6
≤140 ml	33	18% (6)			

Abbreviations: LVEF, left ventricular ejection fraction (%); *LVEDV*, left ventricular end-diastolic volume (mL).

*Indicates a statistically significant differed (*P* < .001) between the patients with LVEF inside or outside the discrimination values.

†Patients with clinical symptoms of left ventricular insufficiency.

‡Left ventricular volumes were not measured in 8 patients.

(Courtesy of Pedersen T, Kelbaek H, Munck O: *Acta Anaesthesiol Scand* 34:183–189, 1990.)

mitted for major surgery. Estimates of left ventricular end-diastolic volume are not warranted clinically.

▶ This study demonstrates that the odds ratio of cardiopulmonary complications increases by eightfold when the left ventricular ejection fraction is abnormal before surgery, especially if it is less than 50%. Because such data can be obtained from a plain chest x-ray film, according to the report of Mangano et al. (1), it appears that, in high-risk surgical patients, all one has to do is look at the chest film and, if an increased cardiothoracic diameter is seen, the risk of complications is elevated and the odds ratio for mortality greatly increased. But I think we knew this from the data of Goldman and others (2) before this study was done.

Can you improve the outcome with excellent perioperative care? Some of the things we don't know from this study are how good the perioperative care was, how monitoring in postoperative care was instituted, and whether anything special was done for high-risk patients. This study helps us in great measure to understand risk; it does not do anything to help us understand how to decrease risk. This appears to be the next major step needed, using large databases such as are available in Scandinavia. In small controlled studies in isolated populations in which care can be rigorously controlled, it appears that normalizing hemodynamics, maintaining cardiac filling volumes in normal ranges, and intensive sympatholysis can improve outcome. Whether or not this will happen in larger populations in which cardiovascular control may be less is not clear.—M.F. Roizen, M.D.

References

1. Mangano DT, et al: *Anesthesiology* 63:65, 1985.
2. Goldman L, et al: *N Engl J Med* 297:845, 1977.

A Computer-Assisted Medical Diagnostic Consultation Service: Implementation and Prospective Evaluation of a Prototype
Bankowitz RA, McNeil MA, Challinor SM, Parker RC, Kapoor WN, Miller RA
(Univ of Pittsburgh; VA Med Ctr, Pittsburgh)
Ann Intern Med 110:824–832, 1989   3–4

The accuracy of a computer-aided consultation service using academic general internists and the Quick Medical Reference diagnostic program was evaluated. The program functions at several levels, including direct viewing of any disease profile, differential diagnosis of more than 4,000 findings, comparison of profiles or differential diagnoses on an electronic spreadsheet, and use of a scoring algorithm to provide ranked diagnostic hypotheses for a given set of patient findings. At this advanced level, the program functions as a medical expert consultant system.

The diagnostic accuracy of computer-aided consultation was examined prospectively in 31 patients seen as diagnostic challenges. A diagnosis was established in 20 of these patients. Computer-assisted diagnoses were

85% sensitive, compared with a diagnostic sensitivity of 80% for consult service physicians and 60% for ward teams. In 26 patients the consultation influenced the postconsultation differential diagnosis of ward teams. House officers considered the service to have been educationally helpful in 25 patients.

The Quick Medical Reference system provides reasonable diagnostic suggestions that may alter the differential diagnosis. It is very often helpful to the diagnostic process, as well as having educational value.

▶ This article is interesting because of what it says about preoperative evaluation and consultation. Although the computer was not used for that in the study, it was used for diagnostic dilemmas. It is apparent that diagnostic accuracy is a more complex issue than is determining the relative possibilities of disease. The article shows the tremendous accuracy of the computer, and it does better than the usual admitting physician in coming to differential diagnoses. It doesn't, however, show the efficacy of the computer system in helping to speed the process of arriving at the correct diagnosis. Nevertheless, this study indicates that computers can aid physicians to become better at what physicians do. The computer functions in this process, I believe, as a very large memory system for linking key symptoms to possible differential diagnoses.—M.F. Roizen, M.D.

Risk

Angina and Other Risk Factors in Patients With Cardiac Diseases Undergoing Noncardiac Operations
Shah KB, Kleinman BS, Rao TLK, Jacobs HK, Mestan K, Schaafsma M (Loyola Univ, Maywood, Ill; Hines VA Hosp, Hines, Ill)
Anesth Analg 70:240–247, 1990   3–5

Previous studies have shown a correlation between a history of recent myocardial infarction (MI) and the incidence of a perioperative MI in patients who undergo noncardiac operations. However, the relationship between chronic stable angina or ECG signs of ischemia and the incidence of perioperative MI is not known. The present prospective clinical trial was designed to determine the incidence of perioperative MI and cardiac death among patients with a preoperative history of cardiac disease who had noncardiac operations and to identify preoperative risk factors that might help to predict these adverse outcomes.

During the 18-month study period 407 men and 281 women with a history of cardiac disease or who were older than age 70 years underwent noncardiac operations. The mean age of the 688 patients was 67.7 years and 349 were older than age 70. One hundred patients underwent emergency procedures. Twenty-four preoperative patient factors were tested against the outcomes.

Forty patients (5.8%) had perioperative MI or died of cardiac causes. Thirty-two patients had perioperative MI and 7 of them had a cardiac death. Seven of the 8 patients who did not have perioperative MI died of left ventricular failure or documented ventricular dysrhythmias, and 1 patient had a sudden, unexplained death. Thus the total number of cardiac deaths was 15 (2.2%).

The incidence of perioperative MI in patients with chronic stable angina was 11.4%, in patients with unstable angina it was 28%, in patients with signs of ischemia on preoperative resting ECGs it was 9.8%, and in those with a previous MI it was 7.3%. The incidence of perioperative MI or cardiac death among the 100 patients who underwent emergency operations was 18%, compared with a 3.7% among those who had elective operations. The incidence of an adverse outcome was 8.2% in patients who underwent abdominal, thoracic, aortic, or major vascular operations, compared with 3.5% for those had other operations.

Other major postoperative complications included new congestive heart failure or worsening of preexisting congestive heart failure in 3.3%, rhythm disturbances in 7%, and stroke in 1.6%. Eight preoperative risk factors were significantly associated with perioperative MI or cardiac death: emergency operation, chronic angina, ECG ischemia, previous MI, age 70 years or older, hypokalemia, and thoracic, abdominal, aortic, and perivascular operations.

▶ The anesthesiologist must recognize the implications of known risk factors but, at the same time, accept the fact that the benefit of surgery may often outweigh these risks. When this is the case, the anesthesiologist can justifiably take pride in his or her ability to utilize modern anesthetic drugs, monitoring, and knowledge in minimizing physiologic trespass in these fragile patients.—R.K. Stoelting, M.D.

Postsurgical Mortality in Manitoba and New England

Roos LL, Fisher ES, Sharp SM, Newhouse JP, Anderson G, Bubolz TA (Univ of Manitoba, Winnipeg; Dartmouth Med School; Harvard Univ; Univ of British Columbia, Vancouver)
JAMA 263:2453–2458, 1990   3–6

The United States spends up to 50% more on hospitals than Canada does on a per capita basis, but little is known of the comparative outcomes. Insurance databases were used to compare postoperative mortality rates associated with 11 surgical procedures before and after adjusting for case mix in residents of New England and Manitoba older than 65 years.

Patients in Manitoba had somewhat fewer high-risk diagnoses. Mortality rates at 30 days for low- and moderate-risk procedures were similar in the 2 regions, but the 6-month mortality rate was lower in Manitoba. Both 30-day and 6-month rates were lower in New England for the 2 high-risk procedures—coronary bypass with valve replacement and hip fracture repair. Mortality was increased in Manitoba for all types of fracture repair and in all age groups. The finding of similar short-term mortality for low- and moderate-risk operations suggests that increased hospital expenditures in the United States may not result in substantially improved outcomes.

▶ The authors examined 11 specific procedures, before and after case mix adjustment, done in patients older than 65 years old. They found that the increased amount of money spent in the United States probably has no effect with regard to low- or moderate-risk procedures but is associated with lower mortality in high-risk procedures. These results agree with my bias because, if our intensive care unit treatment mentality in the United States makes any difference at all, it is in high-risk patients. Nevertheless, I am bothered because I believe that the risk adjustments the authors used might not have been the most optimal. For instance, they didn't use the ASA status or any equivalent objective ASA status. In addition, data from Manitoba are compared from 1980 to 1986 vs. data from New England for 1984 and 1985. This time difference may make major changes in the absolute risk to patients. Thus, although I see some problems with the data, the findings indicate nevertheless that short-term mortality favors Canadians coming to the United States for hip repair and valve/coronary artery bypass surgery, but not for lower risk procedures.—M.F. Roizen, M.D.

Preoperative Prediction of Postoperative Complications
Oguz M, Sayar A, Yalin R (Cumhuriyet Univ, Sivas, Turkey)
Isr J Med Sci 26:147–149, 1990   3–7

An attempt to predict postoperative complications was made in 100 patients having major surgery, 17 of them under emergency conditions. An age range of 18–85 years was represented; the mean patient age was 47 years. A wide range of risk markers was identified (Table 1).

All high- and middle-risk patients had complications, as did half of the patients in the low-risk group (Table 2). Major complications were more than twice as frequent in high-risk patients as in the middle-risk group. No low-risk patients had major complications. Weight loss was significantly more prevalent in high-risk than in middle-risk patients. Low albumin levels occurred at significantly different frequencies in all risk groups. Careful history taking, combined with physical examination and routine laboratory testing, is a simple and reliable approach to predicting complications after major surgery.

▶ Many persons are looking for a more objective index than the ASA Physical Status Index. Although the Physical Status Index at any one hospital will predict risk, it is not reliable across hospitals because of the variability in grading; i.e., a 3 at one hospital will always be at a lower risk than a 4 at that hospital, but a 3 at one hospital may equal a 4 at another hospital. Thus this is a welcome attempt at an objective index of risk based on history, physical findings, and a few laboratory tests. Unfortunately, the group studied isn't large enough to tell how well it predicts, and the indices may need to be reworked to give better discrimination between high-, middle-, and low-risk groups.—M.F. Roizen, M.D.

TABLE 1.—Risk Markers and Their Scores

Risk markers	Score
Weight loss (kg)	
None	0
1-5	1
5-10	2
$>$ 10	3
Minor risk factors	
Bronchitis	1
Smoking	1
Treated hypertension	1
Mild angina	1
Past rheumatic fever or tuberculosis	1
High alcohol intake	1
Diabetes	1
History of jaundice	1
Major risk factors	
Severe obstructive airway disease	4
Current chest infection	4
Recent myocardial infarction	4
Arrhythmias requiring treatment	4
Obstructive jaundice	4
Renal, respiratory or cardiac failure	4
Thrombocytopenia	4
Clinical metastatic cancer	4
Clinical sepsis	4
Albumin level (g/dl)	
3-3.5	1
$<$ 3	2
Lymphocyte count (/mm^3)	
1,500-2,000	1
$<$ 1,500	2
Obesity ($>$ 20% optimal weight)	1

(Courtesy of Oguz M, Sayar A, Yalin R: *Isr J Med Sci* 26:147–149, 1990.)

TABLE 2.—Distribution of Postoperative Complications Among Patients According to Risk

	Complications			
	Present			
Risk	Major	Minor	Total	Absent
High (n=14)	11	14	25	0
Middle (n=32)	9	32	41	0
Low (n=54)	0	27	27	27

(Courtesy of Oguz M, Sayar A, Yalin R: *Isr J Med Sci* 26:147–149, 1990.)

A Prospective Study of Mortality Associated With Anesthesia and Surgery: Risk Indicators of Mortality in Hospital

Pedersen T, Eliasen K, Henriksen E (Herlev Hosp, Univ of Copenhagen)
Acta Anaesthesiol Scand 34:176–182, 1990   3–8

Causes of anesthesia-associated and surgical deaths were sought in a series of 7,306 patients undergoing abdominal, urologic, gynecologic, and orthopedic operations in 1986–1987. Overall hospital mortality was 1.2 deaths per 100 anesthesias. Four patients died during anesthesia, 3 of surgical bleeding and 1 after epidural bupivacaine administration. Seven of 10 deaths occurring during recovery were related to cardiopulmonary failure.

Abdominal surgery was associated with the highest mortality. The odds ratio for death after emergency anesthesia compared with elective

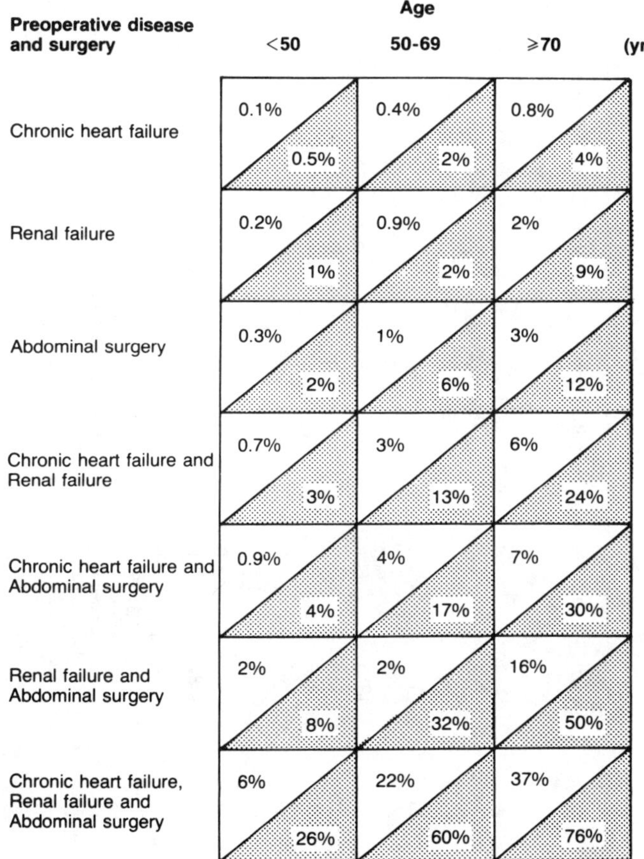

Fig 3–1.—Estimated risk of hospital mortality in relation to age, pre-operative disease, and surgery. Elective surgery = *unshaded area:* emergency surgery = *shaded area.* (Courtesy of Pedersen T, Eliasen K, Henriksen E: *Acta Anaesthesiol Scand* 34:176–182, 1990.)

TABLE 1.—Incidence of In-Hospital Mortality in 7,306 Anesthetics in Relation to Demographic Variables

Demography	No.	In-hospital mortality					
		Minor surgery		Major surgery			
		Elective	Emergency	Elective	Emergency	Total	(n)
Age (yr)							
< 20	405	0.0	0.0	0.0	6.7	0.3	(1)
20–39	2532	0.2	0.3	0.4	0.7	0.2	(6)
40–59	1955	0.0	0.3	0.9	4.3	0.6	(12)
60–69	1116	0.4	2.3*	1.1	12.3*	2.2*	(26)
70–79	886	0.2	4.1**	1.8*	11.0*	2.9**	(27)
≥ 80	293	0.0	7.0†	5.6*	10.3†	5.8††	(18)
Sex							
Male	2634	0.3 (3.2)	1.0 (1.3)	2.5§ (5.8)	13.0§§ (4.5)	2.2§§ (3.2)	
Female	4587	0.0	0.8	0.4	3.2	0.7	
Total incidence of mortality		0.1	0.8	1.0	6.3	1.2	

The mortality rate per 100 anesthetics is given. Numbers in brackets indicate odds ratios. $*P < .05$, $**P < .01$, $†P < .001$, and $‡P < .0001$ indicate a statistically significantly higher rate of mortality in age compared to the patients with lower age, and $§P < .01$ and $§§P < .001$ indicate a significantly higher rate of mortality in males.
(Courtesy of Pedersen T, Eliasen K, Henriksen E: *Acta Anaesthesiol Scand* 34:176–182, 1990.)

anesthesia was 6.8. The risk of death increased with patient age (Table 1), male gender, and the presence of clinical congestive failure (Table 2). Mortality was higher when cardiopulmonary complications occurred postoperatively than when they occurred during anesthesia (Table 3).

TABLE 2.—Incidence of In-Hospital Mortality in Relation to Preoperative Diseases

| | | In-hospital mortality | | | | |
| | | Minor surgery | | Major surgery | | |
Disease	No.	Elective	Emergency	Elective	Emergency	Total
Chronic heart failure	199	0.0	7.4† (11.2)	4.3 (5.0)	28.9†† (7.7)	9.0†† (9.9)
Hypotension (SBP<90 mmHg (12 kPa))	127	0.0	6.5* (10.1)	0.9	31.3†† (6.8)	9.4†† (9.8)
Previous MI						
≥1 yr	125	0.0	14.3†	0.0	15.4*	4.4**
<1 yr	26	0.0		9.1*	16.7*	7.7**
Chronic obstructive lung disease	201	0.0	0.0	4.5* (5.3)	25.0* (5.5)	5.0† (4.7)
Diabetes	141	0.0	0.0	6.1* (7.3)	3.1 (0.6)	2.1 (1.8)
Renal failure	153	0.0	16.7† (25.8)	0.0	12.1†† (2.1)	5.9†† (5.2)
Cancer	1257	0.1 (1.0)	0.0	2.5* (5.0)	16.7† (2.8)	1.1 (1.0)

Total number of anesthetics = 7,306. The mortality rate per 100 anesthetics is given, and numbers in brackets indicate odds ratios. *$P < .05$, **$P < .01$, †$P < .01$, and ‡$P < .001$ indicate a statistically significantly higher mortality rate compared to the total incidence of mortality.
(Courtesy of Pedersen T, Eliasen K, Henriksen E: *Acta Anaesthesiol Scand* 34:176–182, 1990.)

Hospital mortality is related to age, preoperative diagnoses, and surgical factors in Table 4 and Figure 3–1.

Overall mortality associated with anesthesia and surgery was low in this study. In only 30 of more than 7,000 cases was death the result of

TABLE 3.—Incidence of In-Hospital Mortality in Relation to Cardiopulmonary Complications

| | | In-hospital mortality | | | | |
| | | Minor surgery | | Major surgery | | |
Complications	No.	Elective	Emergency	Elective	Emergency	Total
Intraoperative cardiovascular	266	0.0	11.5†† (20.1)	2.2 (2.5)	24.0†† (5.8)	6.8†† (7.0)
Postoperative cardiovascular	241	3.0** (34.4)	19.2** (46.0)	8.6†† (16.3)	36.7†† (21.6)	20.7†† (46.0)
Intraoperative pulmonary	65	0.0	22.2* (40.4)	0.0	12.5 (2.1)	4.6* (4.6)
Postoperative pulmonary	296	4.0** (46.0)	19.4†† (52.9)	5.8† (10.3)	27.6†† (11.5)	15.9†† (30.6)

The mortality rates are given in percent and numbers in brackets indicate odds ratios. *$P < .05$, **$P < .01$, †$P < .001$, and ‡$P < .0001$ indicate a statistically significantly higher rate of mortality compared to the total incidence of mortality.

(Courtesy of Pedersen T, Eliasen K, Henriksen E: *Acta Anaesthesiol Scand* 34:176–182, 1990.)

TABLE 4.—Significant Indicators of In-Hospital Mortality
Following Anesthesia

| | In-hospital mortality | | | |
| | Regression coefficient (β) | Standard errors (SE) | Odds (e^β) | P value |
Risk factors				
Patient factors				
Age ≥ 70 yr	2.20	0.37	9.03	<0.0001
50–69 yr	1.45	0.37	4.26	<0.0001
CHF	1.15	0.35	3.16	<0.0001
Renal failure	2.00	0.44	7.39	<0.0001
Surgical factors				
Abdominal surgery	2.29	0.31	9.87	<0.0001
Emergency surgery	1.67	0.30	5.31	<0.0001
Constant	-8.17	0.44	0.00029	

(Courtesy of Pedersen T, Eliasen K, Henriksen E: *Acta Anaesthesiol Scand* 34:176–182, 1990.)

avoidable anesthetic factors. Attempts to predict mortality risk should take both patient- and surgery-related factors into account.

▶ This well-done study, which looked at the mortality associated with 7,306 patients anesthetized between August 1986 and July 1987 at 1 hospital in Copenhagen, included multiple regression analysis to determine the risks from anesthesia and objective indices of risk. This article adds to the cumulating index of articles showing that operative site, emergency surgery, long operations, age, chronic heart failure, myocardial infarction less than 1 year previously, and renal failure are the major risk factors, and that other risk factors (e.g., angina, hypertension, and diabetes) do not add significantly to the mortality risk. The odds ratio of mortaliy in a patient older than age of 70 was more than 9, that of someone with chronic heart failure was more than 3, renal failure more than 7, and abdominal surgery almost 10; emergency surgery posed a fivefold greater risk than in patients without these conditions. I imagine pretty soon in risk discussions with patients we should talk about their individual risk and be able to predict it based on their previous or morbid conditions. From this study, it appears that there aren't many things you have to find out about to have an informed risk discussion.—M.F. Roizen, M.D.

A Prospective Study of Risk Factors and Cardiopulmonary Complications Associated With Anaesthesia and Surgery: Risk Indicators of Cardiopulmonary Morbidity

Pedersen T, Eliasen K, Henriksen E (Herlev Hosp, Univ of Copenhagen)
Acta Anaesthesiol Scand 34:144–155, 1990   3–9

A prospective study was made of data on 7,306 anesthetized patients having major operations to identify the frequency and type of cardiopulmonary complications that occur and the factors associated with them. The patients had gastrointestinal, urologic, gynecologic, or orthopedic surgery.

Cardiovascular complications requiring intervention occurred during surgery in 3.6% of patients, including 8 who had cardiac arrest and 12 with acute myocardial infarction. Thirty-three patients had clinical signs of severe respiratory insufficiency. Cardiovascular complications were more frequent in patients aged 70 and above, and in those with a history of ischemic heart disease or chronic heart failure (Table 1). Pulmonary complications correlated with older age, preexisting chronic obstructive lung disease, and general anesthesia, including muscle relaxants (Table

TABLE 1.—Significant Indicators of Cardiovascular Complications Following Anesthesia

Variables of significant importance	Regression coefficients (β)	Standard errors	Odds (e^{β})	P Value
Patient factors				
Chronic heart failure	1.83	0.23	6.24	<0.0001
Preoperative renal failure (creatinine > 300 mol/l)	0.85	0.39	2.34	<0.05
Ischaemic heart disease	1.00	0.40	2.71	<0.01
Previous myocardial infarction (< 1 year)	1.65	0.29	5.21	<0.0001
Previous myocardial infarction (1 year)	1.33	0.32	3.78	<0.0001
Age (50–69 year)	1.26	0.45	3.52	<0.0001
(70 year)	1.96	0.46	7.10	<0.0001
Surgical factors				
Major surgery	1.36	0.19	3.90	<0.0001
Constant	-5.98	0.48	0.0025	

(Courtesy of Pedersen T, Eliasen K, Henriksen E: *Acta Anaesthesiol Scand* 34:144–155, 1990.)

TABLE 2.—Significant Indicators of Pulmonary Complications
Following Anesthesia

Variables of significant importance	Regression coefficients	Standard errors	Odds (e^β)	P value
Patient factors				
Age (50–69 years)	1.45	0.30	4.22	<0.0001
(≥70 years)	1.74	0.32	5.64	<0.0001
Chronic obstructive lung disease	1.07	0.23	2.91	<0.0001
Surgical factors				
Major surgery	1.58	0.19	4.85	<0.0001
Emergency surgery	0.92	0.15	2.51	<0.0001
Anaesthetic factor				
General anaesthesia involving muscle relaxants	1.04	0.18	2.83	<0.0001
Constant	−6.18	0.31	0.0020	

(Courtesy of Pedersen T, Eliasen K, Henriksen E: *Acta Anaesthesiol Scand* 34:144–155, 1990.)

2). Both types of complication occurred more often in patients having major operations.

These findings do not imply that precautions to reduce risk are not important at low-risk levels. Nevertheless, it is useful to be able to anticipate cardiopulmonary complications in older patients and in those having a history of ischemic heart disease, chronic heart failure, or chronic obstructive pulmonary disease.

▶ I must admit that this article seems remarkably similar to the article and data these authors published under a similar title that identified risk indicators of hospital mortality (Abstract 3–8). I suppose they ought to be congratulated for separating their data into so many portions that it can be useful in so many ways. Nonetheless, the conclusions are the same, i.e., cardiopulmonary complications and morbidity are increased in those over age 70, those with a history of congestive heart failure or ischemic heart disease with myocardial infarction within the previous year, and those admitted for emergency surgery. A small increase in risk was also seen in patients with chronic obstructive lung disease and those with renal failure. Once again, the authors leave us in doubt as to exactly how they diagnosed these preoperative conditions, and whether the risk and the risk ratios can be altered by any preoperative or perioperative management.—M.F. Roizen, M.D.

4 Operating Room Environment

Infection

Human Immunodeficiency Virus Testing and the Risk to the Surgeon of Acquiring HIV
Howard RJ (Univ of Florida)
Surg Gynecol Obstet 171:22–26, 1990   4–1

Physicians and other health care workers are at risk for infection with HIV, hepatitis B virus, and other infective agents through exposure to blood and other body secretions from infected patients. Although surgeons and other health care workers can now protect themselves from hepatitis B infection with hepatitis B vaccine, no such protection against HIV infection is available.

Most authorities have argued against routine screening of hospital patients for HIV infection and support the policy of the Centers for Disease Control, which advocates that universal precautions be used on all patients during operation. The argument against routine screening is based on the belief that routine screening will not prevent or reduce the risk of infection to health care workers because the results of the test may be false negative, screening may miss patients tested in the "window" between the time they became infected and the development of antibodies, and because there is usually not enough time to test patients who have emergency operations.

Although the risk of acquiring HIV from a single needle-stick injury is low, most surgeons are interested in their lifetime risk of infection. In this study a mathematical model was used to predict the risk of acquiring HIV from patients in a given hospital, based on the total number of needle-stick injuries per year.

By using the minimal likely HIV seroprevalence, an average career of 30 years, and an average of 5 percutaneous exposures per year, the mathematical model predicts that a surgeon's risk of HIV infection during his or her career is .0026. Even though this risk may seem small, in reality at least 47 of the approximately 18,000 Fellows of the American College of Surgeons would become infected during their surgical career. Despite the recommendation to use universal precautions for all patients, surgeons generally do behave differently in the operating room if the patient is known to be infected with HIV than if the patient's HIV status is unknown. The policy of routine voluntary testing of all surgical patients for HIV antibodies should perhaps be reconsidered.

▶ For several years, many anesthesiologists and surgeons have been strongly demanding that surgical patients be routinely tested for HIV status. As this opinion becomes increasingly recognized by patients, they logically might ask the reverse: "Why shouldn't we know the HIV status of doctors?" Not surprisingly, this latter opinion is now becoming stronger and stronger in the lay press. Unfortunately, both issues are based on emotionalism rather than on logic and fact.—R.D. Miller, M.D.

HIV, Trauma, and Infection Control: Universal Precautions Are Universally Ignored

Hammond JS, Eckes JM, Gomez GA, Cunningham DN (Univ of Miami/Jackson Mem Med Ctr, Miami)
J Trauma 30:555–561, 1990

4–2

The medical, legal, and ethical problems associated with routine HIV screening have prompted the recommendation that all patients be presumed to be seropositive; protective measures should thus be adopted by all health care workers. However, this philosophy of "universal precautions" has been difficult to adhere to and enforce. In some trauma population subsets, the prevalence of HIV seropositivity can be as high as 19%. To judge compliance with a strict universal precautions protocol, trauma nurse coordinators randomly observed surgical residents engaged in resuscitations in 8 trauma rooms for a 2-month period.

The overall compliance with strict universal precautions procedures was only 16%. The most common variations involved "sharps" technique. Although glove wear was nearly universal, the use of protective eye wear, ankle and foot protection, and body protection (e.g., wearing gowns or aprons) was usually ignored. Compliance was less than 40% even in the presence of invasive procedures such as endotracheal intubation or insertion of chest tubes. Reasons most often given for the lapse in protocol were not knowing the protocol, forgetting it, or not having time to implement it. Even with the 9 patients residents suspected of being in a high-risk group, the protocol was strictly adhered to only once.

Even under the best of circumstances, compliance with universal precautions is difficult to attain. Passive informational measures cannot be assumed to achieve this goal. Active infection control surveillance and ongoing housestaff inservice training are needed to minimize the risk of inadvertent injury or contamination.

▶ It is difficult to break old habits.—R.D. Miller, M.D.

A Survey of Exposures, Practices, and Recommendations of Surgeons in the Care of Patients With Human Immunodeficiency Virus

Mandelbrot DA, Smythe WR, Norman SA, Martin SC, Arnold RM, Talbot GH,

Stolley PD (Univ of Pennsylvania; Albert Einstein College of Medicine; Univ of Pittsburgh)
Surg Gynecol Obstet 171:99–106, 1990   4–3

Health care workers are concerned about the risk of contracting HIV, and care of patients who are at risk or are infected may be compromised, or even denied, as a result. It is difficult to define the present degree of risk of HIV infection and to formulate policies for the surgical care of HIV-infected patients. A total of 1,461 surgeons in New York City and Philadelphia were surveyed about these issues, with responses received from 551 of them.

Only 2% were presently testing all patients for HIV, but 43% of the respondents believe that all patients in their hospitals should be tested. Six percent of the surgeons refuse to treat any patient who is infected with HIV. Fewer than half of respondents recommend barrier precautions for all hospitalized patients, but surgeons in New York City were more inclined to favor separate facilities for HIV-infected patients. Those surgeons who considered themselves to be at relatively high occupational risk were the most likely to favor widespread testing and separate facilities. Policies tailored to individual hospitals may be more effective than national policies for the surgical care of HIV-infected patients.

▶ Although it is usually preferable to have hospitals adopt policies that are appropriate for an individual institution, the nationwide publicity regarding this issue will demand that national policies be developed applying to all hospitals.— R.D. Miller, M.D.

Relationship Between Anesthetic Procedure and Contact of Anesthesia Personnel With Patient Body Fluids

Kristensen MS, Sloth E, Jensen TK (Randers Central Hosp, Frederiksberg, Denmark)
Anesthesiology 73:619–624, 1990   4–4

As of early 1988, data on 15 patients with HIV seroconversion after contact with infected blood or concentrated virus were documented in a laboratory or health care setting. A questionnaire was administered to anesthesia personnel to determine how often they have such contact during standardized procedures.

Catheterization of a peripheral vein led to contact with blood in 18% of 278 episodes. All but 2 of 15 central venous catheter insertions led to contact. Rates for other procedures ranged from 4% for tracheal intubation to 38% for arterial puncture. Lumbar puncture led to contact with fluid in 23% of episodes. Placement or withdrawal of a drip for blood transfusion led to contact in 43% of 14 episodes. Use of gloves would have prevented an estimated 98% of all contact with patient blood. Such contact was more frequent in the emergency ward than in the operating room.

Contact with patient body fluids occurs frequently in the course of routine anesthesia procedures, and there is no way of predicting when it will occur. Procedure-related precautions, such as the use of gloves and a face mask when appropriate, are therefore necessary.

▶ This study states the obvious.—R.D. Miller, M.D.

The Immunologic Profile of Anesthetists

Ziv Y, Shohat B, Baniel J, Ventura E, Levy E, Dintsman M (Beilinson Med Ctr, Petah Tikva; Sackler School of Medicine, Tel Aviv Univ)
Anesth Analg 67:849–851, 1988   4–5

It has been suggested that certain immunologic functions may be suppressed in anesthetists. Immunologic profiles were obtained from 18 anesthetists, all physician anesthesiologists, aged 30–57 years, as well as from 18 age- and sex-matched healthy controls. The mean period of work in operating rooms was 9 years. Volatile and narcotic techniques each were used about 45% of the time, and regional anesthesia in the remaining instances.

No significant differences were found between the anesthetists and controls when counts of T, B, and natural killer lymphocytes, T-active cells, and T-helper/inducer and T-suppressor/cytotoxic cells were estimated. The xenogeneic graft-vs.-host reaction was used to assess T lymphocyte function. No signs of immunosuppression were found in this group of anesthesiologists, who had practiced for nearly a decade on average.

▶ This article gives further proof of the relative occupational safety of anesthetists. Anesthetists are less exposed to needle injuries than surgeons are and less exposed to the chronically ill patients seen in the general practitioner's office; also, the anesthetic agents themselves don't invoke immunologic disorders in the great majority of anesthetists. However, perhaps the stress of our jobs has something to do with our occupational health.—M.F. Roizen, M.D.

Substance Abuse

Success of Reentry Into Anesthesiology Training Programs by Residents With a History of Substance Abuse

Menk EJ, Baumgarten RK, Kingsley CP, Culling RD, Middaugh R (Brooke Army Med Ctr, Fort Sam Houston, Tex)
JAMA 263:3060–3062, 1990   4–6

TABLE 1.—Specific Drugs Abused
(Many Used in Combination)

Drug	No. of Cases
Fentanyl citrate	99
Unspecified opioids	22
Diazepam	16
Alcohol	15
Inhalation agent	10
Unknown	10
Other	8
Ketamine hydrochloride	8
Barbiturates	7
Sufentanil	6
Cocaine	4
Morphine	3
Heroin	1

(Courtesy of Menk EJ, Baumgarten RK, Kingsley CP, et al: *JAMA* 263:3060–3062, 1990.)

In 1983 the American Society of Anesthesiologists concluded that reentry into the anesthesia practice should be encouraged and supported among residents with a history of substance abuse. An anonymous questionnaire was sent to 159 anesthesiology training programs in the United States to determine the incidence and outcome of reentry into anesthesia practice by residents with a history of substance abuse.

In all, 180 cases of substance abuse were reported, for a prevalence rate of 2% among the 8,810 anesthesiology residents. Of these, 26 residents died because of substance abuse and 1 had significant anoxic brain injury, for a mortality/severe morbidity rate of 15%. Further, 73% abused parenteral opioids, usually fentanyl citrate (Table 1). The remainder abused substances other than parenteral opioids.

Of the 82 programs with at least 1 case report, 74% submitted 113 case reports of resident reentry into anesthesiology training. The sucess rate of reentry was significantly higher for nonopioid abusers than for opioid abusers (Table 2). All but 1 of the 14 cases of suicide or lethal overdose after reentry were opioid abusers. Death was the initial relapse symptom in 13 of the 79 opioid abusers who were allowed reentry into anesthesiology training.

Among anesthesiology residents who abuse parenteral opioids, drug rehabilitation followed by redirection into another specialty may be the most prudent course. The fact that two thirds of the reentrants will relapse into opioid abuse, and 1 of 4 of these will die, represents too high a risk in redirecting the rehabilitated anesthesiology trainee back into anesthesia practice.

▶ This article probably represents some of the best data we have on this horrible problem. Clearly, the substance being abused is an important variable in how successful reentry is. These data will certainly heat up the controversy as to whether abuse with the newer narcotics and fentanyl should prevent some-

TABLE 2.—Case Reports of Substance Abuse in Anesthesia Residents

Substance Abused	No. of Case Reports	No. (%) of Cases Allowed to Reenter Training	No. of Cases Excluded (in Training)	No. of Success/Failure Determinations Possible	No. (%) of Reentry Successes	No. (%) of Reentry Failures	No. (%) of Deaths After Reentry
Group 1 (parenteral opioids)	132	87 (70)	8	79	27 (34)	52 (66)	13 (16)
Group 2 (other drugs)	38	26 (76)	3	23	16 (70)	7 (30)	1 (4)
Unknown	10	...	10	0	...	...	...

(Courtesy of Menk EJ, Baumgarten RK, Kingsley CP, et al: *JAMA* 263:3060–3062, 1990.)

one from reentering anesthesia as a career despite an inadequate treatment program.—R.D. Miller, M.D.

Miscellaneous

Fatal Abuse of Nitrous Oxide in the Workplace

Suruda AJ, McGlothlin JD (Natl Inst for Occupational Safety and Health, Cincinnati)

J Occup Med 32:682–684, 1990

4–7

Nitrous oxide has had a reputation for being a safe analgesic and anesthetic in dentistry and its sale and use for these purposes are under the jurisdiction of the Food and Drug Administration. Although intentional inhalation of nitrous oxide is well known, there are no special labeling requirements or restrictions on the sale or use of nitrous oxide in the food and restaurant industry or in laboratories.

Between 1984 and 1987 a total of 11 deaths from on-the-job abuse of nitrous oxide were found in an Occupational Safety and Health Administration investigation and in reports to the Consumer Product Safety Commission. The 11 deaths, all of young men, involved recreational inhalation from tanks or cylinders of nitrous oxide used for legitimate business purposes.

Commercial users of nitrous oxide should be aware of this hazard. Warning labels and tighter controls over the use of nitrous oxide are warranted.

▶ This is another journal that anesthesiologists are not likely to read, but the article emphasizes the danger in the anesthetics we use.—R.D. Miller, M.D.

Noise Pollution in the Operating Theatre
Hodge B, Thompson JF (Royal Prince Alfred Hosp, Sydney, Australia)
Lancet 335:891–894, 1990   4–8

Like other working environments, the operating theater is susceptible to noise pollution, which can lead to impaired concentration and performance, interference with communication, and increased levels of stress among the theater staff and increased anxiety among patients who are conscious during the procedure. To identify the main sources of noise in the operating theater, sound levels were measured during a typical major operation.

Overall sound levels were within the recommended levels for a satisfactory working environment [up to 30 dB(A) as recommended by the Standards Association of Australia]. However, loud intermittent noises of up to 108 dB were emitted by suckers, "intercoms," and alarms on anesthetic monitoring devices. The loudest noises were recorded during the preoperative preparation period. During surgery, noise levels were much greater than levels of normal speech between staff members. Preferred speech interference levels (PSILs) were often exceeded, and a comparison of noise levels during the operation with PSILs showed that reliable communication between any 2 staff members was possible only by shouting.

Excessive noise in the operating theater can impair communication and performance among the theater staff. Even noises of lesser amplitude, particularly those that are unpredictable and/or uncontrollable, and unnecessary background conversation can also interfere with communication and performance in the operating theater.

▶ I completely agree with the results of this study. Operating rooms are too noisy and probably have too many people in them. This is one of the first groups to examine this issue and in an objective manner.—R.D. Miller, M.D.

Work and Rest Cycles in Anesthesia Practice

Gravenstein JS, Cooper JB, Orkin FK (Univ of Florida; Harvard Med School; Univ of California, San Francisco)
Anesthesiology 72:737–742, 1990   4–9

To define the work and rest patterns in anesthesia practice in the United States, a questionnaire on existing and desirable work and rest patterns was published in a newsletter that is mailed to about 22,000 anesthesiologists and anesthesiology residents and 24,000 nurse anesthetists (CRNAs). About 3,000 anonymous replies were received, for a response rate of 6.5%.

During the 6-month study period the mean work week ranged from 47.5 hours among CRNAs to 69.8 hours among residents (table). The longest continuous periods of administering anesthesia without a break ranged from 6.6 hours among CRNAs to 7.7 hours among residents, and the longest continuous period of administering anesthesia with or without a break ranged from 14.1 hours among CRNAs to 20 hours among residents. However, the respondents believed they could work safely without a break for 4.2 hours (CRNAs) to 5.2 hours (anesthesiologists), the respondents believed it was safe to administer anesthesia, with breaks, for 12.8 hours (CRNAs), to 15 hours (residents). About 73% of the respondents worked at least occasionally beyond their perceived self-limitations, and 61% said they had made errors in administering anesthetics that were attributable to fatigue.

Although this survey may not present an accurate pattern of work or attitudes of anesthesia providers in the United States because of the small sample size and potential for bias, these responses deserve attention and further study. Fatigue can affect professional performance, the ability to learn, and family life.

▶ There are multiple problems with this study, making it difficult to reach any definitive conclusions. On the other hand, this issue is extremely important, as it is widely recognized that vigilance is an important factor in preventing unexpected adverse outcomes. Anesthesia practice will increasingly have to take into account whether it is in the private practice or the university setting.—R.D. Miller, M.D.

Professional Hours in a Typical Week, by Gender and Job

Job Category	Female	Male	Both Genders
Anesthesiologist	53.8 ± 1.03 (218)	56.5 ± 0.40 (1,106)	56.0 ± 0.38 (1,324)
Resident	67.3 ± 2.59 (38)	70.7 ± 1.38 (117)	69.8 ± 1.22 (155)
CRNA	46.2 ± 0.56 (597)	49.2 ± 0.68 (468)	47.5 ± 0.44 (1,065)
All categories	49.1 ± 0.52 (853)	55.5 ± 0.36 (1,691)	53.3 ± 0.30 (2,544)

Note: Values are mean ±SEM; numbers of respondents are given in parentheses.
(Courtesy of Gravenstein JS, Cooper JB, Orkin FK: *Anesthesiology* 72:737–742, 1990.)

Measuring the Workload of the Anesthesiologist
Gaba DM, Lee T (Stanford Univ; Palo Alto VA Med Ctr)
Anesth Analg 71:354–361, 1990   4–10

Workload is an important factor in performance during any set of complex dynamic tasks. The mental workload of 9 anesthesia residents was measured during treatment of 19 patients using a secondary task paradigm in which performance on an extra task (addition problems, in this instance) served as a probe of "spare capacity." The surgical procedures ranged from hernia repair to cardiac valve replacement.

An excessive response time correlated with such activities as "manual task" and speaking with the attending anesthesiologist. In 40% of all presentations, the addition problem was skipped or took a relatively long time to complete. Complexity of a given case and the resident's experience level both contributed to the overall workload. Subjective ratings confirmed that induction of anesthesia and emergence from it were the times of the greatest workload.

Studies of this type, applied to various anesthesia personnel, patient situations, and stress conditions, should help to define workload patterns in anesthesia. The role of workload in errors and in problems of human-machine interaction then can be assessed.

► I agree that induction of anesthesia and subsequent emergence are the times of greatest mental and physical activity for the anesthesiologist. Clearly, from the patient's perspective, the time in between is equally important.—R.K. Stoelting, M.D.

Thermoregulatory Vasoconstriction Decreases Cutaneous Heat Loss
Sessler DI, Moayeri A, Støen R, Glosten B, Hynson J, McGuire J (Univ of California, San Francisco; Univ of Chicago)
Anesthesiology 73:656–660, 1990   4–11

When patients are given cold intravenous fluids or receive lavage of internal cavities with large volumes of fluid, their central temperature is decreased. To compensate for that decrease, thermoregulatory vasoconstriction reduces heat loss to the environment by diminishing blood flow in cutaneous arteriovenous shunts and capillaries. The distribution of cutaneous heat loss and the extent to which thermoregulatory vasoconstriction decreases thermal flux were investigated.

Five healthy volunteers (mean age, 28 years), minimally clothed, received central venous infusions of cold lactated Ringer's solution. Shivering was observed in all volunteers throughout the infusion despite an ambient temperature of 30.8° C. Peripheral cutaneous blood flow was measured with venous-occlusion volume plethysmography and skin surface temperature gradients. Vasoconstriction in centrally located skin was measured by laser Doppler flowmetry.

Fingertip blood flow decreased by approximately tenfold shortly after

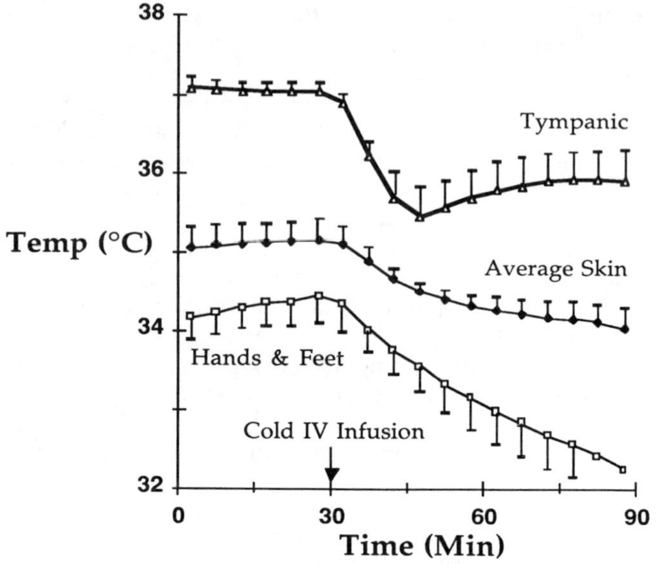

Fig 4–1.—Tympanic membrane temperature decreased approximately 1.5° C in the first 15 minutes after cold fluid infusion began *(arrow)*. During the rest of the study, when the infusion rate was lower, central temperature decreased further to approximately 1° C below control. Average skin-surface temperature decreased slowly to approximately .7° C below control. The most prominent decrease in skin temperature occurred in the hands and feet (consistent with the known distribution of thermoregulatory arteriovenous shunts). All values obtained for epochs >35 minutes differed significantly from control. (Courtesy of Sessler DI, Moayeri A, Støen R, et al: *Anesthesiology* 73:656–660, 1990.)

the cold fluid infusion began. Skin temperature gradients increased to ≥4° C at approximately the same time. In the first 15 minutes after the infusion began, the tympanic membrane temperature decreased by 1.5° C but recovered in part when the infusion rate was lower (Fig 4–1). Skin temperatures in the hands and feet decreased more prominently than in the head and trunk. Flow in capillaries of centrally distributed skin fell by 40%. Total heart flux decreased by about 25%; heat flow from arms and legs decreased by 25%; from trunk and head, 17%; and from hands and feet, 50%.

The data provided evidence that thermoregulatory vasoconstriction decreases cutaneous loss of metabolic heat by about 25%. The most prominent decrease seems to occur in skin with arteriovenous shunts, but capillary constriction in skin without these shunts is also an important source of conservation of metabolic heat.

▶ These data would seem to support the use of insulating materials to cover the limbs and scalp during anesthesia in "cold" operating rooms.—R.K. Stoelting, M.D.

5 Anesthetic Techniques and Complications

Induction of Anesthesia

Anaphylaxis During Induction of General Anesthesia: Subsequent Evaluation and Management

Moscicki RA, Sockin SM, Corsello BF, Ostro MG, Bloch KJ (Harvard Med School; Massachusetts Gen Hosp, Boston)
J Allergy Clin Immunol 86:325–332, 1990   5–1

Anaphylaxis to intravenous drugs, which occurs once in every 5,000–15,000 general anesthesias, is associated with a mortality of 4% to 6%. Data on 27 patients referred for evaluation of anaphylaxis during general anesthesia were reviewed. Of the patients, 12 had a history of atopy, 3 had urticaria, and 5 had a history of drug reactions. Most patients were evaluated a month or more after the anaphylactic event.

Skin test results were positive in 13 patients, most frequently with thiobarbiturates or muscle relaxants. There was a reaction to antibiotics in 2 patients, and 2 dermatographic patients had ambiguous skin test results. General anesthesia was administered to 11 patients in conjunction with prednisone and diphenhydramine for premedication. Of 3 patients with negative skin test results, 1 had arrhythmia. There was no reaction in 1 dermatographic patient. Positive skin tests implicated an agent that was avoided in 7 patients, 1 of whom had delayed urticaria/angioedema after the end of general anesthesia.

An alternative method of anesthesia is preferred, if feasible. Skin testing with appropriate agents is critical, and any agent that is implicated should be strictly avoided. In addition, prednisone and diphenhydramine may be given preoperatively. Patients with positive skin test results should wear a Medic-Alert bracelet.

▶ I am unconvinced that a patient known to be highly sensitized to a drug would benefit from routine pretreatment with corticosteroids and antihistamines before the subsequent induction of anesthesia. Such an approach may introduce a false sense of security. Also, failure of an allergic reaction to occur does not prove that the pretreatment was useful.—R.K. Stoelting, M.D.

Rapid Sequence Anesthesia Induction for Emergency Intubation

Yamamoto LG, Yim GK, Britten AG (Univ of Hawaii; Kapiolani Med Ctr for Women and Children, Honolulu)
Pediatr Emerg Care 6:200–213, 1990   5–2

Rapid sequence induction (RSI) is an expeditious, controlled means of inducing anesthesia to facilitate intubation and limit its complications in the emergency setting. Data were reviewed on the use of RSI in the airway management of 19 patients in the emergency department who required emergency intubation.

First, reliable intravenous access was assured. Preoxygenation was mandatory. Atropine prevents bradycardia from vagal stimulation. If a nondepolarizing muscle relaxant is to be used, a priming dose is helpful. Pressure on the cricoid ring to occlude the esophagus limits the risk of passive gastric regurgitation and aspiration. A muscle relaxant and sedative are given simultaneously or in rapid sequence.

Vecuronium has desirable properties for RSI. The sedative used more frequently is thiopental. If hypovolemia is suspected in a head-injured patient, fentanyl, diazepam, or low-dose thiopental may be used in conjunction with volume resuscitation.

The most frequent indication for intubation was hypoventilation secondary to seizures or anticonvulsants. Intubation with RSI proved to be less difficult than anticipated. No complications from intubation significantly influenced the outcome.

Rapid sequence induction can be carried out safely in the emergency department by the emergency physician. This is most useful, because most hospitals do not have 24-hour in-house anesthesiologists. The needed equipment is listed in the table.

Equipment Necessary for RSI

Uncuffed endotracheal tubes, sizes 2.5 to 6.0
Cuffed endotracheal tubes, sizes 6.0 to 8.5
Endotracheal tube stylets
Laryngoscopes, straight blade sizes 0 to 3, curved blade sizes 2 to 4
Oral airways
Ventilation masks in all sizes for bag-valve-mask ventilation
Large and small self-inflating ventilation bag with oxygen reservoir
   (tail) and positive end expiratory pressure (PEEP) valve attachment
Oxygen source
Suctioning source
Large bore stiff suction tips
Flexible suction catheters
Nasogastric tubes
Pulse oximeter
Electrocardiogram monitor
Tracheostomy tubes
Tracheostomy surgical instrument set
Large bore needle catheter for needle cricothyrotomy
Preassembled transtracheal ventilation setup
Having a spare for each of the above will reduce the likelihood of
   problems caused by misplaced or malfunctioning equipment

(Courtesy of Yamamoto LG, Yim GK, Britten AG: *Pediatr Emerg Care* 6:200–213, 1990.)

▶ I included this article for 2 reasons: (1) It is a nice review of RSI of anesthesia in the emergency situation, and (2) it raises the issue of 24-hour in-house coverage by the anesthesia care team to respond to emergencies with the most skilled personnel available. We all know the horrible feeling that occurs when we are unable to intubate a patient after RSI. A table presented in an article by Malan and Johnson (1) succinctly outlines the management of the failed intubation.—R.K. Stoelting, M.D.

Reference

1. Malan TP Jr, Johnson MD: *J Clin Anesth* 1:104, 1988.

Seizures During Opioid Anesthetic Induction: Are They Opioid-Induced Rigidity?
Smith NT, Benthuysen JL, Bickford RG, Sanford TJ, Blasco T, Duke PC, Head N, Dec-Silver H (Univ of California, San Diego; VA Med Ctr, San Diego; Northwestern Univ; Univ of Manitoba, Winnipeg; Pomerado Hosp, Poway, Calif)
Anesthesiology 71:852–862, 1989   5–3

Several episodes of alleged grand mal seizure after fentanyl, sufentanil, or alfentanil anesthesia induction have been reported. However, electroencephalographic (EEG) confirmation was not available for any of these patients. Tape-recorded EEG and electromyographic (EMG) data obtained during induction of opioid anesthesia in a number of drug trials were reviewed retrospectively for evidence of opioid-induced seizures.

Bilateral EEG leads were obtained in 40 patients undergoing cardiac operations, of whom 20 received fentanyl and 20 received sufentanil anesthesia. The EEG leads in 87 patients who received alfentanil for noncardiac operations also were studied. Electromyographic recordings were obtained in 69 patients who received a higher dose of alfentanil to quantitatively assess rigidity during anesthesia induction. The tapes were played back into an EEG chart recorder and the EEG charts were examined independently by 3 investigators for epileptiform activity.

Of the 127 patients, 93 exhibited mild to intense muscle activity as determined clinically and by the EMG when recorded. Rigidity occurred in 7 of the 20 fentanyl-treated patients, 7 of the 20 sufentanil-treated patients, and 79 of the 87 patients who received alfentanil anesthesia; 46 episodes of rigidity were classified as intense and were associated with movements that could be interpreted as seizures (Fig 5–1). However, the EEG changes associated with these episodes consisted of small sharp waves related to muscle noise or other artifacts and never revealed true electrical seizure activity (Fig 5–2). Thus the phenomenon reported as

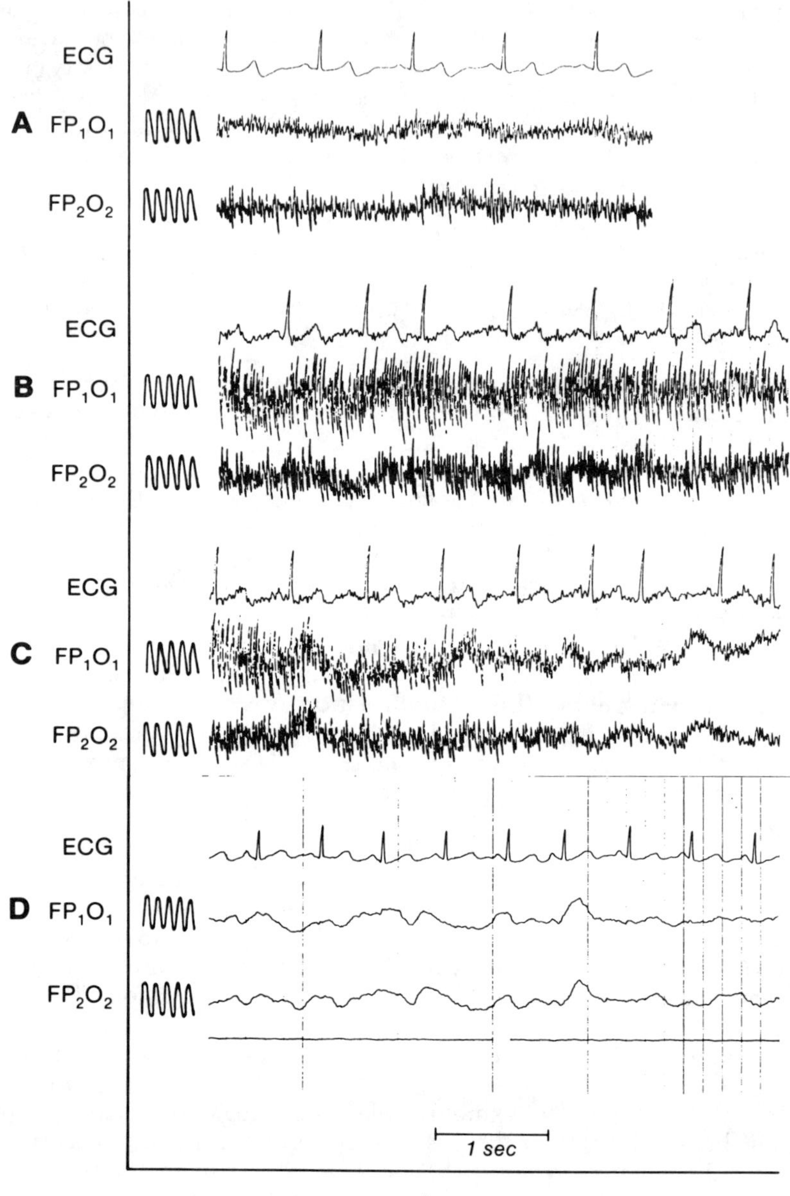

Fig 5–1.—Electroencephalographic changes during anesthetic induction with alfentanil. The awake state *(A)* is followed by loss of consciousness *(B)* with intense rigidity and sharp waves in the EEG. After muscle relaxants are administered *(C)*, rigidity is rapidly extinguished *(C–D)*, with concomitant loss of sharp wave activity. Reference sine waves are 10 Hz and 10 μV peak-to-peak. Elapsed time between beginning of *A* and the end of *D* was 8 minutes. (Courtesy of Smith NT, Benthuysen JL, Bickford RG, et al: *Anesthesiology* 71:852–862, 1989.)

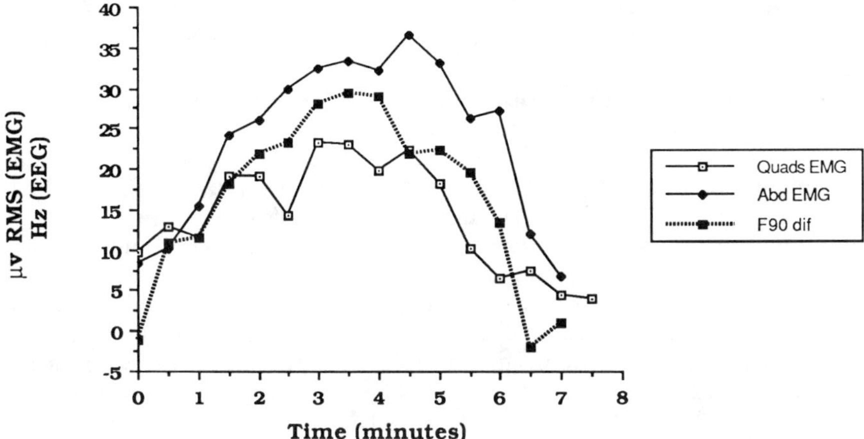

Fig 5–2.—A comparison between changes in the EMG and that portion of the EEG that may be related to muscle noise, as recorded before, during, and after alfentanil-induced rigidity (F90 dif indicates F90 difference, F90 is the frequency below which 90% of the EEG activity lies). To compute the F90 difference, the mean F90 values obtained in patients who received alfentanil but had no rigidity (n = 18) was subtracted from the mean EEG values obtained in patients during severe alfentanil-induced rigidity (n = 10). Each mean represented a 30-second period. The difference reflects at least qualitatively the influence of EMG activity on the EEG recording, as the EEG was essentially subtracted from the EEG plus muscle noise. That difference was then plotted as a function of time. On the same graph, the EMGs from 2 muscle groups were plotted as a function of time. Although the EEG differences and the EMG represent different recordings, different computations, and different units, these plots follow each other reasonably closely, including the rapid changes during the onset and resolution of rigidity. Other differences calculated from other variables derived from the EEG showed the same pattern as the F90 difference. The similarity between the EEG difference and the root mean square (RMS) of the EEG suggests that the EMG noise in the EEG closely tracks the EMG recorded from other sources. *Quads,* quadriceps; *Abd,* abdominal. Alfentanil was administered at time 0 minutes and the neuromuscular blocking agents between minute 4 and minute 5. (Courtesy of Smith NT, Benthuysen JL, Bickford RG, et al: *Anesthesiology* 71:852–862, 1989.)

seizures may have represented severe opioid-induced rigidity, rather than true grand mal seizures.

▶ This is an excellent study that attempts to distinguish between seizures vs. rigidity after induction of anesthesia with narcotics. From a practical point of view, both seizures and rigidity are characteristics that one would rather not have with a drug used to induce anesthesia.—R.D. Miller, M.D.

Neuromuscular and Cardiovascular Effects of High-Dose Vecuronium
Tullock WC, Diana P, Cook DR, Wilks DH, Brandom BW, Stiller RL, Beach CA (Univ of Pittsburgh; Organon Inc, West Orange, NJ)
Anesth Analg 70:86–90, 1990   5–4

Vecuronium bromide is a nondepolarizing muscle relaxant that has a relatively short duration of action and minimal cardiovascular effects. The effects of large bolus doses of vecuronium on the onset and duration of neuromuscular blockade, histamine release, and cardiovascular parameters during fentanyl-nitrous oxide anesthesia was investigated in 40 patients aged 18–59 years undergoing low-risk operations of at least 2-hour expected duration.

The patients were randomly divided into 4 study groups. General anesthesia was induced with thiopental, midazolam, and fentanyl, and maintained with inspired nitrous oxide and additional thiopental, midazolam, and fentanyl. After induction, the ulnar nerve was stimulated with surface electrodes and the evoked compound electromyogram (EMG) of thumb adduction was monitored. Patients were given vecuronium, either .1, .2, .3, or .4 mg/kg injected rapidly through a catheter T-port.

The time from vecuronium injection until peak EMG signal reduction was taken as the onset time. The degree of neuromuscular blockade was defined as the ratio of the height of the first response (T_1) of the train-of-four to the height of the control EMG (T_c). The interval between vecuronium injection and return of the first twitch (T_1) to 25% of control was taken as the clinical duration of neuromuscular blockade. Residual neuromuscular blockade was antagonized with edrophonium and atropine. Neuromuscular recovery was referenced to the final EMG baseline when the response to the train-of-four was stable and T_4/T_1 was greater than .9. Venous blood samples for the measurement of plasma histamine levels were collected immediately before and 1, 3, and 5 minutes after vecuronium administration.

The time to anesthesia onset decreased, and the clinical duration of neuromuscular blockade increased, with increasing vecuronium doses. The difference in reduced onset time between the .2 mg/kg dose and the .3 and .4 mg/kg doses was statistically significant, whereas the difference between the .1 and .2 mg/kg doses was not. Edrophonium was necessary in 30 patients for antagonism of residual blockade at completion of the operation. In the average patient, neuromuscular transmission had recovered to 84% of baseline by 2 minutes after edrophonium and to 90% of baseline by 5 minutes. There was no evidence of a dose-related change in blood pressure or pulse. Changes in histamine plasma levels were not dose related. No side effects (e.g., bronchospasm, flushing, or hives) occurred. Large bolus doses of vecuronium can be used safely to speed the onset of neuromuscular blockade, but the duration of action is significantly prolonged.

▶ The concept of utilizing extremely large doses of a nondepolarizing muscle relaxant to quicken the onset time of neuromuscular blockade is well known, of which this study is an excellent example. However, this approach turns a neuromuscular blocker of intermediate duration into a long-acting one. We obviously are still not close to a replacement for succinylcholine.—R.D. Miller, M.D.

Lower Oesophageal Reflux During Priming With Vecuronium
Martin C, Guillen J-C, Dupin B, Ragni J, Aknin P, Gouin F (Hôp Sainte Marguérite, Marseille, France)
Br J Anaesth 64:33–35, 1990   5–5

Vecuronium has a relatively slow onset time, which limits its usefulness in rapid-sequence anesthesia induction. The onset time to complete neuromuscular block may be decreased by administering the drug in divided doses. The lower esophageal sphincter is the major barrier to regurgitation of acid gastric contents into the esophagus. Drugs that decrease the sphincter's tone may increase the risk of acid regurgitation and subsequent aspiration into the lungs. To assess the effects of vecuronium, given in divided doses, on the occurrence of acid reflux into the lower esophagus, 32 patients undergoing elective thoracic operations were studied. None had a clinical history of gastroesophageal reflux.

After anesthesia induction with thiopental and fentanyl, 16 patients were given vecuronium .01 mg kg^{-1} as a priming dose, followed by an intubation dose of .1 mg kg^{-1} 4 minutes later; the other 16 patients were not given a priming dose. Neuromuscular function was monitored by electromyography. The lower esophageal pH was monitored through a soft plastic pH probe inserted into the esophagus and connected to a programmable pH meter.

Administration of a priming dose of vecuronium significantly shortened the time to tracheal intubation. The lower esophageal pH ranged from 1 to 6.9 at the different stages of anesthesia induction, but there was no difference between the 2 groups in pH values at similar stages. One patient in each group had acid reflux during anesthesia induction, but in neither patient was the acid reflux related to the injection of vecuronium. The use of the recommended priming dose of vecuronium, .01 mg kg^{-1} does not increase the risk of gastric acid reflux into the esophagus.

▶ There is no question that the "priming" can hasten the onset time of vecuronium. This study suggests that there is an element of safety with this approach. Conversely, there are multiple reports of anesthesiologists who are uncomfortable with this approach. The widely varying opinions regarding this approach dictate that clinicians will have to make their own decisions on an individual basis about the desirability of this approach.—R.D. Miller, M.D.

Lower Esophageal Sphincter Integrity Is Maintained During Succinylcholine-Induced Fasciculations in Dogs With "Full" Stomachs
Cook WP, Schultetus RR (Univ of Florida)
Anesth Analg 70:420–423, 1990   5–6

Succinylcholine increases intragastric pressure, with a magnitude that is directly related to the intensity of muscle fasciculations; this increased pressure might cause regurgitation of gastric contents. However, the major barrier to gastric regurgitation is the tone of the lower esophageal sphincter (LES). Barrier pressure is the difference between LES and intragastric pressure. To examine whether succinylcholine can overcome barrier pressure, the latter was assessed in dogs with fasted and full stomachs by esophageal manometry before and after treatment with succinylcholine.

After fasting, fasciculations did not significantly increase either mean intragastric pressure or LES pressure. When the stomachs of the dogs were filled with saline solution, 300 mL, the mean intragastric pressure and mean LES pressure were both significantly increased. Fasciculations did not increase either pressure further. Barrier pressure remained positive in all animals and under all conditions, creating a barrier to passive regurgitation.

Intragastric pressure increased when stomachs were filled; however, LES pressure increased simultaneously. Therefore, barrier pressure was maintained under conditions of full stomachs and during succinylcholine-induced fasiculations. Regurgitation did not occur.

▶ This study attempts to attenuate the fear of increased intragastric pressure associated with succinylcholine administration. Although this study is nicely done, it has several deficiencies that prevent application of the data to clinical medicine. First, the magnitude of fasciculations were not quantified. Second, and far more important, is that clinical studies have shown that the extent to which an increase of intragastric pressure occurs in patients varies considerably. This marked variability dictates the study of a large number of subjects. Whether the increased intragastric pressure seen with succinylcholine is important clinically remains controversial and speculative.—R.D. Miller, M.D.

Rapid Induction Sequence With Vecuronium: Should We Intubate After 60 or 90 Seconds?

Boulanger A, Hardy J-F, Lepage Y (Univ of Montreal)
Can J Anaesth 37:296–300, 1990   5–7

Although succinylcholine is often used for rapid sequence induction of anesthesia, it has many side effects. Results with succinylcholine were compared with those of vecuronium at 60 seconds' and 90 seconds' delay before intubation in 123 patients to optimize the rapid induction sequence.

Patients in groups I and II were given d-tubocurarine, .05 mg/kg^{-1}, 4 minutes before the administration of succinylcholine. Patients in groups III and IV were given vecuronium instead of succinylcholine. In groups I and III an apneic delay of 60 seconds was allowed before intubation; in groups II and IV this delay was 90 seconds. There was no significant difference in intubating conditions between groups I and IV. Intubating conditions in group III were significantly worse than those in the other groups. A 90-second delay after succinylcholine administration improved the intubation conditions in male patients.

Vecuronium is an acceptable alternative for rapid tracheal intubation if delays of 90 seconds are used. However, a clinically significant proportion of men were in unacceptable intubation conditions despite the use of generally acceptable regimens for rapid sequence induction of anesthesia.

The optimal dosage or ideal delay may have to be redefined for these men.

▶ This is another of the many "intubating" studies. This is a particularly well-performed one, especially recognizing that the investigators were blinded as to which muscle relaxant was actually given. Although the authors state that a delay of 90 seconds allows vecuronium to be just as effective as succinylcholine for intubation of the trachea, there can be no doubt that vecuronium, no matter how manipulated, cannot match the quick onset time of succinylcholine.—R.D. Miller, M.D.

Endotracheal Intubation and Tracheostomy

Bronchial Cuff Pressures of Double-Lumen Tubes
Brodsky JB, Adkins MO, Gaba DM (Stanford Univ)
Anesth Analg 69:608–610, 1989

5–8

The double-lumen endobronchial tubes (DLTs) frequently used in thoracic surgery may cause bronchial rupture, a rare but devastating complication. Overinflation of the bronchial cuff can result in ischemic pressure damage to the respiratory mucosa. The pressure/volume characteristics of the bronchial cuffs of 4 commercially available DLTs were compared.

Size 41-F polyvinylchloride (PVC) DLTs from 3 manufacturers and a red-rubber Robertshaw tube of equivalent size were tested under experi-

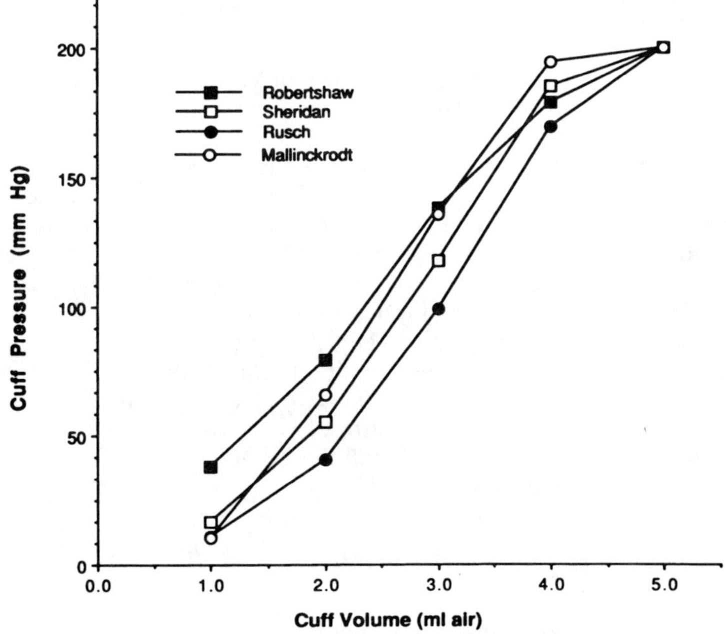

Fig 5–3.—Pressure/volume relationships of bronchial cuffs of the 4 left double-lumen tubes. The Mallinckrodt, Rusch, and Sheridan tubes were size 41F and the red-rubber Robertshaw tube was a size larger. (Courtesy of Brodsky JB, Adkins MO, Gaba DM: *Anesth Analg* 69:608–610, 1989.)

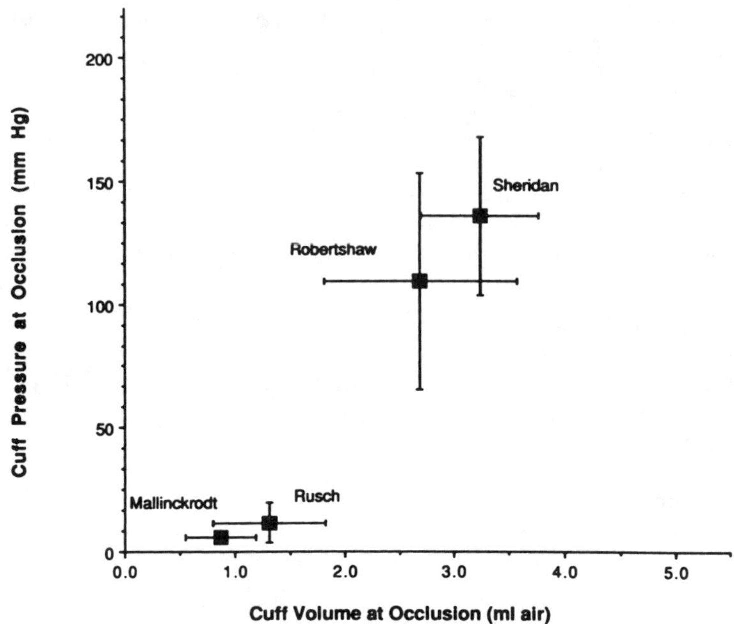

Fig 5–4.—Bronchial cuff pressure at the volume necessary to occlude the model airway. Average values for occlusion pressure (mm Hg) and occlusion volume *(mL air)* are shown ± SD. There were no significant differences in either pressure or volume between the Mallinckrodt and Rusch tubes, but both tubes had occlusion pressures and volumes that were significantly lower *(P < .05)* than those of the Sheridan and Robertshaw tubes. (Courtesy of Brodsky JB, Adkins MO, Gaba DM: *Anesth Analg* 69:608–610, 1989.)

mental conditions. The bronchial lumen of each tube was connected to the breathing circuit of an anesthesia machine that delivered 10 liters of oxygen per minute.

Three milliliters of air resulted in a pressure increase to 100 mm Hg or greater in the bronchial cuffs of all 4 DLTs (Fig 5–3). The bronchial cuff pressure at the volume necessary to occlude the model airway was the important relationship to be examined. Occlusion volume and pressure with 1 of the PVC tubes (Sheridan) and the red-rubber Robertshaw (Leyland) tube were significantly higher than with the other 2 PVC tubes (Mallinckrodt and Rusch) (Fig 5–4).

When distended with volumes of air greater than needed to seal the model airway, all PVC cuffs produced high and potentially dangerous bronchial cuff pressures. The pressure of the bronchial cuff of the Rusch PVC DLT remained lowest at all volumes. The risk of ischemic pressure injury to the bronchus should be less with proper use of the Rusch or Mallinckrodt PVC tube. High-pressure cuffs (e.g., the red-rubber tube) have a tendency to dilate asymmetrically, thus requiring greater volumes to seal the bronchus.

▶ We've known for years that endotracheal tube cuffs have markedly different performance characteristics. Thus it should come as no surprise that such variation occurs with endobronchial cuffs. Because such cuffs usually are in use for less time than tracheal cuffs, most of us pay little attention to how well they work and what damage they may do.—R.R. Kirby, M.D.

Effects of Short-Term Endotracheal Intubation on Vocal Function
Beckford NS, Mayo R, Wilkinson A III, Tierney M (Univ of Tennessee, Memphis; Memphis State Univ)
Laryngoscope 100:331–336, 1990   5–9

Patients often report transient hoarseness and dysphagia after endotracheal intubation, and the morbidity can exceed that associated with surgery itself. Vocal changes were assessed in 10 patients who had short-term outpatient surgery under general anesthesia with endotracheal intubation and compared with changes in 10 age-matched controls who did not have surgery or general anesthesia. The average intubation time was 66 minutes. Fundamental frequency, frequency perturbation, electroglottography, laryngeal videoendoscopy and videostrobolaryngoscopy, and subjective speech analysis were all used before and after surgery in the study group and at 8-hour intervals in controls.

There were no consistent differences in fundamental frequency, but jitter (cycle-to-cycle fundamental frequency variation) increased significantly in most intubated patients. Electroglottography and endoscopic studies failed to show consistent changes in glottic mucosal function in the surgical group. Subjective judgments indicated a less intense, rougher voice after surgery, without consistent changes in pitch. Listeners believed that there was a lowered affect in postintubation speech. Most patients had some tightness in voice quality.

Vocal changes are noted consistently after short-term endotracheal intubation, but the changes do not appear to result solely from damage to the vocal folds. The multisystemic effects of general anesthesia can disturb the fine harmony required for normal voice production.

▶ This article can teach us more about vocal function than most anesthesiologists know existed. I've never heard of general anesthesia, per se, being a major factor in the determination of normal voice production, and because the subject is so foreign to me, I'm unable to decide whether this study proves that it is. Nevertheless, the data are well presented and worth considering. Perhaps electroglottography, jitter, and stroboscopic laryngoscopy are destined to be added to the airway lexicon.—R.R. Kirby, M.D.

Massive Gastric Distention in the Intubated Patient: A Marker for a Defective Airway
Tessler S, Kupfer Y, Lerman A, Arsura EL (State Univ of New York, Brooklyn; Maimonides Med Ctr, Brooklyn)
Arch Intern Med 150:318–320, 1990   5–10

Tracheal intubation is associated with few complications. A clinical sign enabling physicians to detect complications early may improve management of mechanically ventilated patients. Two potentially lethal complications were signaled by massive gastric distention.

Woman, 71, was hospitalized in status asthmaticus. She needed endotracheal intubation, mechanical ventilatory assistance, and treatment with antibiotics, corticosteroids, and β_2-adrenoreceptor agonists. Nasogastric feedings were initiated. During her hospital course, the endotracheal tube (ETT) cuff pressures were greater than 30 mm Hg. Chest radiographs showed a cuff-to-trachea diameter ratio of more than 1.5. Subsequent films showed this to be increasing despite maintenance of ETT cuff pressures of less than 25 mm Hg. Three weeks after intubation, pronounced abdominal distention was noted. On physical examination the patient's abdomen was distended without tenderness, guarding, rebound, or rigidity. Her bowel sounds were normal. Radiographs showed massive gastric dilation and dilated loops of small bowel. A few hours later, increasing respiratory distress developed. Gurgling in the stomach synchronous with ventilation was noted on physical examination. Esophagoscopy revealed the ETT balloon through a 1.5-cm wide tracheoesophageal fistula located 16 cm distal to the incisors. Bronchoscopy through the ETT showed the tip of the tube to be 2 cm above the carina. The patient was extubated and reintubated; the new tube position was confirmed by bronchoscopy. The patient improved initially, but died 3 days later.

The second patient, a woman aged 76 years with myasthenia gravis, had similar findings. She was able to be extubated and discharged. The data underscore the importance of monitoring ventilated patients radiographically. Massive gastric distention may be a warning of a possible communication between the ventilator and gastrointestinal tract. In such cases, the position of the ETT should be confirmed endoscopically.

▶ High-volume, low-pressure cuffs have not solved the problems of cuff-induced tracheal damage despite their widespread use. Improved design and/or application is necessary. Unfortunately, most clinicians believe that if a problem such as that reported here occurs, it must represent inadequate care. This is not always the case. For an interesting review of the subject, see Guyton's article (1).—R.R. Kirby, M.D.

Reference

1. Guyton DC: *Crit Care Update* 1:1, 1990.

Tears of the Trachea and Main Bronchi Caused by Blunt Trauma: Radiologic Findings
Unger JM, Schuchmann GG, Grossman JE, Pellett JR (Univ of Wisconsin; Univ of Tennessee, Knoxville)
AJR 153:1175–1180, 1989

The role of chest radiography in diagnosing acute injury to the airway was analyzed in a retrospective review of chest films in 9 patients with confirmed tears of the trachea or main bronchi. The following signs of air leak were seen at radiography: subcutaneous emphysema and pneumomediastinum in 7 patients, pneumothorax in 6, and air surrounding the bronchus in 1. Fractures involved the upper part of the thorax in 4 patients. Specific signs of tracheobronchial damage were abnormalities of the endotracheal tube such as an extraluminal tip or overdistention of the balloon cuff in 2 patients and the fallen lung sign, indicating peripheral lung collapse, in 2. Although the major importance of chest radiography in cases of tracheobronchial tears may be to verify the existence of air leak, the presence of the fallen lung sign and endotracheal tube abnormality are more specific indications of airway injury.

▶ Many anesthesiologists may practice a lifetime without seeing a traumatic airway disruption. Even those who work in critical care medicine may not see this problem often. Thus few of us have wide-ranging clinical experience in this area, and articles such as this are valuable to remind us of what we knew in the past.—R.R. Kirby, M.D.

Self-Extubations: A 12-Month Experience
Coppolo DP, May JJ (The Mary Imogene Bassett Hosp, Cooperstown, NY)
Chest 98:165–169, 1990   5–12

Unplanned patient removal of an endotracheal airway tube can result in a life-threatening incident. A prospective study of inadvertent extubations was done to determine the frequency of this occurrence and to define factors that may represent special risks.

During a 1-year period, 112 intubated adults were seen in an intensive care unit. Twelve of these patients extubated themselves, for an overall incidence of 11%. No risk factors could be identified. The proportion of patient-hours was comparable when the 2 groups were assessed for tube size, tube site, ventilation mode, and ventilator type. The mean number of hours of intubation was lower in the group that extubated themselves. Of the extubations, 69% were deliberate and most of these incidents occurred despite the use of sedation and restraints. None of the patients died as a result of extubation, but complications occurred in 31%. The reintubation rate in patients who deliberately extubated themselves was 11%.

Self-extubation was a common occurrence in this series. Despite obvious hazards, this event was well tolerated by these adults. Adult patients who deliberately extubate themselves can be safely observed rather than automatically reintubated.

▶ Perhaps the message is that patients often are better able to judge when they should be extubated than are the physicians caring for them. I applaud the decision to observe such individuals before making the knee-jerk decision to reintubate.—R.R. Kirby, M.D.

Oral Intubation in the Multiply Injured Patient: The Risk of Exacerbating Spinal Cord Damage

Rhee KJ, Green W, Holcroft JW, Mangili JA (Univ of California, Davis, Med Ctr, Sacramento)
Ann Emerg Med 19:511–514, 1990   5–13

The use of oral intubation during the resuscitation of seriously injured patients has been discouraged because of the possibility of cervical cord damage. Data were evaluated concerning an 18-month experience in an emergency department in which oral intubation was the usual method of airway control for victims of blunt trauma. The series included 237 intubated patients.

Twenty-one patients (8.9%) had cervical cord or bone injury. A neurologic loss did not follow an airway maneuver in any case. In 213 patients, oral intubation was the definitive airway maneuver. No significant differences were found in the type of definitive airway maneuver between patients with cervical injuries and those without such injuries. The risk of spinal cord injury from oral intubation was low.

The issue of how best to manage the airway in an unstable injured patient can be definitively settled only in a large, prospective trial. Until such a study is done, decision on the technique of airway management should be based on the operator's skill, confidence, and experience with various methods rather than on fear of inflicting spinal cord damage.

▶ To this article I can only respond, Bravo!—R.R. Kirby, M.D.

The Laryngeal Mask Airway: Clinical Appraisal in 250 Patients

Maltby JR, Loken RG, Watson NC (Univ of Calgary, Alta)
Can J Anaesth 37:509–513, 1990   5–14

The laryngeal mask (LM) airway is intermediate in design and function between an oropharyngeal airway and a tracheal tube. It consists of a tubular oropharyngeal airway fused at its distal end to an oval silicone mask that lies in the hypopharynx (Fig 5–5). An inflatable rim around the mask provides an airtight seal around the larynx when inflated after insertion.

Its efficacy was proven in spontaneously breathing patients. To assess its efficacy during semiclosed and basal flow anesthetic techniques, the LM airway was used in 250 nonobstetric patients (mean age, 42 years) who underwent a variety of procedures lasting for 10–280 minutes. Sur-

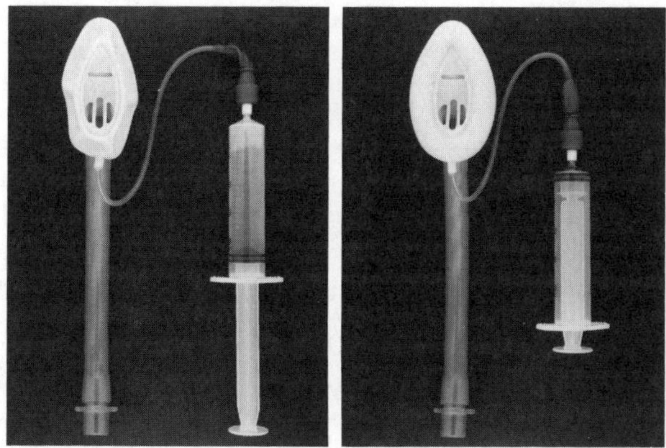

Fig 5–5.—Laryngeal mask airway. **Left,** deflated for insertion. **Right,** cuff inflated. (Courtesy of Maltby JR, Loken RG, Watson NC: *Can J Anaesth* 37:509–513, 1990.)

gery ranged from minor gynecologic and urologic procedures to major abdominal and orthopedic operations performed with either spontaneous respiration or intermittent positive pressure ventilation. Anesthetic techniques and drugs were similar to those that would have been used with face-mask intubation or with tracheal intubation. The LM airway was passed under light inhalational anesthesia.

Of the 250 patients, 238 completed the study. Positioning of the LM airway was perfect in 69% and satisfactory in 31%. Blind insertion was successful at the first attempt in 187 patients, required some manipulation in 61, and was impossible in 2 patients, both of whom had small mouths. Because of airway obstruction or a large gas leak, tracheal intubation was required in 10 patients. The device was so well tolerated that some patients tried to talk while it was still in place. Postoperative dryness of the throat was reported by 36% of the patients and a sore throat by 8%.

The LM airway does not require laryngoscopy for insertion, it relieves the anesthetist's hands from holding a face mask, it cannot be misplaced in the esophagus, and it is well tolerated during emergence from anesthesia. It costs approximately $80 and can be autoclaved for multiple use. Even after autoclaving the device more than 40 times, none of the 10 samples used in this study showed any deterioration. The LM airway will probably have an important role in anesthetic practice.

▶ The LM airway is an interesting concept designed to circumvent placement of a tracheal tube. The future acceptance of this device will depend on multiple factors, including (1) the perceived and/or real dangers of tracheal intubation, (2) the need to provide positive pressure ventilation, and (3) whether aspiration is reliably prevented. The reusable nature of the airway in this day of concern about cross-contamination between patients is unlikely to be perceived as an advantage.—R.K. Stoelting, M.D.

Cardiovascular Response to Insertion of Brain's Laryngeal Mask

Hickey S, Cameron AE, Asbury AJ (Western Infirmary, Glasgow; Vale of Leven District Gen Hosp, Alexandria, Scotland)
Anaesthesia 45:629–633, 1990

5–15

Brain's laryngeal mask (LM) airway avoids the need for laryngoscopy and tracheal intubation, which increases arterial pressure and heart rate. These changes may be undesirable in patients with myocardial or cerebrovascular insufficiency. The arterial pressure and heart rate changes associated with LM airway insertion were compared with those associated with Guedel airway insertion in 100 patients undergoing minor elective surgery. All had oral premedication. Patients were randomized into 2 groups; 1 had a Guedel airway inserted after anesthesia and the other had an LM airway inserted after anesthesia. Arterial pressure and heart rate were measured before and after airway insertion. Ease of airway insertion and any complications were also noted.

No significant changes in arterial pressure were seen in the 2 groups. Both had decreased arterial pressure after induction of anesthesia. In both groups, airway insertion was followed by increased systolic and diastolic pressures. Peak arterial pressure occurred sooner in the Guedel airway group. No significant changes in heart rate were seen between the 2 groups. Both had an increased heart rate after induction of anesthesia. The first peak in heart rate occurred sooner in the Guedel airway group, but the time was significantly different than that for arterial pressure. There was a second peak in heart rate that was quicker in the LM airway group.

Insertion of Brain's LM airway, with the anesthetic technique described in this study, increases arterial pressure and heart rate significantly but transiently. Because these changes are identical to those associated with the Guedel airway, the 2 airways appear to be interchangeable and cause no relevant difference in cardiovascular response. Compared to standard oral airways, the LM airway has many advantages.

▶ The similarity in cardiovascular responses between the 2 artificial airways is not surprising, considering the probably similar degree of upper airway stimulation. It is surprising that laryngospasm did not accompany insertion of either airway in these patients lightly anesthetized with propofol, 2.5 mg kg^{-1} and 66% nitrous oxide.—R.K. Stoelting, M.D.

Postoperative Sore Throat: Effect of Oropharyngeal Airway in Orotracheally Intubated Patients

Monroe MC, Gravenstein N, Saga-Rumley S (Univ of Florida)
Anesth Analg 70:512–516, 1990

5–16

The effect of a hard, plastic oropharyngeal airway on the incidence of postoperative sore throat was studied prospectively in 203 adults undergoing general endotracheal anesthesia. Patients were randomly assigned to receive either a hard plastic oropharyngeal airway or a soft, interdental gauze bite-block during anesthesia. All patients underwent orotracheal intubation with cuffed endotracheal tubes with high-volume, low-pressure cuffs.

Based on answers to questionnaires completed the day after surgery, the incidence of postoperative sore throat was 35.2% in the oropharyngeal airway group and 42.5% in the gauze bite-block groups; the difference was not significant. However, the incidence of postoperative sore throat was significantly higher when blood was noted on the airway instrument than when it was not. There was trend toward a higher incidence of postoperative sore throat among anesthesia residents who had less than 1 year of experience in intubation.

The intraoperative use of a hard, plastic oropharyngeal airway, compared with a soft gauze bite-block, does not increase the incidence of postoperative sore throat in orotracheally intubated patients. However, pharyngeal trauma is a significant factor in postoperative sore throat and is probably caused by aggressive oropharyngeal suctioning.

▶ I have always questioned how a tube in the trachea could cause pharyngitis (sore throat). If pharyngeal trauma caused by direct laryngoscopy or suctioning is the true culprit, it may not be possible to avoid the "sore throat" attributed to the endotracheal tube.—R.K. Stoelting, M.D.

The Nasogastric Tube Syndrome

Sofferman RA, Haisch CE, Kirchner JA, Hardin NJ (Univ of Vermont, Burlington; Yale Univ)
Laryngoscope 100:962–968, 1990

5–17

In the past 5 decades, only a few studies have addressed the problem of bilateral vocal cord paralysis resulting from nasogastric tube use. Four diabetic patients with various stages of renal failure experienced sudden and life-threatening postcricoid ulceration and vocal cord paralysis. Autopsy examination of an involved larynx yielded information on the pathophysiology of the nasogastric tube syndrome.

Man, 28, with insulin-dependent diabetes and progressive renal failure, received a cadaveric renal transplant. The patient had a nasogastric tube in place until the fourth postoperative day. He complained of throat pain on day 8, and on day 12 required a tracheotomy after stridor and bilateral vocal cord paralysis were identified. *Staphylococcus aureus* was identified in cultures from a postcricoid ulcer at rigid esophagoscopy. Transplant failure requiring nephrectomy appeared to be a direct result of nasogastric tube syndrome.

Three common factors in these 4 patients and those in previous studies were throat pain, presence of a nasogastric tube, and vocal cord paralysis, usually bilateral. Symptoms may be noted within 24 hours of tube placement or may take days or weeks to become apparent. The pathophysiologic mechanism is thought to be paresis of the postcricoid musculature secondary to ulceration and infection over the posterior lamina of the cricoid.

Throat irritation is common with the nasogastric tube, but the potential for serious complications must not be overlooked. Esophagoscopy is required for correct diagnosis of the nasogastric tube syndrome. The tube should then be removed, and antibiotics administered. Diabetic patients receiving renal transplants are particularly vulnerable and must be carefully observed for development of the syndrome.

▶ This is important information for the anesthesiologist to consider because the trachea and esophagus of many patients are intubated. It seems appropriate to give credit where credit is due.—R.K. Stoelting, M.D.

Acute Airway Management: Role of Cricothyroidotomy
DeLaurier GA, Hawkins ML, Treat RC, Mansberger AR Jr (Med College of Georgia, Augusta)
Am Surg 56:12–15, 1990   5–18

Cricothyroidotomy as a surgical procedure in the management of upper airway obstruction was condemned for several decades until its safe use as an emergency procedure was reconfirmed in 1976. The records of all 34 patients who underwent cricothyroidotomy between September 1984 and January 1988 were reviewed.

Emergency cricothyroidotomy was performed on 31 patients with acute trauma in whom intubation was considered unsafe because of associated head and neck injury or in whom attempts at intubation had failed. Three patients who had not sustained acute trauma underwent the procedure when oral or nasal intubation could not be accomplished. Ten patients had laryngoscopy and 2 had bronchoscopy after cricothyroidotomy or subsequent tracheostomy.

Fourteen patients died of their injuries, 13 of them within the first several hours after injury. The 20 surviving patients were evaluated in 2 groups. The first group included 11 patients whose cricothyroidotomy tube remained in place until decannulation; the second group included 9 patients who underwent formal tracheostomy subsequent to emergency cricothyroidotomy.

One patient in the first group has remained in a vegetative state because of severe head injury, and the cricothyroidotomy has remained in place for 4 months. Decannulation was performed in the other 10 patients after an average of 6.3 days. Six patients had laryngoscopy within 10 days of decannulation. After an average follow-up of 67 days 3 patients were found to have minor complications consisting of stomal granulation and minimal tracheal erosion.

In the second group tracheostomy was performed within 30 minutes to 9 days after cricothyroidotomy, and the tracheostomies were left in place for 8–270 days. During an average follow-up of 83 days 6 patients had complications. Two patients required reoperation because of partial airway obstruction. One patient was never decannulated before his death from oral cancer 9 months after tracheostomy. The other 3 complications were considered minor and included bleeding, supraglottic inflammation, and stomal granulation. In all, only 2 of the 20 survivors experienced significant morbidity as a result of surgical airway management. It appears that tracheostomy subsequent to emergency cricothyroidotomy does not necessarily reduce airway-related morbidity in these patients.

▶ The value of cricothyroidotomy is to provide life-saving oxygen delivery until a more definitive procedure can be accomplished. Every anesthesiologist is encouraged to be familiar with the necessary steps for performance of this procedure.—R.K. Stoelting, M.D.

Percutaneous Tracheostomy: A New Method
Schachner A, Ovil Y, Sidi J, Rogev M, Heilbronn Y, Levy MJ (Beilinson Med Ctr, Petah Tikva, Israel; Sackler School of Med, Tel Aviv Univ)
Crit Care Med 17:1052–1056, 1989   5–19

Tracheostomy is one of the most effective life-saving procedures available, but it is associated with a relatively high rate of complications. A new rapid method of definitive low tracheostomy, based on the percutaneous principle and using a newly designed instrument kit, was evaluated. The kit contains a 5-mL syringe, 21-gauge needle, no. 10 blade scalpel, 12-gauge needle curved at its outer tip with an upper plastic hub, a flexible metal guidewire, a plastic mandrel, and a conventional cuffed tracheostomy cannula. The kit also contains a specially designed percutaneous tracheostomy dilator.

Technique.—After a skin incision has been made in the neck, the 12-gauge needle is introduced into the tracheal lumen, the flexible metal guidewire is gently introduced through the needle, and the needle is removed. The percutaneous tracheostomy dilator is slipped over the guidewire into the trachea. The handles are then squeezed to enlarge the intercartilaginous space, and the cuffed tracheal cannula is secured in place.

After extensive investigation in both cadaver and animal experiments, percutaneous tracheostomy was performed in 47 men and 33 women aged 22–87 years. Thirty-three patients required airway control after neurosurgical procedures or after severe head trauma, 23 underwent percutaneous tracheostomy before radical excision for head and neck cancer, and the remaining 24 had severe cardiorespiratory problems. Twenty-nine procedures were performed in the operating room under standard surgical conditions; the other 51 were performed at bedside, either in the intensive care unit, the emergency department, or on the ward.

Although 21 of the 80 patients died, none of the deaths was attributable directly or indirectly to percutaneous tracheostomy. None of the patients had infection at the stoma site. In 22 patients, x-ray laminography of the trachea revealed no pathologic findings. All 10 patients who underwent tracheoscopy after decannulation had smooth healing of the tracheal opening. No stenosis was detected. Percutaneous tracheostomy appears to be a safe and speedy procedure that is easily learned.

▶ Percutaneous tracheostomy has been advocated and equipment provided for its performance for the past 2 decades. However, it's never really caught on as a preferred method to establish emergency airway control. Each new device/technique seems promising at its inception. We'll have to await further evaluation of this one.—R.R. Kirby, M.D.

Regional Anesthesia—Peripheral Nerve Blocks

A Comparison of Three Methods of Axillary Brachial Plexus Anaesthesia
Baranowski AP, Pither CE (St Thomas' Hosp, London)
Anaesthesia 45:362–365, 1990   5–20

Axillary brachial plexus block is commonly used in outpatient surgery on an upper extremity, and various techniques to produce a satisfactory brachial plexus block have been advocated. In the present study 3 different techniques for producing an axillary brachial plexus block were compared, in 100 patients scheduled for outpatient hand surgery. Fifty patients were randomly allocated to the use of paresthesia to localize the plexus, a peripheral nerve stimulator was used to locate the 4 main peripheral nerves in 25 patients, and a catheter was inserted into the brachial plexus sheath in 25 patients.

Each patient received 40 mL of lidocaine 1.5% solution with epinephrine 1:200,000 added, which was injected in increments according to the number of peripheral nerves that were located. Attempts were made to find up to 3 of the 4 main peripheral nerves. An intravenous cannula was inserted into the contralateral hand. No sedation or intravenous analgesia was given.

Only 2 patients required general anesthesia. There was no statistical difference in the number of successful blocks among the 3 groups. However, the catheter technique blocked the ulnar and median nerves significantly less frequently than the other techniques combined. Because of the technical difficulties encountered with the use of the catheter technique, and in view of a possible risk of neurologic damage associated with the paresthesia technique, the nerve stimulator technique is recommended for routine brachial plexus block.

▶ The evidence is mounting that utilization of a nerve stimulator adds to the success rate of certain regional anesthetic techniques, in this instance, brachial plexus block.—G.W. Ostheimer, M.D.

Thyroidectomy Under Local Analgesia: The Anatomical Basis of Cervical Blocks

Yerzingatsian KL (Univ Teaching Hosp, Lusaka, Zambia)
Ann R Coll Surg Engl 71:207–210, 1989   5–21

The different types of cervical blocks used during thyroidectomy have not been well studied. Even with the most effective deep cervical block, the platysma muscle and midline visceral structures remain vulnerable to pain perception during operation. Superficial, deep, and modified cervical blocks that can be used for regional anesthesia in thyroidectomy have their advantages and disadvantages.

To obtain a superficial cervical block, local anesthetic solution is deposited midway along the length of the sternocleidomastoid muscle overlying an area where all cutaneous branches are distributed in the neck (Fig 5–6). The needle is usually placed superficial to the investing layer of the deep fascia. A superficial cervical block is safe and simple to perform. However, used on its own, it is inadequate for thyroidectomies as it does not densensitize the platysma muscle, strap muscles, or visceral structures.

The purpose of a deep cervical block is to inject local anesthetic in such a way that the solution is distributed in the deep compartment. An interscalene, parascalene, cervical, or paravertebral technique may be used. Although a deep cervical block is effective, it requires attention to detail and great care because of its potential for complications. Furthermore, as with a superficial cervical block, a deep cervical block does not desensitize the platysma muscle or obtund visceral sensation.

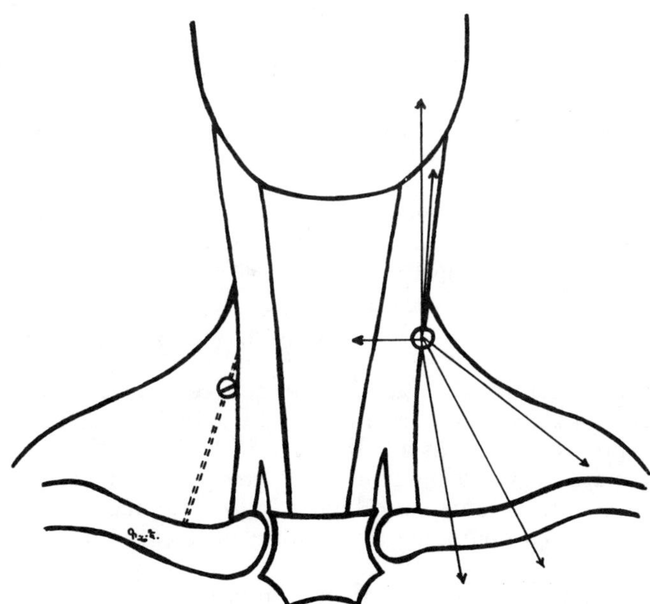

Fig 5–6.—Superficial and deep cervical blocks. (Courtesy of Yerzingatsian KL: *Ann R Coll Surg Engl* 71:207–210, 1989.)

A modified cervical block uses a combination of regional blocks and infiltration. With this technique, the needle is placed at a point midway along the length of the sternocleidomastoid muscle. The injection is then sequenced in 4 steps, depositing a volume of anesthetic solution at each step. One advantage of a modified cervical block is that the platysma and strap muscles are desensitized, and visceral sensation is obtunded. The potential complications associated with a deep cervical block should not occur with this technique. However, the fact that large volumes of solution must be used to obtain an adequate block is a disadvantage. Moreover, muscle damage has been reported. A modified cervical block was used in 19 patients undergoing thyroidectomy, none of whom had respiratory problems. There were no deaths.

A modified cervical block is recommended when general anesthesia in patients undergoing thyroidectomy is contraindicated or cannot be administered. Modified cervical block anesthesia is safe and effective, and the technique is simple to learn.

▶ How many readers have done superficial or deep cervical blocks for thyroidectomies or surgery in that area of the neck? I was taught to do these blocks for thyroidectomies with appropriate intravenous sedation. It is an excellent anesthetic for both the patient and the surgeon. However, it demands that the surgeon handle the tissues of the neck in a gentle manner. I think this is one block that is underutilized for thyroid operations, and it needn't be used only in patients who are ill. In fact, the healthy patient probably will tolerate the blocks and procedure even better than one who is ill.—G.W. Ostheimer, M.D.

Continuous Interscalene Brachial Plexus Block During and After Shoulder Surgery

Haasio J, Tuominen M, Rosenberg PH (Univ Central Hosp, Helsinki)
Ann Chir Gynaecol 79:103–107, 1990   5–22

The efficacy of an interscalene brachial plexus block with a .75% solution of bupivacaine containing epinephrine was assessed for shoulder surgery in 20 patients. Postoperative analgesia was provided by a continuous infusion of .25% bupivacaine. Twenty patients who received general anesthesia with bupivacaine for shoulder surgery served as a control group.

Surgery was performed successfully under regional anesthesia in 16 of the 20 study patients; the other 4 required fentanyl during the procedure. Supplementary sedation was administered in 13 cases. The need for postoperative analgesia was similar in the 2 groups. The mean plasma concentrations of bupivacaine were higher in the regional anesthesia group from 5 minutes to 3 hours, but by 24 hours the concentration was similar between the 2 groups. In 1 patient local anesthesia was discontinued because of side effects. Four patients had mild local anesthetic toxicity. In healthy patients there was no advantage to performing shoulder surgery under interscalene brachial plexus block with the use of bupivacaine, compared to joint surgery with general anesthesia.

▶ In skilled hands, a continuous interscalene brachial plexus block for perioperative patients with shoulder injuries is obviously efficacious and has considerable advantages.—R.D. Miller, M.D.

Regional Anesthesia—Spinal and Epidural

The Effect of Removal of Cerebrospinal Fluid on Cephalad Spread of Spinal Analgesia With 0.5% Plain Bupivacaine

Jawan B, Lee JH (Chang Gung Mem Hosp, Kaohsiung, Republic of China)
Acta Anaesthesiol Scand 34:452–454, 1990   5-23

The spread of local anesthetic solution in the CSF depends on numerous factors. Higher cephalad spread of spinal analgesia may result from increased intra-abdominal pressure. The reason for the higher spread is thought to be a decrease in CSF volume. If that is the correct mechanism, an intentional reduction of CSF volume, without an increase in intra-abdominal pressure, should facilitate the cephalad spread of local anesthetic solutions. This hypothesis was tested in 66 patients.

The patients were undergoing various urologic procedures. None had evidence of increased intra-abdominal pressure. The patients, who were randomly assigned to 3 groups, all received 10 mg of .5% bupivacaine for spinal anesthesia. In group I the anesthetic solution was injected after free drops of CSF. Patients in groups II and III had 3 mL and 5 mL of CSF removed, respectively, before the injection of bupivacaine. The analgesic level obtained 20 minutes after injection was taken as the maximum spread of the anesthetic.

The mean cephalad spread of analgesia at 20 minutes was $T_{10.2}$ for group I, $T_{9.4}$ for group II, and T_7 for group III (table). Although the difference in the level of spread was not significant for groups I and II, fur-

Mean (±1 SD) Cephalad Spread of Analgesia and Number of
Patients With Degree of Motor Blockade According to
Bromage Score 20 minutes After Injection

Group	Level of analgesia	Grade N	I	II	III	IV
I	T10.2 ± 2.0		17	2	1	0
II	T9.4 ± 1.8		14	7	1	0
III	T7.0 ± 2.1		16	5	1	0

Note: I, complete motor blockade; II, almost complete blockade; III, partial blockade; IV, no blockade.
Abbreviation: N, number of patients.
(Courtesy of Jawan B, Lee JH: *Acta Anaesthesiol Scand* 34:452–454, 1990.)

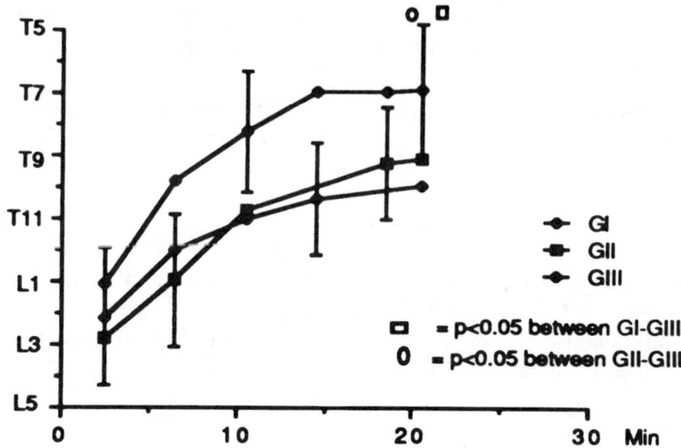

Fig 5–7.—Mean cephalad spread of analgesia. Group I (GI), control; GII, – 3 mL CSF; GIII, – 5 mL CSF. (Courtesy of Jawan B, Lee JH: *Acta Anaesthesiol Scand* 34:452–454, 1990.)

ther reduction of the CSF volume in group III resulted in a statistically significant difference (Fig 5–7).

The reduction of CSF volume before injection of local anesthetic seems to accelerate the spread of analgesia. With less spinal fluid present for mixing with the anesthetic agent, less agent is necessary to bathe the spinal segment. Removal of 5 mL of CSF was necessary for a significantly higher spread.

▶ This study contributes to our knowledge about the spread of spinal anesthesia. I wonder what the incidence of postdural puncture headache was in the 3 groups?—G.W. Ostheimer, M.D.

Continuous Spinal Anesthesia With a Microcatheter Technique: Preliminary Experience

Hurley RJ, Lambert DH (Harvard Univ; Brigham and Women's Hosp, Boston)
Anesth Analg 70:97–102, 1990   5–24

The large diameters of currently available spinal catheters require insertion through large spinal needles. This has limited the use of continuous spinal anesthesia, because this technique results in an unacceptably high rate of postdural puncture headache (PDPH) in young patients. Currently, continuous spinal anesthesia is used mostly in elderly patients and for lengthy operations. A 32-gauge microcatheter for continuous spinal anesthesia that can be threaded through a 26-gauge or larger spinal needle was used in 58 patients aged 17–75 years.

Variety of elective procedures were performed under continuous spinal anesthesia with the new microcatheter. In the first 24 patients, the stylet was removed and a Tuohy-Borst adapter attached to the free end of the catheter. Because of problems with catheter kinking, the catheter stylet was left in place to radiopacify and stiffen the catheter in the next 21 patients. As it was often difficult to advance the catheter/stylet past the tip of the spinal needle into the subarachnoid space, a 20-mm piece of 20-gauge Teflon intravenous tubing was used as a threading aid in the next 13 patients.

In the first phase of the study, spinal anesthesia was successful in 18 of the 24 patients. One 65-year-old woman had PDPH after use of a 26-gauge needle, but this resolved without treatment. One catheter broke during removal, 2 were difficult to thread, and 3 could not be threaded at all. In the second phase, all 21 patients had successful continuous spinal anesthesia with the catheter stylet left in place. None had PDPH. In the third phase of the study, 1 patient had PDPH, 2 had inadequate spinal anesthesia, and another catheter broke when the tape holding it down became stuck to the bed linens. After neurosurgical consultation, it was decided not to retrieve the 2 broken catheter fragments. Neither patient has experienced any untoward effect.

The overall complication rate during the development of this microcatheter method was 20%. The problems of threading and the inability to inject or withdraw the stylet were resolved by integrating the catheter and the stylet, and by using a threading aid. The incidence of inadequate anesthesia and PDPH with the microcatheter technique did not appear to differ from that encountered with single-injection spinal anesthesia. A catheter with increased tensile strength now being used in the fourth phase of this study is expected to eliminate the complication of broken catheters.

▶ Continuous spinal anesthesia is a tool that should be in the armamentarium of every anesthesiologist. The technique has fallen into disuse because of the purported high incidence of PDPH after puncture of the dura with a large-bore epidural needle. However, some studies have shown that the incidence of headache is not as great as one would presume, and this may be because of the development of a fibrin matrix around the catheter, which helps to seal the dural hole when the catheter is removed.

In an effort to eliminate the problem of increased PDPH, a variety of small-gauge or "micro" catheters have been developed. The authors delineate their experience with a 32-gauge micro catheter that is inserted through a 26-gauge spinal needle. Other small-gauge catheters presently available will pass through spinal needles ranging in size from 22 to 25 gauge. The method is not without its technical difficulties, and there have been a few disturbing reports that repeated dosing with 5% hyperbaric lidocaine has resulted in arachnoiditis in some instances. Information is spotty at the present time, but you can be assured that the YEAR BOOK will continue to report developments in the field of continuous spinal anesthesia with small-gauge or microcatheters in the future.—G.W. Ostheimer, M.D.

Use of a Chlorhexidine Dressing to Reduce Microbial Colonization of Epidural Catheters
Shapiro JM, Bond EL, Garman JK (Stanford Univ; Vitaphore Corp, Menlo Park, Calif)
Anesthesiology 73:625–631, 1990   5–25

Epidural catheters are used increasingly to infuse analgesic agents. However, epidural abscess is a rare but recognized complication that may produce meningitis, paralysis, or death. The efficacy of a chlorhexidine gluconate patch in preventing proliferation of skin flora at the site of catheter insertion was examined in vitro and in a clinical trial. The patch consists of chlorhexidine gluconate chemically bound to a urethane composite that is held in place by a urethane film with acrylic adhesive.

A bioassay showed that the chlorhexidine dressing, in vitro, delivered drug in a biphasic mode: higher levels in the first 3 days and, subsequently, for up to 10 days at a lower level. Dressings were well tolerated by nonwounded skin. In a pilot study of 17 patients, 29% had positive culture results. Catheters remained in place for a mean of nearly 4 days. Nine of 31 control catheter cultures in the clinical study proper were positive, compared with 1 of 26 cultures in the test group. *Staphylococcus epidermidis* was the predominant isolate. Use of a chlorhexidine patch to deliver antiseptic to epidural catheter wound sites limits catheter colonization and might reduce the risk of catheter-related infection.

▶ I think the idea of a chlorhexidine dressing to reduce microbial colonization at the insertion site of the epidural catheter through the skin is an acceptable concept. This prophylactic approach should be used in larger numbers of patients to see if there are any adverse reactions to the patch. Epidural abscesses are extremely rare and are almost unheard of in the nonimmunocompromised patient. We are all concerned about the possible occurrence of an epidural abscess, but meticulous attention to technique plus the bacteriostatic or bacteriocidal action of the local anesthetics and/or opioids add a further measure of protection for patients receiving a continuous epidural block.—G.W. Ostheimer, M.D.

Test Doses: Optimal Epinephrine Content With and Without Acute Beta-Adrenergic Blockade
Guinard J-P, Mulroy MF, Carpenter RL, Knopes KD (Virginia Mason Med Ctr, Seattle; Centre Hosp Univ Vaudois, Lausanne, Switzerland)
Anesthesiology 73:386–392, 1990   5–26

In the past decade, the use of a test dose containing 15 μg of epinephrine to detect intravascular placement of a needle or catheter has become standard practice before epidural anesthesia. To determine the sensitivity and specificity of this approach, as well as the lowest effective dose, studies were made both in healthy volunteers and in the presence of β-adrenergic blockade.

TABLE 1.—Subjects With Heart Rate Variation ≥20 bpm
After Injection of Saline, Lidocaine 1%, or Lidocaine 1%
Plus Epinephrine

| | | Loading or Infusion | |
Injections	Saline	Esmolol	Propranolol*
Saline	0/9	0/9	0/8
L	0/9	0/9	0/8
L + E (5 μg)	8/9	6/9	5/8
L + E (10 μg)	9/9	8/9	8/8
L + E (15 μg)	9/9	7/9	7/8

Abbreviations: L, lidocaine 1%; L + E, lidocaine 1% + epinephrine.
*Heart rate changes with propanolol were bradycardia.
(Courtesy of Guinard J-P, Mulroy MF, Carpenter RL, et al: *Anesthesiology* 73:386–392, 1990.)

Nine healthy volunteers received 3 series of 5 infections of test doses after infusion of either saline, esmolol, or propranolol. The 5 injections comprised saline, 1% lidocaine, or 1% lidocaine containing 5, 10, or 15 μg of epinephrine. All subjects completed the first 2 series of injections during saline and esmolol infusions; 8 received the series of 5 test injections after propranolol infusion.

Epinephrine injections during saline infusion significantly increased the heart rate by an average of 31–38 beats per minute and increased systolic blood pressure (SBP) by an average of 17–26 mm Hg. With esmolol, epinephrine injections increased the heart rate by an average of 23–31 beats per minute and SBP by an average of 18–30 mm Hg. After propranolol injection, epinephrine caused a decrease in the heart rate by an average of 21–28 beats per minute, whereas SBP increased by an average of 22–35 mm Hg (Tables 1 and 2).

The findings indicate that a test dose containing 10 μg or 15 μg epinephrine is a reliable marker of intravascular injection in young, healthy,

TABLE 2.—Subjects With SBP Increase ≥15 mm Hg After
Injection of Saline, Lidocaine 1%, or Lidocaine
1% Plus Epinephrine

| | | Loading and/or Infusion | |
Injections	Saline	Esmolol	Propranolol*
Saline	0/9	0/9	2/8
L	2/9	1/9	1/8
L + E (5 μg)	4/9	7/9	7/8
L + E (10 μg)	7/9	9/9	8/8
L + E (15 μg)	8/9	9/9	8/8

Note: See Table 1 for explanation of abbreviations.
(Courtesy of Guinard J-P, Mulroy MF, Carpenter RL, et al: *Anesthesiology* 73:386–392, 1990.)

nonpregnant subjects. Further, a positive response can be detected reliably by an absolute increase in heart rate of at least 20 beats per minute. Tachycardia is no longer a reliable sign of intravascular injection in the presence of acute selective or nonselective β blockade. During acute β-adrenergic blockade, an increase in SBP of at least 15 mm Hg is a sensitive, although not entirely specific, indicator of the intravascular injection of epinephrine.

▶ The last paragraph of the summary of this well-done study summarizes where we stand with the use of epinephrine as a test dose and demonstrates that it is a reliable marker of intravascular injection in young, healthy, nonpregnant patients.—G.W. Ostheimer, M.D.

The Air Test as a Clinically Useful Indicator of Intravenously Placed Epidural Catheters

Leighton BL, Norris MC, DeSimone CA, Rosko T, Gross JB (Thomas Jefferson Univ; Univ of Connecticut, Farmington)
Anesthesiology 73:610–613, 1990   5–27

This study was performed to determine whether a precordial Doppler probe placed over the lower maternal sternum without confirmation can reliably detect the intravenous placement of an epidural catheter in labor. The probe was used in 313 patients after insertion of an epidural catheter, attempted aspiration, and a test dose of .25% bupivacaine. An injection of 1 mL of air then was made through the catheter while heart tones were monitored continuously.

No patient had new symptoms that were attributable to the air test. All but 8 of 281 patients with a negative test had segmental analgesia after injection of bupivacaine (table). The 8 remaining had no evidence of toxicity even though they received 12 mL or more of .25% bupivacaine within 4 minutes. The intravenous location of the catheter was confirmed

Results of Air Test After Placement of Epidural Catheter

Clinical Outcome	Air Test Result	
	Negative	Positive
Epidural anesthesia demonstrated	273	6*
No epidural level but no evidence of iv placement	8	0
Intravenous catheter placement confirmed	0	16 †
Total	281	22

*Two patients had tinnitus after subsequent doses of local anesthetics.
†P < .01, compared with negative air test groups.
(Courtesy of Leighton BL, Norris MC, DeSimone CA, et al: *Anesthesiology* 73:610–613, 1990.)

in 16 of 22 patients who had positive air test results. The air test yielded false positive results in 6 (2%) cases.

The air test is a useful and safe means of detecting the intravenous placement of an epidural catheter during labor. Nevertheless, the present findings should be confirmed by further investigation before the test is widely used in clinical practice.

▶ The results of this study are interesting but will not be useful in clinical practice. After our group demonstrated that embolic phenomena could be detected more than 50% of the time at cesarean delivery by precordial Doppler detection, I know of no Department of Anesthesiology in the United States in which this technique is routinely used. After reading this study, I feel as if I'm answering the question on an examination where the answer is true (yes, intravenous air can be detected by the use of a precordial Doppler sensor), true (yes, precordial Doppler sensors should be available in every Department of Anesthesiology), and unrelated (I know of no department that uses a precordial Doppler sensor during the routine administration of epidural anesthesia).—G.W. Ostheimer, M.D.

Motor and Sensory Blockade After Epidural Injection of Mepivacaine, Bupivacaine, and Etidocaine: A Double-Blind Study

Axelsson K, Nydahl P-A, Philipson L, Larsson P (Örebro Med Ctr Hosp, Örebro; Linköping Univ, Linköping, Sweden)
Anesth Analg 69:739–747, 1989   5–28

The Bromage scale is widely used to estimate motor blockade in epidural anesthesia. However, motor blockade can be measured more accurately by quantitative dynamometry or isometric muscle force methods. A double-blind study was conducted to quantify motor blockade in healthy volunteers given 1 of 3 commonly used local anesthetics for epidural anesthesia, and to assess the accuracy of the Bromage scale compared with quantitative methods.

The 30 healthy men were randomly assigned to receive epidural injection of either 20 mL of 2% mepivacaine, .5% bupivacaine, or 1.5% etidocaine. All solutions contained epinephrine 1:200,000. Muscle force measurements for hip flexion, knee extension, and plantar flexion of the big toe to measure the degree of motor blockade during anesthesia were obtained at baseline and during the onset and regression of epidural anesthesia. The Bromage scale was also used to estimate motor blockade.

There was no significant difference between analgesia onset after the epidural injection of mepivacaine and bupivacaine. However, etidocaine had a significantly faster onset of sensory blockade than the other 2 agents. The onset of motor blockade for hip flexion and knee extension was significantly faster than that of plantar flexion of the big toe, regardless of which local anesthetic was used. However, men who received etidocaine had complete motor blockade, whereas those who were given mepivacaine or bupivacaine retained 5% to 33% of baseline muscle force. The L5–S2 segment, which controls plantar flexion of the big toe, had the least motor blockade.

The duration of maximal motor blockade was significantly longer after etidocaine than after bupivacaine, and was shortest for mepivacaine. During regression, the isometric muscle force returned at the same time in the knee, hip, and big toe in each group. Complete restoration of muscle function occurred after 600 minutes with etidocaine, after 360 minutes with bupivacaine, and after 180 minutes with mepivacaine. The Bromage scale corresponded to motor blockade only for the first half of the regression phase, as the muscle force of all movements was not restored until 1–3 hours after Bromage grade 0 was reached.

The spread of sensory blockade was identical with all 3 local anesthetics tested, but etidocaine produced more effective motor blockade. The isometric quantitative method for assessing onset, degree, and duration of motor blockade was superior to the Bromage scale, which reflected motor function accurately only during the first half of the regression phase.

▶ This study comparing quantitative dynamometry or isometric muscle force to the Bromage scale, which is widely used to quantify motor block from spinal/epidural anesthetics, reminds me of the comparison between the Brazelton Neonatal Behavior Assessment Scale and the screening neonatal neurobehavioral examinations, i.e., the Early Neonatal Neurobehavioral Scale and the Neurologic and Adaptive Capacity Score. The Brazelton examination is the gold standard in neonatal neurobehavior, and it would appear that quantitative assessment of muscle force may be the silver standard to quantify motor block.—G.W. Ostheimer, M.D.

Motor Blockade and EMG Recordings in Epidural Anaesthesia: A Comparison Between Mepivacaine 2%, Bupivacaine 0.5% and Etidocaine 1.5%
Nydahl P-A, Axelsson K, Philipson L, Leissner P, Larsson PG (Örebro Med Centre Hosp, Örebro; Linköping Univ, Linköping, Sweden)
Acta Anaesthesiol Scand 33:597–604, 1989   5–29

Two different quantitative methods of evaluating motor block during epidural anesthesia were compared when 3 different local anesthetics were used in 27 healthy young men in a double-blind study. Ten were randomly allocated to epidural anesthesia with 20 mL of mepivacaine 2%, 9 received 20 mL of bupivacaine .5%, and 8 received 20 mL of etidocaine 1.5%. Epinephrine 1:200,000 was added to all 3 anesthetic solutions.

Motor block of the rectus abdominis muscles was quantitatively assessed by rectified integrated electromyographic recordings (RIEMG) and as number of turns (TURNS) in EMG recordings from 3 different segmental levels, T7, T9, and T11. Motor block of the quadriceps muscles was estimated by EMG recordings simultaneously with muscle force measurements at maximal isometric knee extension. The results were compared with those of the Bromage scale.

There was good correlation between RIEMG values and muscle force in knee extension during epidural anesthesia; TURNS added no further information. Etidocaine gave more profound and longer motor block at T11 than did mepivacaine or bupivacaine. For quadriceps muscle function motor block was almost complete with all 3 drugs. The duration of maximum motor block was 45–60 minutes with mepivacaine, compared with about 5 hours with etidocaine. When the Bromage scale indicated complete regression of motor block, the muscle force of knee extension was still only 30%, and the quadriceps RIEMG was still only 35% of control values.

Etidocaine provides good motor block spread over more spinal segments from the injection site than either bupivacaine or mepivacaine. However, motor block outlasted sensory block by 150 minutes. The RIEMG measurements are useful for quantitative assessment of motor block of the abdominal and quadriceps muscles during epidural anesthesia.

▶ This study demonstrates that another method of evaluating motor block by RIEMG recordings, as well as changes in the direction (rise/fall) of the electromyograph, offers a more sensitive evaluation of motor block in the regression phase than the Bromage scale does. We are indebted to Dr. Bromage for devising a screening motor block scale. However, as with all screening evaluations, more in-depth analysis of motor block by a variety of methods gives more in-depth information about the duration of the regression of motor block. Interestingly, with etidocaine, motor block outlasted sensory block by 150 minutes according to the RIEMG evaluation. Studies with etidocaine over the years have shown controversial results. Some studies have documented that motor block wore off before the regression of sensory anesthesia, and in others the regression of sensory and motor block appeared to be within the same time frame. This study supports clinical observations reported by a number of investigators that patients perceive pain before they recover from motor block with etidocaine.—G.W. Ostheimer, M.D.

Shivering During Epidural Anesthesia
Sessler DI, Ponte J (Univ of California, San Francisco; King's College School of Medicine and Dentistry, London)
Anesthesiology 72:816–821, 1990   5–30

Shivering during epidural anesthesia is commonly attributed to normal thermoregulatory shivering, but nonthermoregulatory etiologies have also been proposed. To further investigate the etiology of shivering during epidural anesthesia, an epidural catheter was inserted into 6 healthy men and 4 healthy women aged 25–38 years. Six of the 10 were randomly assigned to skin-surface warming below the T_{10} dermatome and 4 did not receive extra warming.

After a 15-minute control period each volunteer was given 1 cold and 1 warm 30-mL epidural injection of 1% lidocaine without epinephrine at a rate of 15 mL/min in random order. The injections were at least 3 hours apart. Tympanic membrane skin-surface temperature gradients and average skin temperatures were measured with thermocouples and electronic thermometers. Overall thermal comfort was evaluated at 5- to 10-minute intervals using a 100-mm visual analog scale (VAS). At the end of the study each volunteer was asked to guess which epidural injection was warm and which was cold.

Tympanic membrane temperatures decreased significantly in the 6 unwarmed volunteers. Tremor occurred after 10 of 12 epidural injections in unwarmed volunteers, but after only 1 of 8 injections given to warmed volunteers. There was no significant difference in integrated electromyographic intensity after either warm or cold injection of lidocaine, and the volunteers were unable to guess whether epidural injections were warm

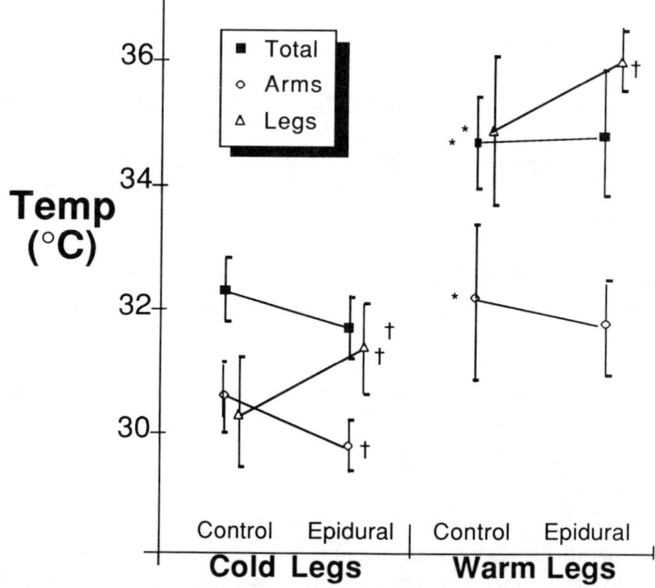

Fig 5–8.—Skin-surface temperatures (mean of 10, area-weighted sites) in volunteers with unwarmed legs (left side: 12 injections in 6 volunteers) and unwarmed legs (right side: 8 injections in 4 volunteers). Average total skin temperatures in each group are subdivided into average leg temperature (3 sites) and average arm temperature (4 sites). Control points (on left of each data set) are connected with points that indicate maximum change after epidural injection of lidocaine (usually occuring approximately 45 minutes after injection). Skin temperatures during control periods were significantly higher in warmed than in unwarmed group. *$P \leq .01$. Leg skin temperature increased significantly after epidural injection in both groups. However, arm (and head, back, and chest) temperatures decreased enough in unwarmed group that total skin temperature decreased significantly. †$P \leq .05$. (Courtesy of Sessler DI, Ponte J: Anesthesiology 72:816–821, 1990.)

or cold. Thermal comfort as assessed on the VAS increased significantly in all volunteers after epidural injection, with maximal comfort occurring at the lowest central temperatures. Tremor was always preceded by hypothermia and vasoconstriction in the arms.

Skin surface temperatures during control periods were significantly higher in warmed than in unwarmed volunteers. Average leg skin temperature increased significantly after epidural injection in both groups. However, average arm (and back, chest, and head) temperatures decreased enough in the unwarmed group to decrease the average total skin temperature significantly (Fig 5–8).

These findings suggest that tremor during epidural anesthesia is primarily normal thermoregulatory shivering. The temperature of the injected epidural solution does not influence tremor intensity, nor does central hypothermia necessarily produce a subjective sensation of cold.

▶ This nicely done study expands our knowledge of shivering during epidural anesthesia. Because we know that the pregnant patient responds in the same manner, it would be interesting to add the next step in this evaluation, which is the use of warmed intravenous solutions immediately before initiation of the epidural block.—G.W. Ostheimer, M.D.

Postmortem Findings After Epidural Anaesthesia
Wulf H, Striepling E (Univ Hosp, Kiel, Germany)
Anaesthesia 45:357–361, 1990   5–31

The advantages and complications of continuous postoperative epidural analgesia have been well reported, but only a few postmortem studies of pathologic sequelae of epidural anesthesia have been published. The postmortem findings in patients with continuous epidural analgesia were compared with those in a control group.

Of 497 patients who had received epidural analgesia with bupivacaine .25% to .5% for postoperative pain relief for at least 24 hours, 24 died of causes unrelated to the analgesia. Permission for autopsy was granted for 10 patients. Nine patients had septic complications after epidural catheter insertion. Nine patients had received low-dose heparin prophylaxis. Duration of epidural analgesia ranged from 2 to 21 days (table). Autopsy specimens from 10 patients without epidural catheters also were examined.

Nonspecific hyperemia, observed in both groups, was attributed to the general hyperemia that occurs when right ventricular failure is the cause of death. Slight epidural hemorrhage occurred in 6 patients with epidural catheters. A macroscopically visible hematoma was present in 1 patient with thrombocytopenia. The inflammatory alterations may have resulted from local irritation by the catheter or from solution injected into the epidural space. Signs of epidural infection were present in the specimens from 7 patients who died of systemic infection. None of the patients

Patients in Epidural Group (With Epidural Catheter)

Patient number	Age (years)	Sex	Diagnosis	Infection	Duration of epidural (days)	Interval—end of epidural till death (days)
01	45	F	Ovarian carcinoma	None	2	0
02	20	M	Acute myeloid leukaemia, bone marrow transplantation, thoracotomy	Mycotic infection	21	3
03	78	M	Perforated colonic tumour	Chronic peritonitis	9	21
04	56	M	Ruptured spleen, ileus, caecal perforation	Chronic peritonitis	14	0
05	85	M	Pleural carcinoma	Bronchopneumonia	7	0
06	75	F	Metastatic uterine carcinoma, enterostomy	Purulent peritonitis	2	47
07	71	M	Metastatic bronchial carcinoma, bowel resection	Fibrinous peritonitis	3	0
08	63	F	Pancreatic carcinoma	Purulent peritonitis	11	3
09	67	M	Cholecystectomy	Bronchopneumonia	12	0
10	38	F	Squamous cell carcinoma of the thigh	Purulent peritonitis	16	0

(Courtesy of Wulf H, Striepling E: *Anaesthesia* 45:357–361, 1990.)

without epidural catheters had those findings. No other pathologic alterations were seen in bone, spinal cord, pia mater, or nerve roots.

These results support the reluctance of most anesthetists to insert epidural catheters in the presence of systemic infection or immunodeficiency.

Consideration should be given to discontinuing its use if infective complications develop in a patient who already has an epidural catheter in place. The strictest attention must be paid to asepsis, and antibiotic prophylaxis is strongly recommended if an epidural catheter is deemed essential. A platelet count should be performed before catheter insertion in patients with a predisposition to thrombocytopenia, e.g., cancer or preeclampsia among others. The epidural catheter should not be used or moved if coagulopathies develop. Patients receiving continuous epidural analgesia should always be closely monitored for signs of spinal pressure (back pain, pain on injection, local tenderness, fever, neurologic deficits), because these may indicate spinal abscess or hematoma formation.

▶ I am in complete agreement with the conclusions of the authors of this paper.—G.W. Ostheimer, M.D.

Extravascular Absorption of Irrigating Fluid During TURP: The Role of Transmural Bladder Pressure as the Driving Pressure Gradient
Hultén JO, Sundström GS (Sundsvall Hosp, Sundsvall, Sweden)
Br J Urol 65:39–42, 1990   5–32

A pressure head driving solution into the prostatic veins or gland tissue always is a risk during transurethral prostatic resection (TURP). The critical intravesical pressure range for extravascular absorption of irrigating fluid depends on the perivesical tissue pressure. The pressure gradient underlying extravascular absorption is the transmural bladder pressure, or detrusor pressure, which is the intravesical pressure less perivesical pressure.

Transmural pressure was measured before and during epidural anesthesia in 6 patients undergoing TURP. Both conventional medium-fast-fill cystometry and "free flow" cystometry were performed. Transmural pressure increased early but slowly during medium-fast-fill cystometry. After epidural block the bladder filled more at a higher pressure level, but the pressure curve did not change. The rise in pressure in patients was similar whether the filling rate was constant or whether free-flow cystometry was done through the resectoscope. In the latter case, flow closely reflected intravesical pressure.

A pressure gradient for extravascular absorption is present in the very early phase of bladder filling. Substantial extravascular absorption may occur even if the intravesical pressure is below the pressure in the prostatic veins. Absorption probably is influenced by incomplete perforation of the prostatic capsule, clotting, and accumulation of irrigating fluid in the perivesical tissues.

▶ For the anesthesiologist, the important message is that epidural anesthesia does not influence the transmural pressure response produced by filling the bladder with fluid.—R.K. Stoelting, M.D.

Malignant Hyperthermia

Localization of the Malignant Hyperthermia Susceptibility Locus to Human Chromosome 19q12– 13.2

McCarthy TV, Healy JMS, Heffron JJA, Lehane M, Deufel T, Lehmann-Horn F, Farrall M, Johnson K (Univ College, Cork, Ireland; Children's Hosp, Univ of Munich; Technical Univ of Munich; St Mary's Hosp Med School, London)
Nature 343:562–564, 1990   5–33

Malignant hyperthermia (MH) is an inherited skeletal muscle disorder that is triggered in susceptible persons by commonly used inhalational anesthetics. An almost identical animal disorder, porcine MH, exists in pigs. The locus controlling expression of porcine MH is linked genetically to the glucose phosphate isomerase locus. In humans, this linkage maps to chromosome 12q12–13.2. Because of the phenotypic similarity of human and porcine MH, it was hypothesized that the human MH locus would map to 19q.

To test this hypothesis, the genetic linkage between susceptibility to MH (MHS) and markers that span 19q12–13.2 was studied in 3 large Irish families in which MHS was segregated as an autosomal dominant trait. Linkage between MHS and DNA markers from the glucose phosphate isomerase locus region of human chromosome 19 was seen with a maximum log likelihood ratio (lod score) of 5.65 at the CYP2A locus.

The locus controlling expression of human MHS maps to chromosome 19q12–13.2, similar to that in porcine MH. Human MH and porcine MH are most probably caused by mutations in homologous genes.

Ryanodine Receptor Gene Is a Candidate for Predisposition to Malignant Hyperthermia

MacLennan DH, Duff C, Zorzato F, Fujii J, Phillips M, Korneluk RG, Frodis W, Britt BA, Worton RG (Univ of Toronto; Hosp for Sick Children, Toronto; Children's Hosp of Eastern Ontario, Ottawa; Toronto Gen Hosp)
Nature 343:559–561, 1990   5–34

Predisposition to malignant hyperthermia (MH) is presently determined through a halothane- and/or caffeine-induced contracture test on a skeletal muscle biopsy. Because Ca^{2+} is the chief regulator of muscle contraction and metabolism, the primary defect in MH may be in Ca^{2+} regulation. This is supported by several studies that indicate a defect in the Ca^{2+} release channel of the sarcoplasmic reticulum. Complementary DNA and genomic DNA encoding the human ryanodine receptor (the Ca^{2+}-receptor release channel of the sarcoplasmic reticulum) have been cloned and the ryanodine receptor gene *(RYR)* mapped to region q13.1 of human chromosome 19 in close proximity to genetic markers that map near the MH susceptibility locus in humans and halothane-sensitive gene in pigs.

To determine whether the *RYR* gene is a likely candidate for the human MH phenotype, a linkage study was undertaken in families with MH to learn if the MH phenotype segregates with chromosome 19q markers, including markers in the *RYR* gene. In each of the 9 families studied, the affected parent was heterozygous for the *RYR* polymorphism and the unaffected parent was homozygous for this marker, making all children fully informative. In each family there was complete cosegregation of 1 *RYR* allele with the MH phenotype, resulting in a lod score of 4.20 at a linkage distance of 0 centimorgans.

These findings, combined with the physiologic data that a Ca^{2+} release channel defect exists in individuals predisposed to MH, suggest strongly that the basic defect in MH results from mutations in the *RYR* gene. Because the porcine halothane-sensitive gene segregates with the *GPI* locus, and this locus maps in human beings to 19q, very close to the *RYR* gene, it is possible that mutations in the *RYR* gene may be responsible for the halothane-sensitive phenotype in pigs.

▶ These studies illustrate the progress being made to develop a test for MH. On a broader basis, molecular biology techniques are being used by multiple groups to solve the problems associated with MH, including identification of a specific receptor responsible for this disease.—R.D. Miller, M.D.

Masseteric Muscle Spasm as a Normal Response to Suxamethonium
Leary NP, Ellis FR (St James's Univ Hosp, Leeds, England)
Br J Anaesth 64:488–492, 1990   5–35

An increased jaw muscle tone may be a normal response to suxamethonium. About 50% of patients with masseter spasm, masseteric muscle spasm, and masseteric muscle rigidity may be susceptible to malignant hyperthermia (MH). Using a unique myotonometer, the myotonic response of the masseter muscles after various doses of suxamethonium was measured in 50 healthy adults undergoing elective surgery under thiopental-nitrous oxide anesthesia. The doses of suxamethonium used were .25, .5, .7, 1, and 2 mg/kg.

Most patients had a myotonic response lasting for less than 100 seconds. In 5 patients there was a maximum increase in masseter tone of more than 1 kg, whereas a maximum tone greater than 500 g developed in 12. The dose of suxamethonium correlated negatively with increased tone onset, offset, peak and duration times. There was no correlation between suxamethonium dose and magnitude of increases in jaw tone, but 50% of patients were still generating an increased tone 10 seconds after the offset of fasciculations. None of the patients had signs of a hypermetabolic state.

It can be predicted that 1 in every 20 patients will have a masseteric muscle tone increase of more than 1,500 g and 1 in every 100 will have an increase of more than 2,000 g. An increased masseter tone of this degree may be interpreted as "masseteric muscle spasm" and the patient referred erroneously for MH screening. The value of masseteric muscle spasm as an early sign of MH is questionable.

▶ This study emphasizes that masseter muscle spasm cannot be used as an early sign of MH.—R.D. Miller, M.D.

Safety of General Anesthesia in Patients Previously Tested Negative for Malignant Hyperthermia Susceptibility
Allen GC, Rosenberg H, Fletcher JE (Hahnemann Univ)
Anesthesiology 72:619–622, 1990   5–36

The in vitro contracture test has been used for 2 decades to determine susceptibility to malignant hyperthermia (MH), but there have been no reports of anesthetic challenge of patients believed previously to be MH negative. To determine whether patients with a negative in vitro contracture test had adverse anesthetic outcomes when subsequently exposed to triggering anesthetic agents, the medical records for 54 anesthetic exposures in 42 MH-negative patients were examined. Contracture testing was done in a standard manner with 3% halothane alone and incremental doses of caffeine alone.

Sixteen patients were given anesthesia with known MH-triggering agents on 23 occasions without incident. In 6 patients with previous masseter muscle rigidity, volatile anesthetic agents produced no adverse reactions. In these patients succinylcholine was avoided. Eleven MH-negative patients were managed as if they were MH susceptible, even though they had tested negative. Two patients were also given prophylactic injections of dantrolene.

"Triggering" anesthetic agents may be given safely to patients who test MH negative by in vitro contracture testing. However, these findings should be interpreted cautiously. The anesthetic experience of larger numbers of MH-negative patients needs to be analyzed.

▶ These data are reassuring with respect to the usefulness of contracture tests in patients considered to be possibly MH susceptible. Nevertheless, I suspect that most clinicians would attempt to avoid all known triggering drugs in a patient who previously manifested symptoms suggestive of MH despite a subsequent negative contracture test.—R.K. Stoelting, M.D.

Malignant Hyperthermia Susceptibility in Adult Patients With Masseter Muscle Rigidity
Allen GC, Rosenberg H (Hahnemann Univ)
Can J Anaesth 37:31–35, 1990   5–37

Masseter muscle rigidity (MMR) after succinylcholine exposure may be an early sign of malignant hyperthermia (MH). To determine the incidence of MH susceptibility in patients older than age 15 years with a previous episode of MMR, medical records and in vitro contracture test results of 24 adults were evaluated. For comparison, the number of children younger than age 16 years tested for MH because of previous MMR also was determined.

During the 4-year study, 6 of the 24 adult patients tested for MH susceptibility because of previous MMR proved MH susceptible by in vitro contracture testing. In contrast, during the same period, 44 of 75 children tested for MH susceptibility because of previous MMR had positive in vitro contracture tests. There was no clinical sign predictive of MH susceptibility. Two of the 6 MH-susceptible adults had acute MH after MMR.

The coincidence of MMR and MH susceptibility is lower in adults than in children, but episodes of MH can occur in 25% of adult patients. The development of MH after MMR may be delayed. Conservative management should be undertaken when MMR occurs in adult patients. These patients should undergo diagnostic muscle biopsy and in vitro contracture testing to determine MH susceptibility.

▶ See comment for Abstract 5–36.—R.K. Stoelting, M.D.

Azumolene Reverses Episodes of Malignant Hyperthermia in Susceptible Swine

Dershwitz M, Sréter FA (Massachusetts Gen Hosp, Boston; Harvard Med School; Boston Biomed Research Inst)
Anesth Analg 70:253–255, 1990   5–38

Dantrolene is an effective drug in the treatment of malignant hyperthermia (MH), but its lack of water solubility and the difficulty in preparing a solution suitable for intravenous use are major disadvantages. Azumolene is a dantrolene analogue with much greater water solubility than dantrolene. In vitro studies on strips of skeletal muscle tissue obtained from MH-susceptible patients have shown that azumolene has physiologic effects similar to those of dantrolene.

To determine whether azumolene could reverse episodes of MH in susceptible swine, 10 pigs bred to be susceptible to MH were given 2% halothane and 67% nitrous oxide in oxygen via an anesthesia face mask and allowed to breathe spontaneously. The animals were then observed for signs of MH. Once the diagnosis of MH has been made, the pig was given 100% oxygen by face mask, and azumolene was administered intravenously in 5-mg increments at 2-minute intervals until the hind limbs were supple.

In each episode of MH, rigidity was terminated by a dose of azumolene of less than 2 mg/kg. There was an inverse relationship between the time it took for hind limb rigidity to develop and the total dose of azumolene required to terminate the episode of MH. Thus pigs that were more sensitive to the triggering effect of halothane required larger doses of azumolene to reverse MH. Azumolene appears to be approximately equipotent with dantrolene in terms of reversing episodes of MH. Azumolene may be a candidate for investigations of MH in human beings, but further studies are needed to determine the toxicity of the drug in laboratory animals and its stability in solution.

▶ Assuming this drug is as effective as dantrolene and no more toxic, it is likely that greater water solubility will become a determining factor in its selection.—R.K. Stoelting, M.D.

Prediction of Malignant Hyperthermia Susceptibility: Statistical Evaluation of Clinical Signs

Hackl W, Mauritz W, Schemper M, Winkler M, Sporn P, Steinbereithner K (Univ of Vienna)
Br J Anaesth 64:425–429, 1990

5–39

Data were reviewed concerning 61 patients who had adverse reactions interpreted as malignant hyperthermia (MH) to determine whether symptoms can aid in recognizing this disorder. Susceptibility for MH was determined by in vitro testing of a sample of quadriceps femoris muscle.

Thirty-eight patients (62%) were identified by the in vitro contracture test as susceptible to MH. Symptoms, including generalized rigidity, masseter spasm, tachycardia, cyanotic skin mottling, and fever, were more frequent in these 38 patients. Significant differences were found for generalized rigidity and cyanosis as well as for ventricular arrhythmia, postoperative myoglobinuria, intraoperative temperature, and the postopera-

Diagnostic Relevance of Clinical Signs Occurring Alone or In Combination

Clinical sign	n	n (MHS)	Univariate analysis		Multiple regression	
			Odds ratio	P	Odds ratio	P
Generalized rigidity						
Absent	42	20	19.8	0.0001	26.4	0.0001
Present	19	18				
Arrhythmia						
Absent	43	23	4.3	0.036	6.2	0.024
Present	18	15				
Cyanosis						
Absent	33	15	5.5	0.005	5.4	0.018
Present	28	23				

Total number of patients *(n)*, a number of malignant hyperthermia susceptible (MHS) patients in whom the clinical sign was absent or present.
$n = 61$.
(Courtesy of Hackl W, Mauritz W. Schemper M, et al: *Br J Anaesth* 64:425–429, 1990.)

tive creatine kinase concentration. Generalized rigidity was an especially helpful finding (table).

No clinical symptoms are specific features of MH, and prediction of susceptibility on clinical grounds alone is limited to relatively few fulminant cases. The in vitro contracture test is necessary to confirm or exclude MH in less marked or abortive cases.

▶ It's interesting that this study evaluating clinical signs says that the clinical signs are not as good as the in vitro contracture test. The article could have said that from the start, because the authors use the in vitro contracture test as the gold standard. Obviously, nothing will be as good as what is acknowledged to be the gold standard. Nevertheless, the article does give good indications that generalized rigidity, dysrhythmia, and cyanosis, as well as a body temperature higher than 38°, had good sensitivity and specificity when the in vitro contracture test was used as the gold standard. One wonders how good the in vitro contracture test would be in relation to the actual event of MH in patients. I don't believe we have the knowledge of how good the in vitro contracture test is as an ideal test of MH at this time. Nonetheless, I believe that this study greatly advances the science pertaining to MH evaluation and comes to the conclusion that masseter spasm and sinus tachycardia are not of much value, whereas generalized rigidity, ventricular arrhythmia, cyanosis, and fever exceeding 38°C are very useful signs.—M.F. Roizen, M.D.

Additional Reading

Wiswell TE, Bent RC, Solenberger R: Malignant hyperthermia in infancy. *South Med J* 82:1451–1452, 1989.

NPO and Aspiration of Gastric Contents

▶ ↓ In this group of papers there is further exploration of the administration of fluids in the immediate preoperative period. Splinter et al. (Abstract 5–40) concluded that drinking large volumes of clear apple juice 2.5 hours before scheduled surgery did not have any measurable effect on gastric volume pH and may offer benefits such as improved patient comfort. However, the gastric pH averaged 1.7 ± .6, well below the magical pH of 2.5. Subsequently, Splinter et al. in another study (Abstract 5–41), reported that drinking clear fluid up to 3 hours before scheduled surgery in unlimited amounts did not have any measurable effect on the gastric volume pH of healthy children aged 2–12 years. Again, the gastric pH was 1.7 ± .4. Schreiner et al. (Abstract 5–42), who allowed clear liquids up to 2 hours before induction of anesthesia, believe that there was no substantial effect on the volume of gastric contents or the percentage of patients with a fluid pH of less than 2.5. More than 90% of the study and control groups had a gastric pH of less than 2.5.

The overall conclusion from these 3 papers is that, although the risk of aspiration of fluid with a gastric pH of less than 2.5 is not diminished, giving clear liquids appears to present no additional risk of aspiration of gastric contents and may provide some psychological benefit, as evidenced by the decreased irritability before induction of anesthesia. Pulmonary aspiration of gastric contents is uncommon in children. However, I wonder, if we allow children to drink whatever they want until 2 hours before surgery, why we don't give a palatable clear antacid or H_2 antagonist within the hour before induction of anesthesia? I know of no studies in which a clear antacid or 1 dose of an H_2 antagonist has produced any harm in the preoperative pediatric patient. I would think that the effect of the clear antacid and/or oral H_2 antagonist is the next logical step in our reappraisal of maintaining children on a "nothing by mouth" status after midnight.— G.W. Ostheimer, M.D.

Large Volumes of Apple Juice Preoperatively Do Not Affect Gastric pH and Volume in Children

Splinter WM, Stewart JA, Muir JG (Izaak Walton Killam Hosp for Children, Halifax, NS)
Can J Anaesth 37:36–39, 1990

5–40

The appropriate length of time that children should abstain from food and drink before anesthesia is not known. Previous studies have shown that ingestion of specific amounts of clear fluid 2–4 hours before induction of anesthesia is safe.

The effect on gastric pH and gastric volume of giving a large volume of apple juice to children late in the preoperative period was assessed in a prospective, randomized, single-blind study of 93 children aged 5–10 years who were scheduled for elective procedures under general anesthesia. Thirty were given clear apple juice, 6 mL kg, 2.5 hours before operation; 32 were given clear apple juice, 10 mL/kg, 2.5 hours before operation; and 31 were kept fasting. Gastric contents were aspirated immediately after induction of anesthesia.

There was no significant difference in gastric volume or pH among the 3 groups after induction of anesthesia (table). Children who were given apple juice were less thirsty and less irritable and upset before induction of anesthesia than children who had not been given anything to drink. A large volume of clear apple juice given to healthy children aged 5–10 years at 2.5 hours before scheduled surgery did not affect gastric contents immediately after induction of anesthesia and improved patient comfort.

Percent of Patients With Risk Factors for Pulmonary Acid
Aspiration Syndrome

Group	Gastric vol $>0.4\,ml\cdot kg^{-1}$	Gastric vol $>0.4\,ml\cdot kg^{-1}$ and pH <2.5	Gastric vol $>1.0\,ml\cdot kg^{-1}$
A	47	47	17
B	59	56	25
C	55	55	10

(Courtesy of Splinter WM, Stewart JA, Muir JG: *Can J Anaesth* 37:36–39, 1990.)

Clear Fluids Three Hours Before Surgery Do Not Affect the Gastric Fluid Contents of Children

Splinter WM, Schaefer JD, Zunder IH (Children's Hosp of Eastern Ontario, Ottawa)

Can J Anaesth 37:498–501, 1990   5–41

Administration of specific volumes and types of clear fluids to children up to 2–3 hours before operation appears to be safe and reduces the thirst, hunger, and poor behavior associated with overnight fasting. In a prospective, randomized, single-blind study the effect of an overnight fast on volume of gastric fluid and pH was compared with the effect of allowing unlimited clear fluid ingestion up to 3 hours before operation.

Sixty-four children (mean age, 5.7 years) were randomly allocated to fasting from midnight until elective operation. Fifty-seven children (mean age, 5.6 years) did not consume solid food on the day of operation but were allowed to drink unlimited volumes and types of clear fluids up to 3 hours before scheduled elective operation. Parents or nursing staff accurately monitored the amount of fluid ingested on the day of operation. In all children the gastric volume and pH was measured immediately after induction of anesthesia.

The mean amount of clear fluids ingested up to 3.3 hours before induction of anesthesia was 203 mL. The fluids ingested included clear fruit juices, water, soda pop, Popsicles, Kool Aid, and Jello. The volume of fluids ingested varied considerably, primarily because of the differences in the children's appetite.

Neither volume of gastric fluid nor gastric pH was affected by the ingestion of clear fluids. The volume of gastric fluid increased significantly with increasing age in both control and study children.

Gastric fluid contents immediately after induction of anesthesia in healthy children between the age of 2 and 12 years are not adversely affected by the ingestion of unlimited types and volumes of clear fluids up to 3 hours before operation. Thus the policy of restricting the clear fluid intake for more than 3 hours before operation under general anesthesia does not benefit children.

Ingestion of Liquids Compared With Preoperative Fasting in Pediatric Outpatients

Schreiner MS, Triebwasser A, Keon TP (Children's Hosp of Philadelphia)

Anesthesiology 72:593–597, 1990   5–42

Clinically important aspiration of gastric stomach contents as a complication of anesthesia is uncommon in children. Furthermore, studies in adults have shown that clear liquids are emptied from the stomach with a halftime of 10–20 minutes. Because the preoperative fast is often an unpleasant experience for children, the effects of liberal intake of clear liquids up to 2 hours before anesthesia induction on gastric fluid volume and pH were examined.

The study was done with 121 ASA physical status 1 or 2 patients aged 1–18 years scheduled for operations requiring tracheal intubation. Before operation, children were randomly assigned to either the control or the study group. Neither group was allowed solid foods, milk products, orange juice, or other pulp-containing juices after 8 PM. Children in the control group were permitted unlimited quantities of clear liquids until 6 hours before anesthesia induction if 1–5 years of age, and until 8 hours before operation if older than 5 years of age. All children in the study group were allowed clear liquids in unlimited quantities until 2 hours before anesthesia induction, except that the final liquid ingestion was limited to 8 oz. After tracheal intubation, gastric fluid was aspirated, the volume measured, and the pH determined. Parents were asked to complete a questionnaire while waiting to rate the preoperative experiences with their children.

Fifty-three children (mean age, 5.9 years) were assigned to the study group, and 68 children (mean age, 7.3 years) were assigned to the control group. There were no significant differences between the groups with regard to volume of gastric fluid aspirated, the proportion with a gastric fluid content of .4 mL/kg or more, the proportion with a gastric fluid pH of 2.5 or less, or the proportion with a pH of 2.5 or less and a gastric volume of .4 mL/kg or more (table). All inductions were uneventful, and no complications occurred. Questionnaires completed by parents revealed that children in the study group were less irritable and had a better overall preoperative experience compared with children in the control group.

Children undergoing operation at this institution are now allowed to drink clear liquids until 2 hours before anesthesia induction. A child who inadvertently drinks clear liquids should have surgery delayed no longer than 2 hours and, if the anticipated delay is 2 hours or longer, clear liquids should be allowed.

Gastric Fluid Analysis

	Study	Control	P
Gastric fluid volume			
mean ± SD (ml/kg)	0.44 ± 0.51	0.57 ± 0.51	0.12
Gastric fluid volume*			
≥ 0.4 ml/kg (%)	23/48 (48)	39/67 (58)	0.77
[H+] mean ± SD	0.015 ± .008	0.017 ± .01	0.47
(*p*H)	(1.81)	(1.77)	
Gastric *p*H ≤ 2.5 (%)†	34/35 (97)	44/48 (92)	0.57
Gastric *p*H ≤ 2.5 (%) and			
volume ≥ 0.4 ml/kg	22/48 (46)	33/67 (48)	0.86

*Gastric fluid volume was not measured in 5 study patients and 1 control.

†An insufficient quantity of fluid was obtained for pH analysis in 13 additional study patients and 19 controls.

(Courtesy of Schreiner MS, Triebwasser A, Keon TP: *Anesthesiology* 72:593–597, 1990.)

Effects of Duration of Fasting on Gastric Fluid pH and Volume in Healthy Children
Crawford M, Lerman J, Christensen S, Farrow-Gillespie A (Hosp for Sick Children, Toronto)
Anesth Analg 71:400–403, 1990   5–43

Although children are expected to fast before elective surgery to minimize the risk of regurgitation, the proper duration of fasting after drinking clear fluids is uncertain. In randomized study the duration of fasting was related to gastric fluid pH and volume in 100 unpremedicated children aged 1–14 years who were scheduled for elective surgery. All were in ASA physicial status I or II. Each child received water, 2 mL/kg, and then fasted for 2, 4, or 6 hours before surgery. Gastric fluid was aspirated after tracheal intubation.

Neither gastric fluid pH nor fluid volume correlated with the duration of fasting, nor did they correlate with age or body weight. The mean gastric fluid pH was 1.8 and the mean fluid volume, .56 mL/kg. Children may receive water, 2 mL/kg, up to 2 hours before elective surgery without lowering the gastric pH or raising the gastric fluid volume beyond values obtained in those who fast for up to 6 hours.

► This study fills in the blanks left by the preceding studies (Abstracts 5–40 and 5–42). We now know that unlimited fluids up to 2 hours before induction of anesthesia have no effect on raising the gastric pH or altering the gastric fluid volume in the pediatric patient. I still like the idea of using an oral H_2 antagonist, with or without a nonparticulate antacid, prior to induction. Certainly, the pharmaceutical companies could make such a concoction palatable for our young patients.—G.W. Ostheimer, M.D.

Effects of Oral Cimetidine and Ranitidine on Gastric pH and Residual Volume in Children
Guay J, Santerre L, Gaudreault P, Goulet B, Dupuis C (Sainte-Justine Hosp, Montreal; Univ of Montreal)
Anesthesiology 71:547–549, 1989   5–44

The preoperative administration of cimetidine or ranitidine to adults reportedly increases gastric pH and decreases gastric residual volume. In another series, when given to children before anesthesia, ranitidine increased the pH without affecting gastric volume, whereas cimetidine increased the pH and also decreased gastric volume.

To compare the effects of preoperatively administered ranitidine and cimetidine on gastric pH and residual volume in children, 60 ASA physical status 1 and 2 children aged 2–6 years scheduled for elective anesthesia and operation were randomly divided into 4 groups of 15 children each. All children had been fasting for 8 hours or longer. Between 1 and 2 hours before anesthesia induction, children were given either cimeti-

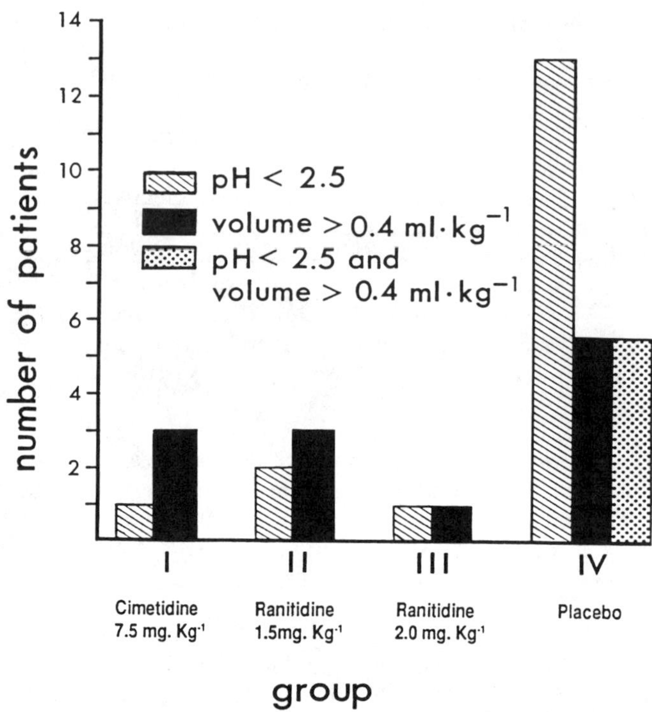

Fig 5–9.—Number of patients having either a pH less than 2.5, a volume greater than .4 mL/kg, or both. Group IV was statistically different from groups I, II, and III for the gastric pH and for the combination of both factors ($P < .001$). (Courtesy of Guay J, Santerre L, Gaudreault P, et al: *Anesthesiology* 71:547–549, 1989.)

dine, 7.5 mg/kg; ranitidine, 1.5 mg/kg; ranitidine, 2 mg/kg; or placebo. All preparations were given orally in a total volume of 5 mL. After anesthesia induction the gastric contents were aspirated, the residual gastric volume was measured, and the gastric pH was determined.

Neither ranitidine nor cimetidine decreased the gastric residual volume compared with placebo. However, both dosages of ranitidine and cimetidine effectively increased the gastric pH compared with placebo. The mean gastric pH did not differ significantly among the 3 study groups, but the control group had a significantly lower mean pH than the other 3 groups. None of the drug-treated children had both a pH of less than 2.5 and a gastric volume of more than .4 mL/kg, whereas 5 (33%) of the placebo-treated children had this combination, which is considered a risk factor for the acid aspiration syndrome (Fig 5–9).

► The fact that oral cimetidine and ranitidine would raise the gastric pH is not unexpected. The important message from this study is that an orally administered H_2 antagonist does raise gastric pH and may decrease residual volume (although that was not demonstrated in this study) in children. A corollary to this study would be consideration of an oral H_2 antagonist in ambulatory surgical patients whether they be children or adults. Aspiration of gastric contents remains a problem in the surgical patient, and the utilization of an oral H_2 antagonist will decrease that risk during general anesthesia, with or without endotracheal intubation.—G.W. Ostheimer, M.D.

Metoclopramide Reduces the Incidence of Vomiting Following Strabismus Surgery in Children

Broadman LM, Ceruzzi W, Patane PS, Hannallah RS, Ruttimann U, Friendly D (Children's Natl Med Ctr; George Washington Univ)
Anesthesiology 72:245–248, 1990   5–45

Strabismus surgery in children is associated with a high incidence of postoperative nausea and vomiting that may significantly delay their discharge from the ambulatory surgical unit. Although droperidol is an effective antiemetic, it can cause profound and protracted somnolence, which may also delay discharge.

To assess the efficacy of metoclopramide given at completion of ambulatory strabismus surgery in young persons, 126 healthy patients aged 2–18 years were assessed. All had general anesthesia with halothane and nitrous oxide in oxygen in an ambulatory setting. None of the patients was given preoperative sedation and none received intraoperative opioids or droperidol.

During a 1-minute period at completion of the operation 62 patients received metoclopramide, .15 mg/kg, intravenously, and 64 were given saline solution intravenously. Severe postoperative vomiting was treated with IV droperidol given intravenously.

The incidence of postoperative vomiting was 35% in the metoclopramide-treated group and 59% in the placebo-treated group. The difference was statistically significant. Patients given metoclopramide reached discharge criteria after a mean of 207.4 minutes, compared with 248.8 minutes for the controls, also a statistically significant difference. Eight placebo-treated patients required the adjunctive administration of droperidol, but none of the metoclopramide-treated group had protracted or severe postoperative nausea and vomiting. There were no adverse effects attributable to metoclopramide, and none of the children was drowsy or sedated.

▶ Metoclopramide appears to be effective in reducing the incidence of postoperative vomiting in children undergoing eye surgery. I hope that this study emphasizes the decreasing need for droperidol in children. Although it is an excellent antiemetic, droperidol can cause major side effects in children as well as in adults.—G.W. Ostheimer, M.D.

Effect of I.V. Metoclopramide on Gastric Emptying After Opioid Premedication

McNeill MJ, Ho ET, Kenny GNC (Royal Infirmary, Glasgow)
Br J Anaesth 64:450–452, 1990

5–46

Opioid premedication reduces the rate of gastric emptying, which results in an increased volume of gastric contents at anesthesia induction and a subsequent increased risk of regurgitation and aspiration. Metoclopramide is commonly used to increase the rate of gastric emptying. However, 2 previous studies reported that intramuscularly administered metoclopramide did not antagonize the effects of opioids on gastric emptying. There is some evidence that the effectiveness of metoclopramide may depend on the route of administration. The effects of intravenously administered metoclopramide on the rate of gastric emptying were investigated in patients premedicated with morphine.

Of 40 patients aged 18–65 years undergoing elective procedures, 10 were randomly assigned to receive diazepam, 10 mg orally; 10 received morphine, 10 mg intramuscularly; 10 received morphine, 10 mg intramuscularly, plus metoclopramide, 10 mg intravenously, 20 minutes later; and 10 received morphine, 10 mg intramuscularly, and metoclopramide, 10 mg intramuscularly, at the same time. Because diazepam does not affect gastric emptying, the diazepam-treated patients served as controls. Paracetamol is not absorbed from the stomach, so 1.5 g was given orally 20 minutes after administration of the preoperative medications to assess gastric emptying indirectly. Paracetamol levels were measured in venous blood samples, taken at 15-minute intervals for up to 90 minutes after administration.

The diazepam-treated control patients, as well as those given morphine plus metoclopramide intravenously, had significantly greater plasma paracetamol concentrations than patients given morphine with or without the concomitant intramuscular administration of metoclopramide. There was no significant difference in plasma paracetamol concentrations between the diazepam-treated patients and those treated intravenously with metoclopramide. The intravenous administration of metoclopramide appears to antagonize the reduction in paracetamol absorption caused by morphine, whereas its intramuscular administration does not.

▶ Conceptually, the pharmacologic effects of drugs are presumed to be caused by their receptor concentrations. If this is true, the route of administration becomes important only by virtue of the amount of drug that reaches the responding receptors. If the effect of metoclopramide is different after intramuscular than after intravenous injection, the presumed explanation is related to the plasma concentration that is achieved following each route of administration.—R.K. Stoelting, M.D.

6 Anesthesia for Certain Types of Surgery and Procedures

Urologic

Severe Hemorrhage After Extracorporeal Shock-Wave Lithotripsy
Stoller ML, Litt L, Salazar RG (Univ of California, San Francisco)
Ann Intern Med 111:612–613, 1989   6–1

Catastrophic renal hemorrhage is a rare complication of extracorporeal shock-wave lithotripsy. Severe hemorrhage occurred in 2 patients soon after lithotripsy.

Case 1.—Woman, 76, underwent uncomplicated lumbar anesthesia after lithotripsy. In the recovery room, hypotension, tachycardia, and cardiac arrest occurred. Although severe hemorrhage was suspected, renal ultrasonography did not show changes consistent with subcapsular hematoma and dissection. Consequently, volume resuscitation was delayed while other diagnoses were considered. The patient lost consciousness suddenly and could not be resuscitated. Autopsy showed massive retroperitoneal bleeding that originated from a wedge-shaped hemorrhage in the left renal cortex. In the
Case 2.—Man, 70, received 2,025 shock waves at 18–20 kV. Severe left-aided flank pain developed within 2 hours of treatment. A sudden drop in blood pressure suggested severe bleeding, and resuscitation was begun immediately, including blood transfusion. The injury was appropriately staged with CT imaging, and the patient improved.

Because life-threatening complications can develop after lithotripsy, thorough clinical examinations are necessary after the procedure. This becomes particularly important now that lithotripsy is usually an outpatient procedure. Knowledge of the immediate and delayed complications of lithotripsy is important.

▶ These 2 cases reports illustrate the catastrophic problems that can occasionally occur with lithotripsy. The first case is especially disturbing because ultrasound examinations did not confirm the presence of bleeding. This leads to the inevitable conclusion that when the cardiovascular signs are consistent with bleeding, bleeding is probably occurring.—R.D. Miller, M.D.

Neurosurgical

Fate of Air Emboli in the Pulmonary Circulation

Presson RG Jr, Kirk KR, Haselby KA, Linehan JH, Zaleski S, Wagner WW Jr (Indiana Univ, Indianapolis; Marquette Univ, Milwaukee; Ecole Normale Superieure, Paris)
J Appl Physiol 67:1898–1902, 1989

6–2

Air embolism occurs in various clinical settings, and the lungs serve an important nonrespiratory function by trapping and excreting venous air emboli. The site of trapping and the mechanism of excretion are uncertain. Surface tension theory suggests that bubbles lodge in precapillary vessels and that from there gas either diffuses directly into alveolar spaces or dissolves into blood flowing in contiguous tissue. Alternatively, venous gas emboli may be trapped directly in the pulmonary capillary bed, from which the gas gradually dissipates across the capillary bed.

Venous air emboli were injected into anesthetized dogs and their elimination was videotaped by in vivo microscopy. Small intravenous bubbles lodged solely in pulmonary arterioles and were eliminated from that site. Bubble volume decreased at the same rate under perfused and nonperfused conditions, indicating that it is independent of regional blood flow. Calculations based on the Fick equation for molecular diffusion predicted an elimination rate nearly identical to that observed experimentally.

The bulk of excretion of venous air emboli is accounted for by molecular diffusion across the arteriolar wall into alveolar spaces. Molecular diffusion alone can explain the disappearance of the bubbles that are observed experimentally.

▶ An interesting article. Whether it has any immediate clinical implications is not addressed.—R.R. Kirby, M.D.

Intracranial Volume–Pressure Relationship Following Thiopental or Etomidate

Artru AA (Univ of Washington)
Anesthesiology 71:763–768, 1989

6–3

Thiopental and etomidate are recommended for induction of anesthesia for patients with increased intracranial pressure, based on reports that both drugs reduce the increased pressure. To determine the effects of thiopental and etomidate on intracranial volume–pressure relationships, mock infusions of CSF were performed in 18 anesthetized dogs. Six dogs (time controls) were studied during anesthesia with halothane and nitrous oxide in oxygen, and the remaining dogs were studied before and after 2 doses of thiopental (approximate cumulative doses were 10.5 mg/kg and 25.5 mg/kg) or 2 doses of etomidate (approximate cumulative doses were 1.52 mg/kg and 3.7 mg/kg).

In the time controls CSF pressure before volume infusion (P_0), peak

CSF pressure (P_p), compliance (C, calculated as the ratio of change of intracranial volume [ΔV] to change of CSF pressure [ΔP], volume-pressure response (VPR, a measure of elastance calculated as the ratio of ΔP to ΔV), pressure volume index (PVI, calculated as the ratio of ΔV to log P_p/P_0), and estimated intracranial compliance (C_e, calculated from PVI as .4343 PVI/P_0) remained steady throughout the study period.

Doses of both thiopental and etomidate decreased P_0 and P_p and increased C_e. In both drug-treated groups there were no significant changes in C, VPR, or PVI.

Under these conditions of "normal" CSF pressure and no intracranial pathology, repeated testing of the intracranial volume–pressure relationship is possible, provided the volume of CSF withdrawn exactly matches the volume infused at each trial and at least 15 minutes are allowed for reequilibration between tests. Small doses of thiopental and etomidate produce comparable decreases of P_0 and P_p and increases in C_e, but no changes in intracranial volume–pressure relationships as indicated by C, VPR, or PVI.

▶ The clinician can be reassured to know that both thiopental and etomidate are drugs that seem acceptable for the induction of anesthesia in patients with preexisting elevations of intracranial pressure. If, indeed, etomidate and thiopental produce similar effects on intracranial pressure but the former is less likely to decrease blood pressure, a case could be made for preferentially selecting etomidate over thiopental. In this regard, intravenous injection of lidocaine has been shown to produce decreases in intracranial pressure similar to those produced by thiopental but without the same degree of associated blood pressure decrease (1).— R.K. Stoelting, M.D.

Reference

1. Bedford RF, et al: *Anesth Analg* 59:435, 1980.

Cerebrospinal Fluid Pressure in Patients With Brain Tumors: Impact of Fentanyl Versus Alfentanil During Nitrous Oxide–Oxygen Anesthesia
Jung R, Shah N, Reinsel R, Marx W, Marshall W, Galicich J, Bedford R (Mem Sloan-Kettering Cancer Ctr; Cornell Univ; Pennsylvania State Univ College of Medicine, Hershey)
Anesth Analg 71:419–422, 1990   6–4

Alfentanil and sufentanil are thought to impart greater hemodynamic stability than fentanyl, but a recent study of patients with brain tumors suggested that significant rises in the CSF pressure may occur if those agents are given to supplement nitrous oxide–oxygen ($N_2O\text{-}O_2$) anesthesia when intracranial compliance is compromised. However, alfentanil administration was associated with a significant drop in blood pressure, which made the CSF pressure changes difficult to interpret. The impact of alfentanil and fentanyl on CSF pressure during $N_2O\text{-}O_2$ anesthesia in patients with brain tumors was studied with blood pressure held constant.

Mean CSF Pressure Values at Baseline and During 3 Successive
5-Minute Intervals

Mean cerebrospinal fluid pressure

Anesthetic	t_o	1–5 min*	6–10 min*	7–15 min*
Alfentanil-N_2O	9.5 ± 1.3	10.1 ± 1.2	11.6 ± 1.4[†]	12.7 ± 1.8 [†]
Fentanyl-N_2O	8.9 ± 1.7	8.1 ± 2.4	7.8 ± 2.3	6.7 ± 2.8
N_2O alone	11.0 ± 2.0	10.6 ± 1.7	10.4 ± 2.1	11.5 ± 2.5

Abbreviations: t_o, baseline; N_2O, nitrous oxide.
Note: All values are means ±1 SE.
*Indicates minutes after baseline.
[†]$P < .05$ vs. baseline value.
(Courtesy of Jung R, Shah N, Reinsel R, et al: *Anesth Analg* 71:419–422, 1990.)

Twenty-four patients were included. Cerebrospinal fluid pressure, heart rate from ECG lead II, mean radial arterial blood pressure, and arterial blood gas tensions were monitored. General anesthesia was induced with thiopental, 5 mg/kg given intravenously in divided doses, and maintained with 70% N_2O in O_2. Ventilation was held constant. Sixteen patients were then randomly assigned to receive either fentanyl, 5 µg/kg, as an intravenous bolus or alfentanil, 50 µg/kg, as an intravenous bolus followed by alfentanil infusion at 1 µg/kg/min. An additional 8 patients served as controls. Blood pressure was held constant with an intravenous infusion of .1% phenylephrine as needed.

Cerebrospinal fluid pressure remained unchanged in patients receiving N_2O-O_2 alone and fentanyl–N_2O-O_2. However, patients given alfentanil–N_2O-O_2 had a gradual rise in CSF pressure that reached 30% above baseline values after 10 minutes and stabilized thereafter (table).

Alfentanil may be associated with an increase in CSF pressure in normocarbic neurosurgical patients with intracranial mass lesions. This effect was not observed after fentanyl administration, suggesting that greater caution is warranted when alfentanil is used for potentiating N_2O-O_2 anesthesia.

▶ It is surprising that 2 opioids given in presumed equal potent doses would have differing effects on CSF pressure. The data further suggest that the previous administration of fentanyl blunts or prevents the subsequent effects on CSF pressure of alfentanil administered as a continuous intravenous infusion.— R.K. Stoelting, M.D.

A Comparison of the Effects of Suxamethonium, Atracurium, and Vecuronium on Intracranial Hemodynamics in Swine
Ducey JP, Deppe SA, Foley KT (Brooke Army Med Ctr, Fort Sam Houston, Tex)
Anaesth Intens Care 17:448–455, 1989   6–5

Atracurium and vecuronium are nondepolarizing neuromuscular blocking agents that provide rapid and safe muscle relaxation. The effects of atracurium and vecuronium on intracranial pressure (ICP), heart rate, arterial blood pressure, and cerebral perfusion pressure (CCP) were compared with those of suxamethonium in 16 Yorkshire swines with normal or increased ICP.

In each animal, an ICP–volume curve was produced by inflation of an epidural balloon. Three points on the curve were identified: the baseline ICP (P_0) and the ICP at the inflection point (P_i) and on the steep portion (P_{max}). The animals were randomly assigned to receive suxamethonium, 1 mg/kg; atracurium, .6 mg/kg; vecuronium, .2 mg/kg; or saline placebo, intravenously in 3 conditions: with the epidural balloon deflated at P_0, at P_i, and at P_{max}.

Atracurium, vecuronium, or placebo had no significant effect on ICP, heart rate, blood pressure, or CCP at any baseline ICP. In contrast, suxamethonium produced an early decrease in ICP within 30 seconds of administration, followed by a rapid increase above the preinfusion level. The increase in ICP was accompanied by a decrease in blood pressure, resulting in a significant decrease in ICP. The mean decrease in CPP was 6 mm Hg at P_0, 6 mm Hg at P_i, and 6 mm Hg at P_{max}. This response was transient, lasting less than 90 seconds, and the magnitude of these effects was directly proportional to the baseline ICP. Neither atracurium, vecuronium, nor placebo affected ICP significantly, irrespective of the initial ICP.

In this swine model, atracurium or vecuronium did not affect ICP or hemodynamics, even in the presence of an increased ICP. In contrast, suxamethoniun produced a decrease in blood pressure coupled with an increase in ICP, resulting in a decrease in CCP. The latter, although not large, may compromise cerebral blood flow in the presence of increased ICP, when the ICP is already marginal. Atracurium and vecuronium may be preferred over suxamethonium in patients with known or suspected intracranial hypertension or marginal CCP.

▶ This study emphasizes the ongoing controversy as to whether succinylcholine should be given to patients with an elevated ICP. The readers will have to decide for themselves whether this transient change of ICP with succinylcholine is of clinical significance.—R.D. Miller, M.D.

Effectiveness of the Kinetic Treatment Table for Preventing and Treating Pulmonary Complications in Severely Head-Injured Patients
Clemmer TP, Green S, Ziegler B, Wallace CJ, Menlove R, Orme JF Jr, Thomas F, Tocino I, Crapo RO (Univ of Utah)
Crit Care Med 18:614–617, 1990   6–6

The Kinetic Treatment Table (KTT) can continuously turn a head-injured patient from side to side up to 72 degrees in each direction. To learn whether the early use of the KTT can prevent pulmonary complications or hasten their resolution in the first 10 days after severe head injury, 49 patients were randomized into a prospective study, 23 of whom were treated on the KTT. The 2 groups had comparably severe head injuries.

There were no significant group differences in mortality, CNS morbidity, or length of stay in the intensive care unit or hospital. Rates of pulmonary improvement also were similar in patients treated on the KTT and those treated conventionally. The efficacy of the KTT remains unproved. A larger multicenter study may be able to demonstrate the value of this treatment.

▶ I was sorry to see the results of this study, because I've recommended the kinetic bed since 1976. However, these devices are almost prohibitively expensive, whether purchased or leased, and if they are not effective, we and our patients should be aware of this fact.—R.R. Kirby, M.D.

Remote Places

Panic Attacks During MR Imaging: Treatment With IV Diazepam
Avrahami E (Tel-Aviv Med Ctr, Israel)
AJNR 11:833–835, 1990

6–7

Panic attacks may occur during the course of magnetic resonance (MR) examinations. During a 2-year period, among 3,000 patients aged 19–56 years who underwent MR imaging, 46 (1.5%) had panic attacks. The panic attacks developed within 5–15 minutes after the start of the examination and prevented its continuation. The most common symptoms were fear, hot and cold flashes, palpitations, chest pain, faintness, and vertigo. The panic attack was unexpected in most patients, and 39 experienced it for the first time.

An intravenous bolus injection of diazepam, 7–10 mg, was given. All 46 patients recovered rapidly, became asymptomatic, and were able to complete the examination. Despite high blood levels of diazepam, somnolence, slow reactions, overrelaxation, and breathing difficulties were not observed. The patients agreed to have repeat MR examinations under the same conditions.

Panic attacks occur when there is an abnormal balance between excitation and inhibition of the locus ceruleus. The high blood level of diazepam probably can influence the polysynaptic connections between the locus ceruleus and higher structures on the brain, blocking the pathologic circle that causes panic attacks.

▶ This is another journal that anesthesiologists are unlikely to read. However, anesthesia in remote place (e.g., radiology) often requires the use of a skillful anesthesiologist. Patients who are claustrophobic may have trouble with the various imaging techniques that are now available.—R.D. Miller, M.D.

Ambulatory

Unanticipated Admission to the Hospital Following Ambulatory Surgery
Gold BS, Kitz DS, Lecky JH, Neuhaus JM (Univ of Pennsylvania; Univ of California, San Francisco)
JAMA 262:3008–3010, 1989

6–8

An increasing amount of surgery is done in the ambulatory setting, and unexpected hospital admission has become an important measure of outcome. A case-control study was conducted among 9,616 adults having ambulatory surgery at a university-affiliated hospital in 1984–1986. Ninety-eight patients were admitted 100 times; 1 patient with coagulopathy was admitted after 3 different laparoscopies.

Procedures that lasted for more than 1 hour were associated with a nearly fourfold increase in the risk of admission. Postoperative vomiting and residence more than an hour's drive away were other risk factors for admission. Age was not closely associated with admission after ambulatory surgery. American Society of Anesthesiologists' physical status was not a significant factor when adjusted for age. Patients having such medical problems as asthma, hypertension, or diabetes were not more likely than others to be admitted after surgery. On multivariate analysis, independent risk factors for admission included general anesthesia, emesis, abdominal surgery, a lengthy procedure, and age. It is hoped that these findings will help to better select patients for ambulatory surgery.

▶ Clearly, an unanticipated admission defeats the entire purpose of an ambulatory surgery setting. Studies such as this will allow us to predict preoperatively which patients are more likely to need an unanticipated admission and should perhaps be treated in a formal hospital setting.—R.D. Miller, M.D.

Delayed Side Effects of Droperidol After Ambulatory General Anesthesia
Melnick B, Sawyer R, Karambelkar D, Phitayakorn P, Lim Uy NT, Patel R (Presbyterian-Univ Hosp, Pittsburgh)
Anesth Analg 69:748–751, 1989   6–9

When given immediately before anesthesia induction in outpatient surgical procedures, droperidol can prevent postoperative nausea and vom-

TABLE 1.—Times to Discharge and Number of Patients With
Nausea, Vomiting, or Pain Before Discharge

	Group 1 (1.25 mg droperidol)	Group 2 (no droperidol)
Number	50	50
Time to discharge (min)	129.8 ± 29.4	139.4 ± 38.2
Number of patients with nausea (%)	4 (8%)	7 (14%)
Number of patients with vomiting (%)	1 (2%)	3 (6%)
Number of patients with pain (%)	16 (32%)	16 (32%)

(Courtesy of Melnick B, Sawyer R, Karambelkar D, et al: *Anesth Analg* 69:748–751, 1989.)

TABLE 2.—Number of Patients With Nausea, Vomiting, or Pain After Discharge

	Group 1 (1.25 mg droperidol)	Group 2 (no droperidol)
Number	43	46
Number of patients with nausea (%)	2 (4.7%)	4 (8.7%)
Number of patients with vomiting (%)	2 (4.7%)	3 (6.5%)
Number of patients with pain (%)	12 (27.9%)	13 (28.3%)

(Courtesy of Melnick B, Sawyer R, Karambelkar D, et al: *Anesth Analg* 69:748–751, 1989.)

iting and significantly shorten the time to discharge. However, low-dose droperidol has been suggested as a cause of extrapyramidal reactions occurring after discharge from the ambulatory care unit. Routine postoperative follow-up phone calls to outpatients also revealed that many of those who received droperidol experienced anxiety or restlessness the night after operation. A study was conducted to investigate the incidence of postoperative side effects of droperidol after its use in outpatient surgery.

Of 100 women undergoing minor gynecologic procedures, 50 were given droperidol, 1.25 mg intravenously, immediately before induction of anesthesia, and 50 were given normal saline solution, .5 mL. Patients were evaluated every 15 minutes in the recovery room for pain, nausea, and vomiting, and were discharged home when deemed appropriate by the attending anesthesiologist. All patients were contacted by telephone

TABLE 3.—Number of Patients With Anxiety, Restlessness, or Unusual Physical Sensations After Discharge

	Group 1 (1.25 mg droperidol)	Group 2 (no droperidol)
Number	43	46
Number of patients with anxiety (%)	10 (23.2%)[a]	0 (0%)
Number of patients with restlessness (%)	3 (7.8%)	0 (0%)
Number of patients with unusual physical sensations (%)	0 (0%)	0 (0%)
Total number of patients with above conditions (%)	10 (23.2%)[a]	0 (0%)

*P < .05.
(Courtesy of Melnick B, Sawyer R, Karambelkar D, et al: *Anesth Analg* 69:748–751, 1989.)

within 24–36 hours after discharge and asked about any unusual physical sensations.

There was no significant difference between the 2 groups with respect to time until discharge, postoperative nausea, vomiting, or pain before discharge (Table 1). The administration of droperidol at anesthesia induction did not decrease the incidence of nausea or vomiting before discharge. Evaluable follow-up data were available for 43 droperidol-treated patients and 46 placebo-treated patients. Telephone follow-up revealed that 2 patients in the droperidol-treated group and 3 in the placebo-treated group vomited after discharge (Table 2). The difference was statistically not significant. Ten patients (23%) who received droperidol, but none of the placebo-treated patients, reported anxiety or extrapyramidal reactions after discharge from the ambulatory care unit (Table 3).

The use of droperidol as a prophylactic antiemetic for minor gynecologic procedures performed in an outpatient surgical care unit may cause side effects after discharge. The routine use of droperidol in all outpatient anesthetics may therefore not be appropriate.

▶ Clearly, droperidol is not the ideal agent to be given prophylactically against nausea and vomiting. When used in the study by Harper et al. (1), a number of patients expressed dysphoria so severe that they would not come back to have a second "volunteer" study done. It isn't clear why patients in whom tracheal intubation was deemed necessary were omitted from this study. Are they a different group? Or would these same adverse effects of droperidol occur in such patients with very little benefit? Patients in this series had a very low incidence of nausea and vomiting after minor gynecologic outpatient procedures compared to those generally reported in the literature. Thus this study found no benefit for droperidol. Patients didn't leave earlier and didn't have a lower incidence of nausea and vomiting, and there was a significant side effect. Is this lack of benefit of droperidol limited to this study and not generalizable? If so, why is droperidol use so common.—M.F. Roizen, M.D.

Reference

1. Harper MH, et al: *J Pharmacol Exp Ther* 199:464, 1976.

An Evaluation of Tests of Psychomotor Function in Assessing Recovery Following a Brief Anaesthetic

Cashman JN, Power SJ (Guy's Hosp, London)
Acta Anaesthesiol Scand 33:693–697, 1989   6–10

Minor surgery is being performed increasingly in an outpatient setting. Anesthesia for this type of surgery requires that patients recovery rapidly and return to "street fitness," defined as the aptitude for real life skills. A variety of psychomotor function tests are commonly used before discharge to assess the patient's recovery from anesthesia. To determine the usefulness of 4 commonly used tests, results in 26 women who underwent minor gynecologic procedures in an outpatient facility were evaluated.

The 3 psychomotor tests were the letter cancellation test, the critical flicker fusion test, and a test of simple reaction time. A picture recall test was used to assess return of short-term memory. Patients were randomly allocated to receive premedication with zolpidem, either 5 mg or 20 mg or placebo, administered orally 60 minutes before operation. Anesthesia was induced with either thiopental or methohexital and was maintained with nitrous oxide in oxygen and halothane. The duration of anesthesia was 15 minutes or less. The 3 groups were comparable for age, weight, and baseline values for any of the tests used.

Immediate recovery was fastest in women premedicated with placebo, as indicated by the most rapid wake-up time. All 4 tests showed a similar pattern of recovery in the 3 groups, with an initially large impairment of psychomotor function that gradually decreased over the course of the study. The test of simple reaction time and the picture recall test were both capable of differentiating between the postanesthetic recovery of the highdose group and that of the other 2 groups. The letter cancellation test and the critical flicker fusion test were both too unreliable to be of use in clinical decision making.

Neither picture recall nor simple reaction time had returned to baseline by the end of the study period, even though in simple reaction time the placebo group was close; yet, all patients were deemed fit for discharge on clinical grounds. Strictly speaking, the residual impairment on psychomotor testing suggests that the patients had not fully recovered, but patients in this outpatient facility are usually discharged from 3 hours after completion of surgery. These tests seem to be more sensitive than clinical assessment and should be further evaluated for their use as indicators of fitness for discharge.

▶ Does street fitness correlate with psychomotor recovery? This study doesn't demonstrate that because, despite the differences in reaction time, recall, and so on, all patients were deemed fit for discharge on clinical grounds. Like all good studies, this one leaves us with more questions than it answers. We are left wondering if recovery of psychomotor function correlates with some form of "street fitness." Or, in fact, what is it that most of us term "street fitness," and is there any hope of replacing the judgment of "street fitness" with psychomotor tests of recovery? I think the answers to 2 of these questions will prove to be yes; this study only frames the questions better for us.—M.F. Roizen, M.D.

Cardiac

Effect of Combined Infusion of Nitroglycerin and Nicardipine on Femoral-to-Radial Arterial Pressure Gradient After Cardiopulmonary Bypass

Maruyama K, Horiguchi R, Hashimoto H, Ohi Y, Okuda M, Kurioka T, Konishi K, Muneyuki M, Kusagawa M (Mie Univ, Mie, Japan; Matsusaka Central Gen Hosp, Mie)

Anesth Analg 70:428–432, 1990   6–11

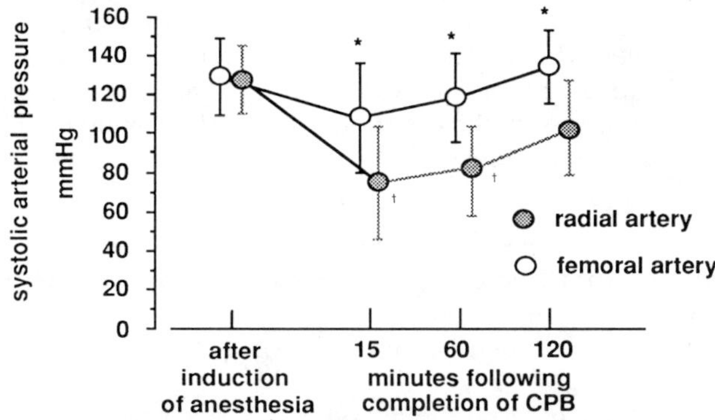

Fig 6–1.—Time-course of changes of systolic arterial pressure in both femoral artery and radial artery in patients with nitroglycerin and nicardipine. In femoral systolic arterial pressure, there was no change throughout study. In radial systolic arterial pressure values at 15 and 60 minutes after completion of CPB were significantly lower than baseline value (repeated-measures analysis of variance followed by Bonferroni *t*-test). There was no difference between femoral and radial arteries in values of systolic arterial pressure after induction of anesthesia. Significant pressure difference between femoral and radial arteries was observed in systolic values at 15, 60, and 120 minutes after completion of CPB. Radial and femoral arterial pressures were compared at each time point using Student's *t*-test, number = 14. Values are mean ± SD. *Significantly different from value of radial artery at same time point ($P < .05$). †Significantly different from baseline value ($P < .05$). (Courtesy of Maruyama K, Horiguchi R, Hashimoto H, et al: *Anesth Analg* 70:428–432, 1990.)

Nitrates and calcium channel blockers are often used during cardiac surgery. Femoral arterial pressure and radial arterial pressure were measured simultaneously to determine whether nitrates combined with calcium channel blockers influence the central-to-peripheral arterial pressure gradient. In 30 adults who were undergoing cardiac surgery the femoral-to-radial arterial pressure gradient was compared in those with and without administration of nitroglycerin and nicardipine; in 14 patients the intraoperative time-course of femoral and radial arterial pressures with nitroglycerin and nicardipine was studied.

Combined nitroglycerin and nicardipine infusion during cardiac surgery that involved coronary artery bypass grafting or valve replacement produced significant increases above baseline in the femoral-to-radial arterial pressure gradient at 60 minutes are cardiopulmonary bypass (CPB). There was no such increase in control patients. The difference in systolic arterial pressure between femoral and radial arteries was seen 15, 60, and 120 minutes after CPB was completed. There was no difference in the mean arterial pressure between femoral and radial arteries throughout the same period (Fig 6–1).

The combined infusion of nitroglycerin and nicardipine intensifies the magnitude and duration of the femoral-to-radial arterial pressure gradient after CPB, at least in chronic users of these drugs. The significant differences between systolic arterial pressures in the femoral and radial arteries were noted at 15, 60, and 120 minutes after bypass.

▶ As the authors mention, failure to recognize that systolic blood pressure as transduced from the radial artery may underestimate central aortic pressure following hypothermic CPB may result in unnecessary administration of vasopressors and/or inotropes. The presumed explanation for this pressure gradient discrepancy is a decrease in peripheral vascular resistance. It is predictable that known vasodilating drugs (nitroglycerin, nitroprusside, isoflurane) might accentuate this gradient.—R.K. Stoelting, M.D.

Cyanide Release From Sodium Nitroprusside During Coronary Bypass in Hypothermia
Lundquist P, Rosling H, Tydén H (Linköping Univ; Univ Hosp, Uppsala, Sweden)
Acta Anaesthesiol Scand 33:686–688, 1989   6–12

There is a risk of cyanide intoxication from sodium nitroprusside (SNP) infusion in patients undergoing open-heart surgery. Simultaneous infusion of SNP and sodium thiosulfate used as an antidote to increase sulfur availability, and thus enzymatic conversion to the far less toxic substance thiocyanate, is recommended by some practitioners. Hypothermia is often used in conjunction with SNP infusion during cardiac bypass operation, but the influence of low body temperature on the release and conversion of cyanide from SNP is not known. Erythrocyte cyanide levels were measured during SNP infusion with and without sodium thiosulfate administered simultaneously during hypothermic cardiopulmonary bypass (CPB) operations.

Of 18 patients undergoing CPB, 9 aged 39–72 years were given plain SNP infusions and 9 aged 48–68 years received SNP plus sodium thiosulfate. Erythrocyte cyanide levels were measured before SNP infusion, before the start of hypothermia, at the end of hypothermia before rewarming, and at the end of the operation. A sensitive fluorimetric method was used to measure the erythrocyte cyanide levels.

The infusion rates of SNP needed to control blood pressure were well below those for which sodium thiosulfate infusion is recommended. At the start of operation, the mean erythrocyte cyanide concentration was .20 μmol/L. In the periods before and after hypothermia, erythrocyte cyanide levels increased slowly but significantly with the infusion rate (Fig 6–2). However, cyanide levels remained well below the levels of 150 μmol/L at which toxic symptoms have been observed. Cyanide levels in 2 of 9 patients receiving SNP alone rose to 8 μmol/L during hypothermia despite the low SNP infusion rates.

The increase in erythrocyte cyanide levels during hypothermia suggests that SNP is also broken down to cyanide under hypothermic conditions, and that cyanide conversion is reduced at low body temperatures. The high cyanide levels found in 2 patients not receiving thiosulfate with the SNP infusion suggests that this antidote should be routinely given with SNP infusion during hypothermic CPB, even when low SNP infusion rates are planned.

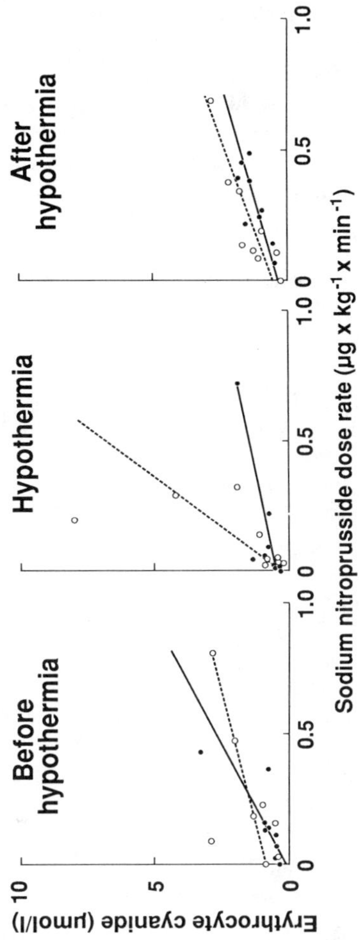

Fig 6–2.—Erythrocyte cyanide in μmol/L at the end of each period of the operation in relation to the infusion rate of SNP in μg × kg⁻¹ × min⁻¹ during preceding period of the operation in cases with *(filled circles)* and without *(open circles)* thiosulfate with corresponding regression lines *(solid lines)* and *(dashed lines)*, respectively. (Courtesy of Lundquist P, Rosling H, Tydén H: *Acta Anaesthesiol Scand* 33:686–688, 1989.)

▶ I do not believe that these data are sufficiently compelling to justify a recommendation that thiosulfate be routinely infused when nitroprusside is administered during hypothermic CPB. Perhaps the value of this article is to alert the clinician to the fact that hypothermia may, in some patients, be associated with unexpected increases in mean erythrocyte cyanide concentrations. Nitroglycerin is an obvious alternative when a vasodilator is required in these patients for prolonged periods. If nothing else, this approach would substitute the remote risk of methemoglobinemia for an equally unlikely occurrence of cyanide toxicity.—R.K. Stoelting, M.D.

Does Cardiopulmonary Bypass Alter Enflurane Requirements for Anesthesia?

Hall RI, Sullivan JA (Victoria Gen Hosp, Halifax, NS)
Anesthesiology 73:249–255, 1990
6–13

The anesthetic level is frequently lowered before the patient is separated from cardiopulmonary bypass (CPB) to reduce the degree of myocardial depression and ease the separation. In a canine study, whether normothermic CPB alone reduces the requirements for enflurane anesthesia was investigated. The null hypothesis was that there were no changes in anesthetic drug requirements after CPB.

Sixteen male dogs were anesthetized with enflurane in oxygen. Cardiopulmonary bypass was initiated in the animals using aortoatrial (group 1) or femoral artery-vein (group 2) cannulation, or none (group 3, control). The minimum alveolar concentration (MAC) was determined by the tail-clamp method before and after CPB.

In group 1 a mean reduction in enflurane MAC of 30% was observed, but the range of reduction was wide. The mean MAC reduction produced by CPB in group 2, about 20%, did not differ statistically from that achieved in group 1, but there was much less variability about the mean. In the control group, the MAC did not differ from the initial value obtained when measured repeatedly over 9 hours.

The degree of variability in groups 1 and 2 did not appear to be explained by hemodynamic differences between the 2 groups. No anesthetic agents other than enflurane were used; thus the influence of other CNS depressants on MAC reduction was eliminated. The reduction in enflurane MAC might then be related to physical factors, but those explanations appear unlikely. Cardiopulmonary bypass itself, therefore, must be responsible for some of the alteration in enflurane requirements.

Because of the wide variability in the reduction of enflurane requirements and lack of knowledge of the mechanism whereby CPB reduces those requirements, the findings cannot be readily applied to humans. A cautious approach to the supplementation of anesthesia during CPB is advisable.

▶ I have often speculated that decreased anesthetic requirements following hypothermic CPB reflect differential rates of rewarming in the brain. These data suggest that normothermic CPB is sufficient to produce a detectable decrease. Perhaps the next step is to determine the additional impact of hypothermia. It is certainly my clinical impression that the decrease in anesthetic requirements after hypothermic CPB is greater than the 19.8% to 30.1% measured in these animals.—R.K. Stoelting, M.D.

Effect of Angiotensin Converting Enzyme Inhibition on Blood Pressure and Renal Function During Open Heart Surgery

Colson P, Ribstein J, Mimran A, Grolleau D, Chaptal PA, Roquefeuil B (Centre Hospitalier Univ, Montpellier, France)
Anesthesiology 72:23–27, 1990   6–14

Renal dysfunction is common after open-heart surgery. Marked activation of the renin-angiotensin system has been observed during cardiopulmonary bypass (CPB), but whether it is beneficial in sustaining blood pressure or deleterious by compromising renal hemodynamics is not clear. In a randomized, double-blind, placebo-controlled trial, the effect of pretreatment with the angiotensin converting-enzyme inhibitor captopril on blood pressure and renal function was evaluated in 18 patients undergoing coronary artery bypass surgery. Patients received either captopril, 100 mg twice a day, or placebo, 2 days before surgery, with the last dose given just about 2 hours before surgery. All patients had no pre-existing cardiac or renal failure.

During CPB, blood pressure and fluid requirements did not differ significantly between captopril- and placebo-treated patients. Effective renal plasma flow and the glomerular filtration rate remained stable in captopril-treated patients but decreased in patients receiving placebo; the difference was significant. Urinary sodium excretion was significantly higher in the group given captopril than in controls. Plasma renin activity increased in the captopril-treated group but remained unchanged in those given placebo group.

Pretreatment with captopril does not impair blood pressure control and attenuates the transient renal dysfunction associated with the CPB in normotensive patients without heart failure. The protective effect of angiotensin-converting enzyme inhibitors in patients at high risk of cardiac surgery-associated renal failure should be evaluated.

▶ These data are encouraging, but it is equally important to recognize that a multitude of factors may be present or interact to cause renal dysfunction following CPB. To treat every patient prophylactically with captopril is clearly not justified on the basis of these data, nor did the authors make such a recommendation.—R.K. Stoelting, M.D.

Determinants of Pulmonary Function in Patients Undergoing Coronary Bypass Operations
Shapira N, Zabatino SM, Ahmed S, Murphy DMF, Sullivan D, Lemole GM (Med Ctr of Delaware, Wilmington; Deborah Heart and Lung Ctr, Browns Mills, NJ; Georgetown Univ)
Ann Thorac Surg 50:268–273, 1990   6–15

The effect of median sternotomy on pulmonary function during coronary revascularization was investigated in 29 generally healthy men aged 42–71 years. Pulmonary function was assessed at discharge an average of 9 days postoperatively and again after 3 months. The peak expiratory flow rate was measured just after extubation. Most patients had internal mammary artery dissection.

All patients recovered uneventfully, and there were no serious pulmonary complications. Most, however, had roentgenographic findings of segmental or subsegmental atelectasis. Abnormalities persisted at the time of discharge in 16 patients, 14 of whom were smokers, but resolved within 3 months postoperatively. The peak expiratory flow rate was reduced by 65% at the time of extubation. Lung volumes were 19% to 33% less than baseline at discharge.

Median sternotomy is associated with significant but short-lived pulmonary dysfunction. Internal mammary artery dissection correlated with more marked changes in function in the present patients. Serious complications could develop in patients with compromised or marginal pulmonary reserve because of preexisting obstructive or restrictive lung disease. It is especially important to minimize chest wall traction and rib trauma in these patients or to avoid internal mammary artery dissection.

▶ Median sternotomy in the absence of skeletal muscle trauma or rib fractures would seem unlikely to limit breathing in a manner that impaired oxygenation and ventilation. In fact, many patients following coronary artery bypass graft operations complain more of pain at the vein harvest site than at the site of the chest incision.—R.K. Stoelting, M.D.

A Comparison of Washed Red Blood Cells Versus Packed Red Blood Cells (AS-1) for Cardiopulmonary Bypass Prime and Their Effects on Blood Glucose Concentration in Children
Hosking MP, Beynen FM, Raimundo HS, Oliver WC Jr, Williamson KR (Mayo Clinic and Found, Rochester, Minn)
Anesthesiology 72:987–990, 1990   6–16

A high blood glucose level may relate to adverse outcomes after cerebral ischemia, possibly because hyperglycemia in brain tissue can promote intracellular lactic acid accumulation, acidosis, the depletion of high-energy phosphates, and structural damage. Removal of glucose-containing solutions just before surgery does not prevent a rise in the blood glucose concentration during cardiopulmonary bypass (CPB).

The effects of packed red blood cells and washed red blood cells on blood glucose, when used as CPB prime, were compared in 20 small infants who required cardiac surgery. The infants, all weighing less than 10 kg, were anesthetized with nitrous oxide/oxygen/isoflurane/fentanyl and received Ringer's lactate before bypass.

Blood glucose levels were significantly higher in infants given packed red blood cells than in those given washed cells at all times after the start of CPB (Fig 6–3). Infants given washed red blood cells had glucose concentrations less than half those of the other infants 10 minutes after the start of bypass, before separation from bypass, and after protamine ad-

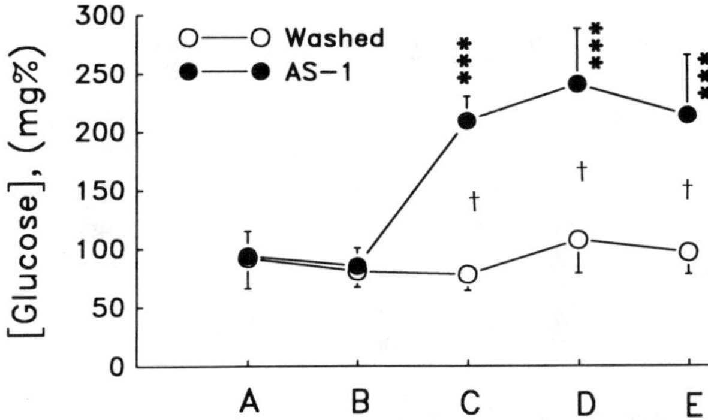

Fig 6–3.—Blood glucose concentrations (mean ± SD) at different stages of anesthesia in the washed red blood cell group *(open circles)* and AS=1 *(filled circles)* group. ***P < .001 (Student's paired *t* test between **B, C, D, E,** and **A,** respectively. †*P* < .001 (Student's *t* test between washed red blood cells and AS=1 groups). **(A)** After start of anesthesia; **(B)** before bypass, **(C)** 10 minutes after start of bypass; **(D)** before discontinuation of bypass; **(E)** after protamine administration. (Courtesy of Hosking MP, Beynen FM, Raimundo HS, et al: *Anesthesiology* 72:987–990, 1990.)

ministration. The use of a washed red blood cell CPB prime significantly lessens the rise in blood glucose that otherwise occurs during CPB.

▶ The authors sought to find out if washing red blood cells before using them for CPB prime would decrease glucose levels. They found that they did. Does this mean we should all go through the extra expense and risk of mismatching and introducing infections to gain the benefit of a lower glucose concentration in children? I think the key question is, "Is there a real correlation between the blood glucose concentration and outcome following neonatal cardiac surgery or neonatal surgery in general?" Clearly, neuropsychiatric complications can follow CPB, are common in children undergoing congenital heart disease repairs, and are hard to detect in this age group. Do we need a randomized outcome study before we accept this increased expense? I don't think we have the answer, and clearly there is a downside to washing the red blood cells—not only the risk of infection and the extra expense, but also the chance of causing hypoglycemia. I don't believe that the data are in yet to establish a guideline, but perhaps this approach is an option that we should consider.—M.F. Roizen, M.D.

Surgical Technique and Operative Mortality in Coronary Artery Bypass: A Postmortem Analysis With Castangiography

Järvinen A, Männikö A, Ketonen P, Segerberg-Konttinen M, Luosto R (Helsinki Univ Central Hosp; Helsinki Univ; Natl Board of Health, Helsinki)
Scand J Thorac Cardiovasc Surg 23:103–109, 1989   6–17

In a series of 1,614 patients undergoing coronary bypass surgery in 1981–1986, the operative mortality was 4%. Postmortem coronary angiography was conducted in 40 men and 14 women (mean age, 55 years). All but 3 patients had triple-vessel coronary artery disease.

Causes of 54 Perioperative Deaths and Incidence of Fresh
Myocardial Infarction

Time of death	n	Cause of death	n	Myocardial infarction
In operating room	25	Myocardial failure Aortic dissection	24 1	6/25 (25%)
Postoperatively ≤7 days	25	Myocardial failure Cerebral damage Pulmonary embolism	21 3 1	21/25 (84%)
8–30 days	4	Myocardial failure Cerebral damage Septicaemia	1 2 1	2/4 (50%)
Total	54		54	29/54 (54%)

(Courtesy of Järvinen A, Männikö A, Ketonen P, et al: *Scand J Thorac Cardiovasc Surg* 23:103–109, 1989.)

Myocardial infarction was present preoperatively in 4 cases and developed perioperatively in 25 (table). Of 215 coronary anastomoses (averaging 4 per patient), 24% were nonfunctioning. Most occlusions were ascribed to technical failure. One fourth of the sequential vein grafts were occluded. Only 15 patients (28%) had complete revascularization, with all stenosed coronary vessels bypassed and all grafts patent. Two of these 15 patients had emergency surgery.

Patient-related risk factors were present in most of the group. The rate of failure was especially high for sequential vein grafts. Myocardial failure was the most prevalent form of operative mortality. If myocardial ischemia is evident shortly after surgery, incomplete revascularization should be suspected and investigated aggressively. Technical failures are a prominent cause of failed coronary bypass surgery.

▶ Of interest, one always relates failure after myocardial revascularization to risk factors such as congestive heart failure, advanced age, emergency operation, female gender, and abnormal ECG preoperatively. Although these factors are contributory, in more than 90% of the patients who did in the early postoperative period, mortality was attributable to technical factors. Thus the common practice of attributing a poor outcome of preexisting (nontechnical) patient risk may not be valid, except when patient risk may make technical revascularization more difficult. Seventy-two percent of these patients had occluded grafts; 10 of the other 15 cases (28%) had myocardial failure in the operating room, suggesting technical problems. Of the other 5 patients, 1 had septicemia, 1 had a pulmonary embolus, and 1 had aortic dissection; 2 others underwent emergency revascularization, in 1 because of failed percutaneous transluminal coronary angioplasty and 1 because of myocardial failure probably resulting from a preoperative infarction. Thus less than 10% of the cases represented patient factors other than those that contributed to the poor technical outcome.

One of the interesting things about this study is relating it to the American experience. The United States spends a lot more on health care costs as a percent of the gross national product than does Finland. One wonders if it is of any benefit. One can take this study and argue that it might be. The death rate was 4% within 30 days in patients whose average age was 55. In the American experience the death rate is about 4.2% in patients aged 65 and older, i.e., an average age, according to Medicare statistics, of approximately 70 years. One would expect that our death rate would be less in patients who are age 55, but that is obviously taking these data too far and speculating. Unfortunately, the authors don't provide us with denominators in their total hospital patient population, so we don't know how sick their patients were in general. But the authors are to be congratulated; at no point in the article do these surgeons blame either the cardiologist for not telling them about the anatomy, nor the anesthesiologist for not maintaining appropriate blood pressure, heart rate, and so on.

The implications of this study are patent; we may in the future confirm graft patency during the operative period before closing the chest and ensure the presence (or absence) of technical factors. Contrast ultrasound offers promise that anesthesiologists will be able to do this in the next 3 years (1).—M.F. Roizen, M.D.

Reference

1. Aronson S, et al: *Anesthesiology* 72:295, 1990.

An Evaluation of the Perioperative Efficacy of Selective β_1-Blockade in Coronary Surgery: Studies With a Late Preoperative Dose of Metoprolol
Wesslén O, Ekroth R, Nyström S-O (Univ Hosp, Uppsala, Sweden)
Scand J Thorac Cardiovasc Surg 23:151–154, 1989   6–18

Long-term β-adrenoceptor blockade now is maintained into the late preoperative period rather than being withdrawn before surgery. Plasma metoprolol levels were measured hourly after oral administration in 9 patients with angina to determine the extent blockade is maintained after a last dose given at 6 AM on the day of coronary artery surgery. All patients had received metoprolol for 6 months or longer in doses of 25–100 mg twice daily.

All patients had an uneventful perioperative course and required no inotropic support. The average time on extracorporeal circulation was 99 minutes and the average aortic cross-clamp time was 53 minutes. The course of the plasma metoprolol concentration is shown in Figure 6–4). The heart rate peaked above 130 beats per minute on the day of surgery and correlated inversely with the plasma metoprolol level.

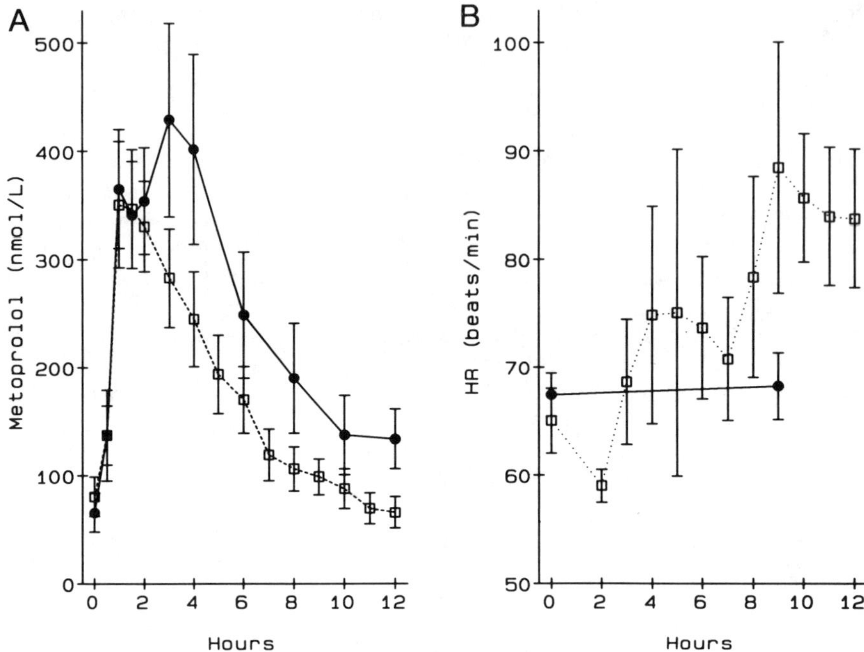

Fig 6–4.—**A,** metoprolol concentrations (means ± SEM) in 9 patients during 12 hours after a per-oral dose of metoprolol on the day before *(circles)* and the day of *(squares)* coronary surgery. **B,** heart rate (means ± SEM) in the same 9 patients. (Courtesy of Wesslén O, Ekroth R, Nyström S-O: *Scand J Thorac Cardiovasc Surg* 23:151–154, 1989.)

Inadequate β–blockade is maintained after a late preoperative oral administration of metoprolol. Apparently, a plasma level that provides full therapeutic effect in other circumstances will be insufficient in the operative setting.

▶ One wonders why physicians don't just go to propranolol infusion when the heart rate increases. Why was there not a propranolol infusion group in this study? I suppose differences in different countries make things more likely. Perhaps this should have been a clonidine patch ala John Ellis. This seems to keep the heart rate down, which may be a major determinant of myocardial ischemia postoperatively. The high incidence of myocardial infarctions says that perhaps these patients weren't completely revascularized. Another factor missing in this study was the absence of commentary about the sedation of the patients postoperatively. Clearly, if one keeps patients sedated, high heart rates might be avoided. Further, although the heart rate peaked at a little over 90, and 1 patient had a heart rate of 130 postoperatively, we aren't told whether the myocardial infarctions occurred in the patients who had high heart rates.—M.F. Roizen, M.D.

Preoperative Plasmapheresis in Patients Undergoing Cardiac Surgery Procedures
Boldt J, von Bormann B, Kling D, Jacobi M, Moosdorf R, Hempelmann G (Justus-Liebig Univ, Giessen, Germany)
Anesthesiology 72:282–288, 1990
6–19

In orthopedic patients, donor plasmapheresis has limited the need for homologous blood and helped to preserve coagulative function. Forty-five patients scheduled for aortocoronary bypass surgery were assigned to undergo plasmapheresis acutely preoperatively, harvesting either autologous platelet-poor plasma (PPP) or platelet-rich plasma (PRP) in a volume of 10 mL/kg. Plasmapheresis began after induction of anesthesia, and the plasma removed was replaced by low-molecular-weight hydroxyethylstarch solution. All patients were heparinized before the start of extracorporeal circulation.

Blood loss on the first postoperative day was significantly greater in the control patients, 2 of whom required red blood cell transfusion. No patients having plasmapheresis were given donor blood or blood products. Changes in laboratory parameters are compared in Figure 6–5. Pulmonary gas exchange was comparable in all groups (table). Platelet-poor plasma and PRP differed only with respect to numbers of platelets, which were greater in the PRP group than in the other groups. Polymorphonuclear leukocyte elastase content increased least in PRP patients and most in controls.

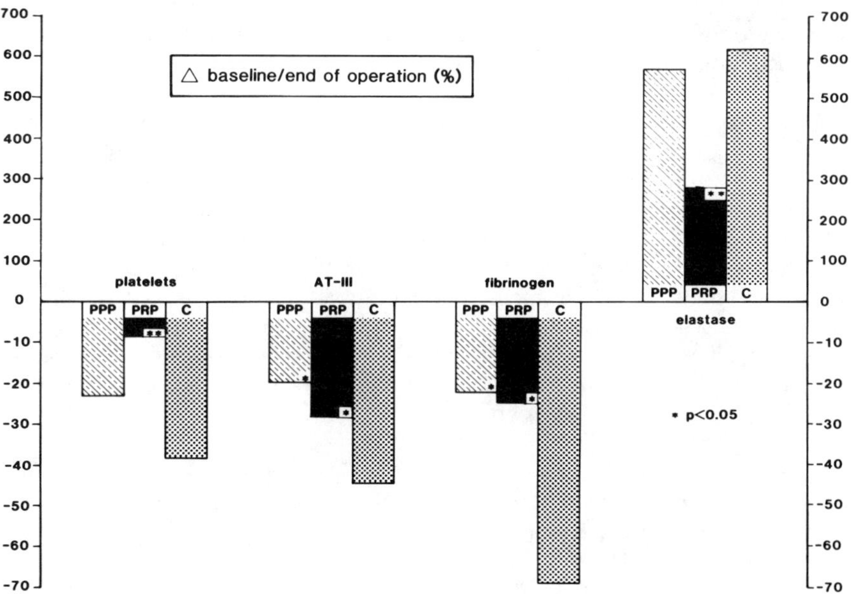

Fig 6–5.—Changes (Δ%) in laboratory variables from the end of the operation to baseline values. *P < .05 vs. control. **P < .05, *versus* **PPP** and control. (Courtesy of Boldt J, von Bormann B, Kling D, et al: *Anesthesiology* 72:282–288, 1990.)

Demographic Data, Data From Preoperative Catheterization, Extracorporeal Circulation, and Postoperative Intensive Care

	PPP	PRP	Control
Age (yr)	62.8 ± 5.1	59.0 ± 3.3	63.7 ± 4.4
Height (cm)	171.2 ± 4.8	168 ± 6.6	175 ± 5.5
Weight (kg)	77.0 ± 5.9	78.7 ± 5.9	72.0 ± 6.1
LVEF (%)	62.3 ± 5.5	62.5 ± 3.6	69.5 ± 4.4
LVEDP (mmHg)	16.4 ± 3.3	14.6 ± 4.4	13.4 ± 6.6
ECC (min)	79.5 ± 12	78.6 ± 4.5	83.5 ± 17.0
Ischemia (min)	46.6 ± 4.8	42.9 ± 4.4	53.5 ± 16.4
Cardioplegia (ml)	1,450 ± 140	1,500 ± 180	1,340 ± 300
Discarded volume at ECC (ml)	845 ± 120	920 ± 140	930 ± 120
Fluid balance after ECC (ml)	812 ± 244	800 ± 210	918 ± 200
Extubation (min)	795 ± 213	790 ± 230	788 ± 202
Maximum temperature (° C)			
Day of operation	37.7 ± 0.8	37.2 ± 0.4	38.2 ± 0.4
First postoperative day	37.5 ± 1.0	37.4 ± 0.4	38.1 ± 0.6
Blood loss (ml)			
Day of operation	298 ± 130	348 ± 170	498 ± 100
First postoperative day	543 ± 230*	500 ± 210*	696 ± 130
Donor blood (patients/units)	0/0	0/0	2/2

Values are mean ± SD.
*$P < .05$ vs. control group.
(Courtesy of Boldt J, von Bormann B, Kling D, et al: *Anesthesiology* 72:282–288, 1990.)

Plasmapheresis, done acutely in conjunction with cardiac surgery, may reduce the need for donor blood and improve coagulation management even in patients with lowered hemoglobin levels. Collection of autologous PRP may be especially helpful.

▶ This well-done study shows that there is decreased blood loss in patients who undergo cardiac surgery procedures in which removal of platelet rich plasma is accomplished right at the start of the operation. The value of this may not be just in giving the platelets back, but in not having the platelets damaged during ECC. While the blood loss is significantly reduced, the blood loss in this operation is so minor that not many patients, in fact only two patients, received any transfusion, and those received a total of two units, not significantly different between groups. Thus, whether the risk of platelet pheresis is worth the benefit is not yet clear in my mind, but I believe that this technique may be better than it's made out to be because of the lack of damaging microthrombi produced by ECC.—M.F. Roizen, M.D.

A Randomized Study of Carbon Dioxide Management During Hypothermic Cardiopulmonary Bypass

Bashein G, Townes BD, Nessly ML, Bledsoe SW, Hornbein TF, Davis KB, Goldstein DE, Coppel DB (Univ of Washington)
Anesthesiology 72:7–15, 1990

6–20

There are 2 approaches to the optimal management of blood gas during delibrate hypothermia. The methods were compared to determine whether the known physiologic responses to CO_2 management during cardiopulmonary bypass (CPB) with moderate hypothermia affect the cerebral or cardiac outcome of patients.

Investigators randomly assigned 86 patients undergoing coronary artery bypass grafting to 1 of 2 groups according to the target value for Pa_{CO_2} during bypass. In 44 patients, the target Pa_{CO_2} was 40 mm Hg, measured at the electrode temperature of 37° C. In 42 patients, the target Pa_{CO_2} was 40 mm Hg, corrected to the patient's rectal temperature. Perfusion was maintained during bypass by bubble oxygenator without artificial filtration. Other variables included mean hematocrit of 23%, and mean arterial blood pressure of 70 mm Hg, which was achieved by infusion of phenylephrine or sodium nitroprusside. Investigators assessed neuropsychological function before surgery, just before discharge, and at 7 months postoperatively.

Neuropsychological scores at 8 days varied widely and showed generalized impairment unrelated to the Pa_{CO_2} group or to hypotension during bypass. At 7 months, there was no significant difference in neuropsychologic performance between the Pa_{CO_2} groups. Nor was there any significant difference in the appearance of new Q waves on ECG, need for inotropic or intra-aortic balloon-pump support, postoperative creatine kinase-MB fractions, or the length of either postoperative ventilation or stay in intensive care.

Carbon dioxide management during CPB at moderate hypothermia has no significant effect on either cardiac outcome or neurobehavior. Because moderate hypothermia is widely used for adult cardiac surgery, these results should have extensive applicability. These results cannot be extrapolated to deeper hypothermia, however. Further research is required to determine whether CO_2 management affects outcome when lower temperatures are used.

▶ This extremely well-done study shows that the question of pH-stat versus α-stat management apparently doesn't make a difference to cardiac or CNS outcome. The power of the study isn't specified, but in doing crude power analysis on my own, if it had made as much as a 20% difference in neuropsychiatric outcome, the authors of this study would have an 80% chance of finding such a difference. The cardiac outcome data are much less definitive because the outcomes are not continuous but discrete variables of myocardial infarction; thus they had only about a 20% chance of finding a difference if one occurred. Nevertheless, I think this is an excellent study. It shows that, at least as far as CNS outcome is concerned, the choice of management doesn't matter, whether based on pH-stat measurement, i.e., the method by which blood gas values are mathematically corrected to the patient's body temperature, or the α-stat method, by which the increased solubility of CO_2 during hypothermia results in a decreased P_{CO_2} producing respiratory alkalosis when blood gas values are corrected for temperature.—M.F. Roizen, M.D.

Vascular

Carotid Artery Stump Pressure: How Reliable is it in Predicting the Need for a Shunt?
Gnanadev DA, Wang N, Comunale FL, Reile DA (San Bernardino County Med Ctr, Calif)
Ann Vasc Surg 3:313–317, 1989   6–21

Whether or not to use a shunt routinely at carotid endarterectomy remains a dilemma. Carotid artery stump pressures were measured prospectively during 84 operations in 71 patients. The only criterion for shunt placement was altered neurologic status during temporary carotid occlusion, as assessed with the patient under local anesthesia. In 2 exceptional patients shunts were placed when neurologic changes developed after carotid occlusion.

Stump pressures were significantly higher in the 15 operations attended by shunt placement than in the 69 unshunted cases (53 mm Hg vs. 34 mm Hg). Only 2 of 41 patients with pressures exceeding 50 mm Hg required a shunt, compared with 22% of 36 patients having stump pressures of 25–50 mm Hg, and 5 of 7 with pressures of less than 25 mm Hg (Fig 6–6). The need for a shunt did not relate to the clinical picture, a history of stroke, or the presence of contralateral carotid disease. There were no deaths, and only 2 patients had a transient neurologic deficit. The 2 shunted patients with high stump pressures had stroke or transient ischemic attack previously.

Monitoring the awake patient for neurologic change remains the best way of determining the need for a shunt at carotid endarterectomy. Stump pressures of 25–50 mm Hg are poor predictors of this need.

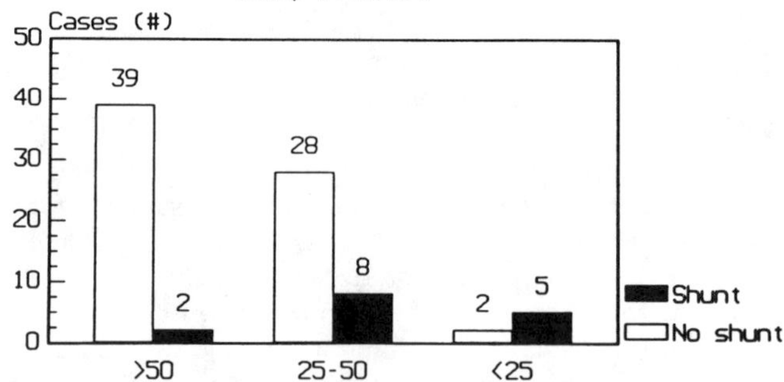

Fig 6–6.—Shunt requirement vs. carotid stump pressure. (Courtesy of Gnanadev DA, Wang N, Comunale FL, et al: *Ann Vasc Surg* 3:313–317, 1989.)

► This study is intriguing from several points of view. It tries to predict and measure accurately how good stump pressure is as a predictor of the need to shunt in patients who are otherwise undergoing local anesthesia for carotid surgery. From the article, I cannot determine how the authors surveyed for morbidity and mortality. They tell us that only 1 patient had a transient ischemic attack, and none had specific CNS deficits postoperatively. If that's so, after the number of shunts they did and the sickness of their patients, they are either the best surgeons in the world or they didn't record all of the morbidity. Next is that their own test, i.e., the ability to understand the neurologic tests they used intraoperatively, was not assessed for its ability to predict which patients would later require a shunt because of poor tolerance of the procedure. Another interesting thing is that, when they failed with local and regional anesthesia, they went to general anesthesia to protect the patient's neurologic function. Why didn't they do that for every case, some would argue? Maybe if general anesthesia is used for the sickest patients, it should be used for all patients. Nevertheless, the predictive value of stump pressure is extremely good, but they don't tell us how they measured it.

Moore and Wylie were very careful to state how they measured stump pressure; it is the diastolic pressure in the carotid artery measured at the brain level when a 22-gauge needle is inserted distal to both common and external carotid occlusion. A key point here is diastolic, and another key point is where it settles—not where it is immediately on insertion, but where it is after approximately 20 or 30 seconds. We aren't told how carefully these authors measured stump pressure or where it was measured. Nevertheless, by their criteria, 5 of 7 patients with stump pressures of less than 25 mm Hg needed shunting, but only 2 of 41 with stump pressures of more than 50 mm Hg required it. Eight of 36 patients with pressures between 25 and 50 mm Hg required shunting. The stump pressure, it should be noted, is not measured during awake states but is measured during halothane anesthesia, according to the Moore and Wylie study; thus the present authors didn't really measure stump pressure in a meaningful way. Nevertheless, they do find some reasonable correlation. At least, it appears that the correlation is as good as their measure of awakeness. We aren't told what the stump pressure was in those 2 patients who eventually required shunting because of neurologic disease.

Thus there are a number of items in this article that leave one in doubt about its validity: (1) We aren't told what the mechanism of follow-up was, or its degree. (2) We aren't told how stump pressure is measured, and it clearly isn't measured in the way described by Wylie and Moore. (3) We aren't given enough data to tell how good their method is at predicting the need for shunt placement.—M.F. Roizen, M.D.

The Processed Electroencephalogram May Not Detect Neurologic Ischemia During Carotid Endarterectomy

Silbert BS, Kluger R, Cronin KD, Koumoundouros E (St Vincent's Hosp, Melbourne)
Anesthesiology 70:356–358, 1989

6–22

Periodic neurologic testing is used to monitor cerebral perfusion during carotid endarterectomy in an awake patient. When carotid endarterectomy is performed in an anesthetized patient, standard or processed electroencephalographic (EEG) monitoring is often used to record cerebral electrical activity (CEA) for the detection of cerebral ischemia. The 2-channel, 5-lead, processed EEG machines provide an attractive alternative to the 16- to 20-lead standard EEG machines because they are easier to apply, use, and read.

To investigate the relationship between the on-line processed EEG and neurologic assessment in the awake state, studies were made in 2 patients undergoing carotid endarterectomy under regional anesthesia who were monitored with a 2-channel processed EEG machine. Both were elderly women, 73 years and 85 years, respectively. Neurologic status during endarterectomy was tested intermittently by asking the patient to squeeze the anesthesiologist's hand.

The first patient lost power in the left hand, and consciousness a few seconds later, at a trial cross-clamping of the internal carotid artery (ICA) and again later when the ICA was clamped while a shunt was inserted. On both occasions, consciousness was recovered immediately on reestablishment of cerebral flow. The transient neurologic changes showed as a noticeable loss of high frequency in the CEA on the processed EEG. On-screen changes associated with the neurologic deficits were reproducible and identical at each point to the decreases in cerebral blood flow.

The second patient also experienced 2 brief episodes (less than 30 seconds) of loss of power in the hand, but she remained conscious and was able to respond verbally. The first episode occurred within 40 seconds of trial ICA clamping, and the second during ICA clamping for removal of the shunt. The awake neurologic evidence of cerebral ischemia was not detected by the 2-channel EEG recorder.

The 2-channel EEG recorder may fail to indicate cerebral hypoperfusion that can be detected by simple neurologic assessment in the awake patient. The ability of this device to record the CEA during carotid endarterectomy performed under regional or general anesthesia should be further investigated.

▶ In rather well-established documents, it is said that the EEG is not very accurate, especially in patients who have previously had either reversible ischemic neurologic damage (i.e., prolonged transient ischemic attacks or stroke) or have actually sustained permanent damage. Both cases discussed in this article appear to fit these categories, although we canot be sure from the description of case 2. The authors state that the lack of sensitivity when an abnormality observed on neurologic examination is present on the EEG is a reason to use local anesthesia with repeated testing of neurologic function. Although this may be so, many surgeons don't like to operate that way and patients become uncontrollable at times. When that happens, usually the surgeon will request induction of general anesthesia. In fact, general anesthesia is protective of neurologic function, a fact that is especially dependent on the type of anesthesia chosen.

Are these 2 cases arguments for local or regional anesthesia? Certainly. But there are an equal number of anecdotal cases that favor general anesthesia and EEG analysis, or general anesthesia and some other form of monitoring.

Another conclusion the authors reach is that, as shown in the second case, adequate cerebral perfusion may be critically dependent on a systolic blood pressure higher than the patient's normal range. There are no data presented to substantiate that this is true. In fact, it has long been known that perfusion and pressure are not equivalent, and that the increase in systolic blood pressure may be caused by the patient's own neurologic response and may do great harm to the heart, the most common organ subject to morbidity and mortality after carotid endarterectomy.

The whole area of carotid endarterectomy has now been thrown open to examination. It is clear that with surgeons doing only a few carotid endarterectomies or doing them in centers that perform fewer than 50 per year, the results of this procedure may be associated with unacceptably high stroke and myocardial morbidity rates. Many would conclude that such institutions (those with a morbidity and mortality rate of more than 3% or 4%) probably should not be engaged in doing carotid endarterectomy at all, no matter what form of monitoring or anesthesia is used.—M.F. Roizen, M.D.

Should Patient Age Be a Consideration in Carotid Endarterectomy?

Pinkerton JA Jr, Gholkar VR (Univ of Missouri-Kansas City School of Medicine; St Luke's Hosp (Kansas City)
J Vasc Surg 11:650–658, 1990   6–23

The prominence of age as a factor in selecting patients for carotid endarterectomy was examined in a series of 607 patients having 685 operations done by a single surgeon. Perioperative results were evaluable in 420 patients younger than 75 years of age and in 115 older patients. Men were more prevalent in the younger group, whereas a greater proportion of the older group had contralateral carotid stenosis and stroke as indications for surgery.

Systemic intraoperative heparinization was used routinely. Patients had partial reversal of heparinization with protamine sulfate after the arteriotomy was closed. Carotid shunts were used selectively on the basis of continuous electroencephalographic monitoring. Patients were in intensive care for 24 hours postoperatively.

Ipsilateral stroke occurred perioperatively in 2% of patients, all in the younger group. Five of 6 perioperative deaths occurred in this group. Elderly patients had a cumulative survival rate of 85% at 2 years and 64% at 5 years. The respective rates of freedom from stroke in survivors were

98% and 87%. Age did not influence stroke morbidity or operative mortality in this series of carotid endarterectomies, despite the fact that medical risk factors are expected to be more prevalent in older patients.

▶ This is incredible undertaking by one surgeon who, in a 15-year period, performed 685 carotid endarterectomies in a group of patients of whom 420 were younger than 75 years of age (560 operations) and 115 were 75 or older (125 operations). The results speak for themselves. An important problem not addressed in the paper is how the morbidity data were collected. There is no mention of a search, whether by neurologists or by surgeons, for ischmic attacks or strokes, or how the mortality and myocardial infarction rates were sought and calculated, or anything about functional status. This paper contains no description of the follow-up process. Yet, as far as one can tell, only 9 of the 115 patients older than 75 years were lost to follow-up.

Thus the article appears to state that patients undergoing carotid endarterectomy are different in that age doesn't make a difference in outcome. On the other hand, age *has* been shown to affect outcome in patients undergoing gastrointestinal surgery, aortic valve replacement, open heart surgery, or coronary artery bypass (1–4). This article also appears to fly in the face of the Rand Study, which listed this age group of patients and this severity of disease as relatively equivocal indications for carotid artery surgery.

I hope someone out there is compiling all of the results on high-risk patients such as these; we'll send them to Rand to show them that their indications, which may have been valid in 1979, no longer hold up—that the Rand description of equivocal indication for surgery because of high risk, which may have been valid in 1979, is no longer valid in 1991.—M.F. Roizen, M.D.

References

1. Greenburg AG, et al: *Arch Surg* 116:788, 1981.
2. Lytle BW, et al: *J Thorac Cardiovasc Surg* 97:675, 1989.
3. Kennedy JW, et al: *J Thorac Cardiovasc Surg* 80:876, 1980.
4. Hibler BA, et al: *Arch Surg* 118:402, 1983.

Combining Clinical and Thallium Data Optimizes Preoperative Assessment of Cardiac Risk Before Major Vascular Surgery
Eagle KA, Coley CM, Newell JB, Brewster DC, Darling RC, Strauss HW, Guiney TE, Boucher CA (Massachusetts Gen Hosp, Boston)
Ann Intern Med 110:859–866, 1989   6–24

Preoperative cardiac evaluation of patients undergoing major surgery is important in identifying those at high risk in whom special monitoring or treatment may help to improve outcomes. Such evaluation is especially important in patients considered for major vascular surgery, in whom the prevalence of severe underlying coronary disease is about 33% and in whom cardiac ischemic events account for more than 50% of postoperative deaths. The ability of clinical features and dipyridamole-thallium imaging in predicting postoperative ischemic events was compared in 200 patients undergoing nonemergent vascular surgery.

Thirty patients (15%) experienced 1 or more postoperative ischemic events. In 6 patients fatal cardiac events occurred. Acute nonfatal myocardial infarction occurred in 4.5%, unstable angina pectoris in 8.5%, and acute ischemia-related pulmonary edema in 4.5%. Of all patients with postoperative ischemic events, 83%, including all 6 who died, had thallium redistribution on preoperative dipyridamole-thallium imaging.

The univariate correlates of the postoperative end points of cardiac death or myocardial infarction included a history of angina, congestive heart failure, and diabetes mellitus. Also, S_3 gallop on evaluation and pathologic Q wave on ECG were correlated with postoperative ischemic outcomes. Two of 4 dipyridamole-thallium test variables correlated with ischemic events—ischemic ECG changes during dipyridamole infusion and thallium redistribution. Of the 64 patients with none of the 5 clinical variables—Q wave on ECG, age greater than 70 years, history of angina, history of ventricular ectopic activity necessitating treatment, and diabetes mellitus requiring treatment—only 2 sustained postoperative cardiac ischemic events. Neither of these patients died. Ten of the 20 patients with 3 or more of these variables had postoperative ischemic events.

Preoperative dipyridamole-thallium imaging appears to be most useful in stratifying patients determined to be at intermediate risk by clinical examination. Thallium redistribution correlates with substantial change in the probability of events in patients with 1 or 2 clinical predictors. However, for almost 50% of patients, thallium imaging may be unnecessary because of very high or low cardiac risk according to clinical assessment.

▶ In this study, the presence of 3 or more clinical variables—Q waves in the ECG, age more than 70 years, history of angina, history of ventricular ectopic activity requiring treatment, and diabetes mellitis requiring treatment—identified a patient group that was at great risk for a cardiac event and had a sizeable risk for coronary artery disease. Ten of the 20 patients in that group had a postoperative cardiac event. On the other hand, those patients with only 1 or 2 of those 5 clinical variables were subject to dipyridamole-thallium imaging, and of those with thallium redistribution, 16 of 54, or 29.6%, had a postoperative cardiac event. Of those without thallium redistribution who had 1 or 2 of the clinical variables, only 2 of 62, or 3.2%, had events. The patients without any of these clinical variables do not need to be studied, according to the conclusions reached by the authors, as only 3.1% (2 of 64) had a postoperative cardiac event.

I think this is one of the hallmark papers in preoperative evaluation, as it indicates the value of taking a history and of segregating patients by clinical variables before doing laboratory testing, especially expensive laboratory testing such as thallium imaging, preoperatively.—M.F. Roizen, M.D.

Pulmonary Edema After Aneurysm Surgery Is Modified by Mannitol

Paterson IS, Klausner JM, Goldman G, Pugatch R, Feingold H, Allen P, Mannick JA, Valeri CR, Shepro D, Hechtman HB (Brigham and Women's Hosp; Harvard Med School; Boston Univ)
Ann Surg 210:796–801, 1989   6–25

Reperfusion of ischemic tissue during abdominal aortic aneurysmectomy (AAA) results in thromboxane (Tx) A_2 generation, increased mean pulmonary artery pressure (MPAP), leukopenia, and noncardiogenic pulmonary edema. To determine whether the hydroxyl radical scavenger mannitol can modify the pulmonary injury in AAA, 26 patients undergoing elective infrarenal AAA were randomly assigned to receive mannitol, .2 g/kg, or saline intravenously before infrarenal aortic clamping. Hemodynamic, hematologic, and pulmonary function studies were obtained.

With saline, 30 minutes after aortic clamping, plasma TxB_2 and MPAP increased significantly, whereas white blood cells and platelets decreased significantly. With removal of the aortic cross-clamp, further increases in TxB_2 and MPAP were noted. Pulmonary dysfunction occurred in all patients within 4–8 hours after surgery, as shown by significant increases in physiologic shunting (Q[sc]S[xsc]/Q[sc]T[xsc]) and peak inspiratory pressure. Chest radiographs showed pulmonary edema in all patients, but the pulmonary wedge pressure remained within normal limits.

Mannitol treatment before aortic cross-clamp application significantly reduced the increase in plasma TxB_2 and MPAP levels compared with saline treatment, and minimized the decrease in white blood cells and postoperative increase in Q[sc]S[xsc]/Q[sc]T[xsc]. Chest radiographs showed no pulmonary edema in any of 11 patients 4–8 hours after surgery. In vitro studies showed that mannitol $1-10^{-4}$ M prevented TxB_2 synthesis by adenosine diphosphate-activated platelets in a dose-dependent manner, whereas dextrose was ineffective in preventing thromboxane synthesis. Mannitol prevents the lung injury that occurs after AAA by inhibiting ischemia-induced thromboxane synthesis.

▶ This is a peculiar study for me to comment on because we just don't see pulmonary edema in our vascular patients after aneurysm surgery. Perhaps the reason is that we average 2.3 L of fluid for aneurysm surgery operations as opposed to their 6.4 L of crystalloid, and more than 3 L of other fluid. Is this difference attributable to the gentleness with which our surgeons handle tissues? Or is the reason we use only 2.3 L, compared to the authors' more than 9 L, related to the fact that our surgeons are much gentler (only in handling tissues, not in interacting with people)? There doesn't appear to be much difference in time.

Another question brought up by this article may relate to why these patients are ventilated postoperatively. But that may be the same problem. If you give a patient 9 L in 6 hours, you may need to ventilate him or pulmonary edema will develop.

Also, why do the authors give mannitol in the way described? If its effect is really experienced postoperatively, perhaps they can give it slower, far earlier in the procedure, and thus not risk increasing preload just as the surgeon is about to clamp the aorta and increase afterload. Why do they stress the heart? Maybe that's why pulmonary edema develops in these patients—because the heart is stressed so much.

In any case, I suppose this article points up the fact that differences in anesthetic practice are necessitated by differences in surgical practice.—M.F. Roizen, M.D.

Aortic Surgery: Effect of Clonidine on Intraoperative Catecholaminergic and Circulatory Stability

Quintin L, Bonnet F, Macquin I, Szekely B, Becquemin JP, Ghignone M (CHU Mondor, Créteil, France)
Acta Anaesthesiol Scand 34:132–137, 1990   6–26

Clonidine reduces catecholamine levels at rest and during exercise, and it may suppress sympathetic and/or circulatory hyperactivity during surgery. The effects of clonidine superimposed on medium-dose narcotic anesthesia were examined in a double-blind study of 28 patients undergoing aortic surgery. Half of the patients received clonidine 4.7 µg/kg, and half received placebo in addition to flunitrazepam 2 hours before anesthetic induction.

In contrast to placebo recipients, patients given clonidine had no marked rise in the plasma level of norepinephrine during aortic surgery and no significant rise in the epinephrine level. Arterial pressure consistently remained lower in clonidine-treated patients. These patients required many fewer anesthetic/circulatory adjustments than did placebo recipients. Clonidine did not alter the need for vasopressors or atropine.

As long as intravascular volume is adequate, administration of clonidine suppresses the rise in plasma catecholamines ordinarily induced by aortic surgery and promotes circulatory stability. Patient management is simplified as a result.

▶ This study furthers the key work of Maze, Ghignone, Quintin, and the Flackes in developing the hypothesis that preoperative sympathectomy is of benefit in sick patients. It should be noted that, in the study, the mean number of anesthetic circulatory adjustments per patient in the clonidine group was 1.8 ± 1.5 vs. 4.1 ± 2.6 in the control group. These circulatory adjustments were needed to keep the systolic blood pressure and heart rate within 30% of baseline values. I am sure from my own feeling, and from this report and others by the same and other authors, that clonidine does confer more intraoperative stability. This group administers more clonidine than we usually do, which is 2–3 µg/kg 120 minutes before induction, but their patients may have a more normal, or even hypervolemic, fluid status preoperatively than do ours.—M.F. Roizen, M.D.

Neonatal

Neonatal Facial and Cry Responses to Invasive and Non-Invasive Procedures

Grunau RVE, Johnston CC, Craig KD (BC Children's Hosp, Vancouver; Univ of British Columbia, Vancouver; Montreal Children's Hosp)
Pain 42:295–305, 1990   6–27

It is difficult to assess pain in neonates. Whether the crying and facial activity induced by an invasive procedure, e.g., an intramuscular injection of vitamin K, can be distinguished from responses to noninvasive tactile events such as applying disinfectant solution to the umbilical cord stump and rubbing the thigh with an alcohol swab, was investigated in 36 infants weighing more than 2,500 g at birth. All infants were considered to be healthy. Crying was analyzed by computer, and facial activity by the Neonatal Facial Coding System. The mean age of the infants was about 2 hours when observed.

Significant procedural effects were found for total facial activity and latency to facial movement. The invasive procedure tended to produce brow bulging, eyes squeezed shut, a deepened nasolabial furrow, and mouth opening. Crying, when it occurred, tended to be higher pitched and more intense after the injection than after the noninvasive procedures.

Acute invasive procedures on newborn infants tend to alter the facial expression and to produce earlier, longer-lasting crying. The facial display may reflect the infant's reaction to pain as predominantly affective and sensory discriminative, with little or none of the cognitive meaning that allows older persons to cope with the experience.

▶ Pain in the neonate has received a great deal of attention in recent years. It is a great relief to this father and clinical investigator to know that babies perceive invasive procedures to be more stressful than noninvasive procedures. That certainly was always my clinical impression.—G.W. Ostheimer, M.D.

Epidurography in Premature Infants

Van Niekerk J, Bax-Vermeire BMJ, Geurts JWM, Kramer PPG (Inst of Anaesthesiology; Univ Hosp for Children and Youth, Utrecht, The Netherlands)
Anaesthesia 45:722–725, 1990   6–28

Epidural anesthesia is used infrequently in premature infants, presumably because of technical problems and concern over toxicity. A caudal epidural catheter was inserted in 20 high-risk premature infants scheduled for abdominal or thoracic surgery under combined caudal epidural and general anesthesia. Epidurography was used to confirm the position of the catheter. The contrast material was iohexol in normal saline in a total volume of .5 mL/kg.

The infants had an average age of 10 days and weighed an average of

1,980 g. Eighteen of the 20 received a single bolus caudal block. Analgesia was considered adequate in all cases. Epidurography showed a misplaced catheter in 3 patients; in 1 the catheter penetrated the dura. The catheter was removed in these cases, and surgery was done, with the bolus caudal block being supplemented by general anesthesia.

Epidurographic control is important when very small infants receive caudal epidural analgesia. Identifying a misplaced catheter can avoid serious complications.

▶ This study further expands our knowledge of regional anesthesia in premature infants. My only question concerning the 3 problems that developed is, What length of catheter was placed in the epidural space? Perhaps by limiting the length of catheter inserted through the needle, these complications might not occur.—G.W. Ostheimer, M.D.

Postoperative Apnea in Former Preterm Infants: Prospective Comparison of Spinal and General Anesthesia

Welborn LG, Rice LJ, Hannallah RS, Broadman LM, Ruttimann UE, Fink R (Children's Natl Med Ctr; George Washington Univ; Natl Inst of Health, Washington, DC)
Anesthesiology 72:838–842, 1990   6–29

Former preterm infants are prone to postanesthetic apnea or bradycardia, or both, when general anesthesia is used. A prospective, randomized study was designed to compare the effects of spinal and general anesthesia on the incidence of postoperative apnea, bradycardia, and periodic breathing in 36 former preterm infants with a postconceptional age of 35–51 weeks who were undergoing repair of inguinal hernias.

Sixteen infants received inhalation anesthesia via an endotracheal tube with neuromuscular blockade, 9 were given spinal anesthesia plus preoperative intramuscular ketamine sedation, and 11 received spinal anesthesia without sedation. Respiration and heart rate were recorded continuously for at least 12 hours after operation.

Five of the 16 infants who received general anesthesia had prolonged

---

Incidence of Postoperative Apnea in Premature Infants With and Without History of Apnea

	Group 1 General Anesthesia (n = 16)	Group 2A Spinal + Ketamine (n = 9)	Group 2B Spinal Anesthesia (n = 11)
No prior history of apnea*	2/10 (20%)	2/3 (67%)	0
Prior history of apnea†	3/6 (50%)	6/6 (100%)	0
Total number of patients	5/16 (31%)	3/9 (89%)	0

*P = .05 (group 2A vs. group 2B).
†P < .02 (group 2A vs. group 2B).
(Courtesy of Welborn LG, Rice LJ, Hannallah RS, et al: *Anesthesiology* 72:838–842, 1990.)

apnea with bradycardia; 2 of them had no history of apnea. Eight of the 9 infants who were given spinal anesthesia with preoperative sedation had prolonged postoperative apnea with bradycardia; 2 of them had no history of apnea. None of the 11 infants who received spinal anesthesia without preoperative sedation had postoperative bradycardia, prolonged apnea, or periodic breathing (table).

None of the apneic episodes was observed clinically; rather, they were detected by analysis of the pneumographic tracings. None of the infants required postoperative tracheal intubation or controlled ventilation. When infants with no history of apnea were analyzed separately, there was no statistically significant increased incidence of apnea among the 3 groups.

▶ This well-defined study expands our knowledge of postoperative apnea in former preterm infants. Does ketamine act like a general anesthetic in these patients? Clearly, there seems to be a relationship between ketamine and general anesthesia and the development of prolonged apnea with bradycardia in the postoperative period. Although the numbers are small, there appears to be increased safety for the former preterm infant who receives a spinal anesthetic. All would agree that standard postoperative respiratory monitoring of these high-risk neonates is recommended after all anesthetic techniques. However, the question that needs to be answered is why these former preterm infants are affected by general anesthetic-like agents.—G.W. Ostheimer, M.D.

Chest Wall Motion of Infants During Spinal Anesthesia
Pascucci RC, Hershenson MB, Sethna NF, Loring SH, Stark AR (Harvard Med School; Harvard School of Public Health)
J Appl Physiol 68:2087–2091, 1990
6–30

In quadriplegic adults with intact diaphragmatic function, the intercostal muscles have a role in moving the rib cage outward during inspiration. Also, there is a paradoxical inward movement of the upper rib cage during tidal breathing in patients with reduced intercostal muscle activity.

The effect of spinal anesthesia on chest wall motion was studied in 7 prematurely born infants who underwent surgical repair of bilateral inguinal hernias when they were about normal term age. The mean postconceptional age at operation was 43 weeks. All infants were assessed while awake, quietly breathing room air, and in the supine position. Chest wall motion was studied before and during spinal anesthesia. Respiratory inductance plethysmography was used to record displacement of the upper rib cage and abdomen.

Spinal anesthesia produced a sensory block at the T2–T4 level with concomitant motor block at the T3–T7 level, which resulted in loss of most intercostal muscle activity. However, diaphragmatic function remained intact. In 6 of the 7 infants the rib cage moved outward during inspiration before spinal anesthesia, but the anesthetic significantly re-

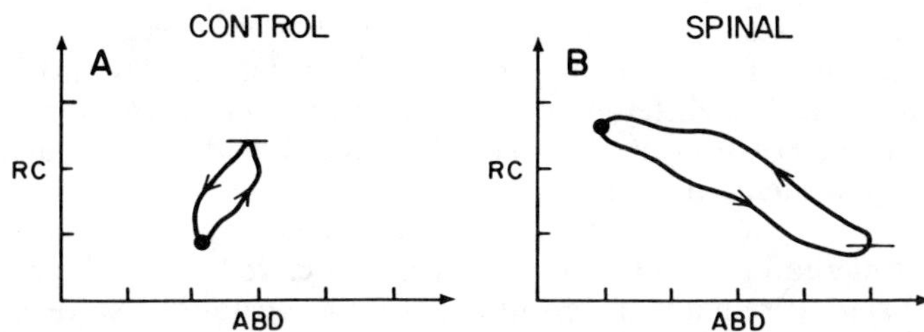

Fig 6–7.—Rib cage vs. abdominal displacement (Konno-Mead) respiratory loops before (**A**) and during spinal anesthesia (**B**). *Circles,* end expiration; *short horizontal lines,* end inspiration. After spinal anesthesia rib cage moves paradoxically and abdominal displacements increase. (Courtesy of Pascucci RC, Hershenson MB, Sethna NF, et al: *J Appl Physiol* 68:2087–2091, 1990.)

duced the outward movement of the rib cage during inspiration in all 6 infants.

Four of the 6 infants had paradoxical inward movement of the rib cage during inspiration (Fig 6–7). The most immature infant had inward movement of the rib cage both before and during anesthesia. Paradoxical rib cage motion resolved as the anesthetic wore off. Six infants had increased abdominal displacement during anesthesia, suggesting increased diaphragmatic motion.

Spinal anesthesia significantly reduced inspiratory rib cage movement in these infants. The findings confirm that, in infants, outward rib cage movement during tidal breathing requires active, coordinated intercostal muscle activity.

▶ For many years the neonate and newborn were not adequately studied during anesthesia. Nicely defined studies such as the current evaluation of chest wall motion of infants during spinal anesthesia will add to our increasing knowledge about the effects of general or regional anesthesia on the newly born.—G.W. Ostheimer, M.D.

Hormonal-Metabolic Stress Responses in Neonates Undergoing Cardiac Surgery

Anand KJS, Hansen DD, Hickey PR (Harvard Med School; Children's Hosp, Boston)
Anesthesiology 73:661–667, 1990   6–31

Hormonal and metabolic responses were examined in 15 neonates undergoing repair of complex congenital cardiac defects with the use of a standardized anesthetic approach. The anesthetic regimen included halothane, ketamine, morphine, pancuronium, and an oxygen-air mixture. All infants survived the surgery, but 4 died in the intensive care unit.

All infants had increases in plasma catecholamines, cortisol, glucagon, and β-endorphin. Insulin levels rose at the end of surgery and remained elevated for 24 hours. Hyperglycemia and lactic acidemia developed during surgery and persisted afterward. The infants who died tended to have more marked stress responses during and after surgery, although they were not distinct from the survivors on the usual clinical and hemodynamic grounds. The differences were apparent before cardiopulmonary bypass and the creation of new hemodynamics could have influenced the hormonal and metabolic responses.

The pattern of neonatal stress response differs from that seen in adults patients undergoing cardiac surgery. It is associated with a high hospital mortality rate. It remains uncertain whether the catabolic state is a cause or an effect of poor outcome when the operation itself seems adequate, but there is some suggestion that extreme stress responses may be associated with poor outcomes.

▶ Although this study is only a preliminary investigation, I believe it gives us enough information to investigate 2 questions: (1) Why are some neonates more stressed than others by these procedures? (2) What alteration in anesthetic administration would decrease this catabolic response.—G.W. Ostheimer, M.D.

Dangers of Neonatal Intubation With the Cole Tube

Mitchell MD, Bailey CM (Hosp for Sick Children, London)
Br Med J 301:602–603, 1990

6–32

Subglottic stenosis appears to be frequent after long-term intubation of the neonatal trachea with a Cole pattern shouldered tracheal tube. Nevertheless, this tube still is widely used, especially by nonanesthetists.

Male infant, 2 weeks, was seen after repeated attempts at extubation had failed. He weighed 1,400 g at birth and had been delivered by emergency section at 37 weeks because of intrauterine growth retardation and a suspected diaphragmatic hernia. The infant was intubated immediately after delivery, but the first attempt at extubation, at age 26 hours, had failed—as did 3 further trials during the next 11 days. A Cole pattern tracheal tube was used in each attempt. This tube was replaced by a 2.5-mm parallel-sided nasotracheal tube. When the latter was removed for bronchoscopy, the upper gum was seen to be severely ulcerated and grooved at the site of the shouldered tube. Severe glottic and subglottic damage was present, with circumferential ulceration conforming to the shape of the Cole tube. Elective tracheostomy proved necessary.

The shoulder of the Cole tube produces an abrupt change from laminar to turbulent air flow and actually increases resistance to air flow. Ulceration and stenosis can develop rapidly if the shoulder impacts in the cricoid region. Similar changes can occur with parallel-sided tracheal tubes, but it is possible to minimize damage through proper tube selection and use. Only that Cole tube specifically designed for neonatal resuscitation should be used—and it should be replaced as soon as possible with a parallel-sided nasotracheal tube.

▶ This case report illustrates the dangers of prolonged intubation of the trachea with a Cole endotracheal tube. I personally like the moderate stiffness of the Cole tube for initial endotracheal intubation and tracheal suctioning, if necessary. However, as soon as the neonate is stabilized, the Cole tube should be removed and replaced with a straight orotracheal or nasotracheal tube. A straight tube that is used orotracheally for a long period of time, however, still presents the problem of pressure ulceration of the hard and soft palate, larynx, and trachea in the premature newborn.—G.W. Ostheimer, M.D.

Pediatric

Recent Experience With Diaphragmatic Hernia and ECMO

Howell CG, Hatley RM, Boedy RF, Rogers DM, Kanto WP, Parrish RA (Med College of Georgia, Augusta)
Ann Surg 211:793–798, 1990   6–33

Extracorporeal membrane oxygenation (ECMO) improves postoperative survival in infants who undergo surgical repair of a congenital diaphragmatic hernia (CDH). However, a substantial number of infants with a CDH repair do not survive the period between surgical repair, transfer to an ECMO facility, and subsequent ECMO therapy.

Sixty-two of 74 infants survived after undergoing ECMO during a 4-year period. Forty-seven infants had meconium aspiration syndrome, 11 had CDH, 9 had persistent fetal circulation, 6 had respiratory distress syndrome-hyaline membrane disease, and 1 had congenital heart disease. Twenty-four of the 27 infants who were referred had respiratory symptoms in the first 12 hours and 3 had become symptomatic after discharge from the newborn nursery. Twenty-five of the 27 had surgical repair. The other 2 infants died in the delivery room afrer referral. Eleven infants were referred for initial surgical repair and 16 were referred for ECMO after successful surgical repair of a CDH elsewhere.

Six of the 27 referred patients (group 1) had successful surgical repair elsewhere and did not require ECMO after transfer; 7 had initial surgical repair as well as ECMO and survived (group 2); 4 had initial surgical repair but died during or immediately after ECMO (group 3); 8 died in transport or on arrival, and 2 died at delivery after referral (group 4) (table). Thus 13 of the 27 referred infants (48%) survived, including 8 of the 11 (73%) referred for initial surgical repair, but only 5 of the 16 (31%) referred for ECMO after surgical repair elsewhere.

Two of the 10 infants who died before ECMO could be initiated were nonviable from the start, but 8 were potential candidates for ECMO. Had ECMO been used in those 8 infants, 4 clearly would have been predicted to survive and the other 4 had a 50–50 chance of survival. Thus the increased survival in the 27 infants referred for ECMO could have been 69%, which is close to the survivial rate in infants who were either delivered at this hospital or referred before undergoing surgical repair of the CDH.

Comparison of Arterial Carbon Dioxide Pressure (Pa_{CO_2}) and
Ventilation Index (VI) Before Surgery and ECMO by Groups

Groups	No.	PaCO$_2$ Before Surgery	VI Before Surgery	PaCO$_2$ Before ECMO	VI Before ECMO
1	6	35 ± 20	513 ± 192		
2	7	41 ± 22	1593 ± 616	51 ± 17	2013 ± 376
3	4	52 ± 4	1025 ± 206	62 ± 26	1895 ± 474
4	10*	53 ± 20	1607 ± 460	68 ± 43	1818 ± 351

Note: PaCO$_2$ is expressed as mm Hg.
*Two patients died before measurements were obtained.
(Courtesy of Howell CG, Hatley RM, Boedy RF, et al: *Ann Surg* 211:793–798, 1990.)

Infants who require surgical repair of a CDH when delivered at a hospital where ECMO is not available should be transferred to a center where surgical and ECMO expertise is available. If they do undergo surgical repair of a CDH where ECMO is not available, they should be transferred to an ECMO center in the early postoperative period before they start to deteriorate.

▶ Those anesthesiologists who anesthetize infants with diaphragmatic hernia, should read this study more as a general review as to the state of art of the use of ECMO.—R.D. Miller, M.D.

Differential Effects of Pancuronium Bromide on Cardiopulmonary Function in the Neonatal Lamb

Wolfson MR, Shaffer TH (Temple Univ)
Pediatr Pulmonol 8:233–239, 1990

6–34

In adults, pancuronium bromide (Panc Br) antagonizes muscarinic receptors, especially those in the heart. Less is known about regional variation in muscarinic receptors and the differential effects of Panc Br in early development. The effects of Panc Br on resting cardiopulmonary function were examined in neonatal lambs, and its effects on cardiopulmonary responses to acetylcholine and histamine also were studied. Physiologic gas exchange and acid-base conditions were maintained. A segment of cervical trachea was bypassed, and its developed pressure response was taken as an indication of airway smooth muscle contraction and bronchoconstriction. The change in pulmonary resistance was a functional indicator of bronchoconstriction.

Pancuronium bromide reduced both the acetylcholine-induced pressure response and pulmonary resistance significantly, but it did not significantly alter the bradycardic and hypotensive responses to acetylcholine. Cardiopulmonary responses to histamine and resting cardiopulmonary function were unaffected by Panc Br administration.

Pancuronium has differential effects on pulmonary and cardiovascular muscarinic receptors in the newborn lamb. Its effect in attenuating airway smooth muscle responses may impair regulation of airway tone and related functions in the neonate.

▶ Although this study was performed in animals, it represents a nice companion to the article of Szeto et al. (Abstract 6–36).—R.D. Miller, M.D.

Comparison of Intraosseous, Intramuscular, and Intravenous Administration of Succinylcholine

Moore GP, Pace SA, Busby W (Madigan Army Med Ctr, Tacoma, Wash; Maricopa Hosp, Phoenix)
Pediatr Emerg Care 5:209–210, 1989   6–35

Intraosseous drug administration is being used more often to resuscitate pediatric patients. This route was compared with the intramuscular and intravenous routes for administering the depolarizing paralyzing agent succinylcholine 1 mg/kg, in sheep that were anesthetized with halothane and subsequently intubated.

Intraosseous access was achieved in less than 30 seconds in all attempts. The average time from succinylcholine administration to respiratory arrest was 31 seconds with intravenous administration, 57.5 seconds with intraosseous administration, and 230 seconds with intramuscular administration. The respective average times to 100% loss of forefoot twitch were 93 seconds with intravenous 101 seconds with intraosseous administration, and 291 seconds with intramuscular administration. All of the group differences were significant.

The intraosseous route appears to be an acceptable alternative to the intravenous administration of succinylcholine. The needle traditionally is directed away from the epiphysis, but studies in pigs have shown no adverse effects from either epiphyseal injection or the infusion of alkaline solution.

▶ This is a journal that most anesthesiologists will not see. The study indicates that the intraosseous administration of succinylcholine is an effective route (at least in sheep).—R.D. Miller, M.D.

Differential Sensitivities of Fetal Muscle Groups to *d*-Tubocurarine

Szeto HH, Hinman DJ (Cornell Univ)
Am J Obstet Gynecol 163:202–209, 1990   6–36

Neuromuscular blockers such as *d*-tubocurarine are used to prevent fetal movement during intrauterine fetal therapies. The dose-response and time-action characteristics of *d*-tubocurarine on the extraocular muscles, nuchal muscles, and the diaphragm were investigated in 9 fetal lambs.

The lambs were instrumented for long-term intrauterine monitoring by electrocortigraphy, electrooculography, electromyography, blood pressure, and heart rate. Increasing doses of *d*-tubocurarine selectively blocked various muscle groups. The extraocular muscles were the most sensitive and the diaphragm was the most resistant. The duration of drug action was directly related to muscle sensitivity to the drug.

Despite total neuromuscular blockade the fetal electrocorticogram continued to cycle, with an increase in synchronized and mixed activity and a decrease in desynchronized activity. There was a significant decrease in heart rate during synchronized and mixed electrocorticographic states but not during desynchronized electrocortigraphic states. This resulted in a loss of the heart rate difference normally displayed between the synchronized and desynchronized states. Fetal blood pressure was not changed with total neuromuscular blockade.

Fetal muscle groups display different sensitivities to the neuromuscular blockade action of *d*-tubocurarine. Therefore, selection of proper dosage may allow adequate suppression of fetal movement without prolonged paralysis of the diaphragm. Even at doses necessary for complete neuromuscular blockade, there are minimal adverse effects on fetal cardiovascular function.

▶ This is an excellent study in a gynecology journal. All pediatric anesthesiologists should read this important study. It is too bad they did not use a neuromuscular blocking drug other than *d*-tubocurarine.—R.D. Miller, M.D.

Preoperative Parental Anxiety Predicts Behavioural and Emotional Responses to Induction of Anaesthesia in Children
Bevan JC, Johnston C, Haig MJ, Tousignant G, Lucy S, Kirnon V, Assimes IK, Carranza R (Montreal Children's Hosp; McGill Univ, Montreal)
Can J Anaesth 37:177–182, 1990   6–37

Earlier studies that assessed the benefit to children of having a parent present at induction of anesthesia have been inconclusive. A study was designed to determine the immediate and late effects on a child's behavior and on parental anxiety of having a parent present at induction of anesthesia for outpatient surgical procedures.

In all, 134 children aged 2–10 years (mean age, 5 years), who underwent a variety of outpatient procedures were divided into a treatment group in which the parent was to be present at induction of anesthesia and a control group in which the parent was not to be in the operating room. Assignment was on an alternate-day basis because random assignment would have caused considerable problems of contamination. The groups were well matched for age, gender, previous hospitalization, and type of surgery performed. The child's fears and behavior and parental anxiety were scored before and at 1 week after operation by using appropriate assessment instruments. No parents refused to be present at induction of anesthesia.

All children became markedly upset in the induction area, and all parents were disturbed after induction of anesthesia. At 1 week after operation parents of both groups had evidence of increased anxiety, and children in both groups showed increased behavioral upset, when compared with baseline values.

Parents were divided into subgroups of anxious or calm parents, based on their anxiety scores in the waiting room. Forty-nine parents had high anxiety levels, 24 of them were present at induction and 25 were not. Children of calm parents behaved in the same way as children of anxious parents who were unaccompanied. However, children of anxious parents were significantly more upset by having a parent present at induction than unaccompanied children of anxious parents.

Highly anxious parents should not be present at induction of anesthesia in their children and should be offered further counseling and support. Assessment of levels of parenteral anxiety should be made part of the routine preoperative evaluation.

▶ I wonder what enterprising anesthesiologist will be the first to set up a counseling and support service for anxious parents of pediatric surgical patients.—G.W. Ostheimer, M.D.

Methaemoglobinaemia in Children Treated With Prilocaine-Lignocaine Cream

Frayling IM, Addison GM, Chattergee K, Meakin G (Royal Manchester Children's Hosp, Manchester, England)
Br Med J 301:153–154, 1990   6–38

A prilocaine-lidocaine (EMLA) cream limits pain from venipuncture and other minor skin procedures in children. It contains 25 g/L of each agent in an oily base. Prilocaine is associated with methemoglobinemia through the action of 2 of its metabolites, 4-hydroxy-2-methylaniline and 2-methylaniline (*o*-toluidine).

Blood methemoglobin levels were measured in 30 healthy children requiring elective surgery and 18 controls aged 1–6 years. The study group had cream applied under occlusion on the arm 2 hours preoperatively; it was removed just before induction of anesthesia. Control children had a mean methemoglobin level of .46%; study children had a peak level of .85% 10 hours after application. After 24 hours the value was .58%, still significantly above the control value.

A small but significant rise in methemoglobin occurs in children receiving an application of EMLA before surgery. It is possible that cumulative effects occur in children who receive the cream daily, and some may be at increased risk because of preexisting anemia, impaired renal excretion, or coadministration of sulfonamide antibiotics. The minimal effective dose should be used when daily applications are necessary.

▶ This study raises the issue of concern over the level of methemoglobinemia that can occur after the use of EMLA in pediatric patients. Interestingly, the investigators did not assess the efficacy of the EMLA patch before induction of anesthesia.—G.W. Ostheimer, M.D.

Effect of Endotracheal Suctioning on Arterial Blood Gases in Children

Kerem E, Yatsiv I, Goitein KJ (Hadassah Univ Hosp, Jerusalem; Bikur Cholim Hosp, Jerusalem)
Intensive Care Med 16:95–99, 1990   6–39

Interruption of ventilation by endotracheal tube suctioning may cause cardiac arrhythmias in patients who already have respiratory compromise. There also is a risk of damaging the tracheal mucosa. The effects of suctioning on arterial blood gas values were examined in 25 consecutive children who required endotracheal intubation. None required a level of inspired oxygen of more than .6. Suctioning was done with the largest possible catheter and lasted for 8 seconds.

Both saturation and oxygen partial pressure (Po_2) fell significantly after suctioning with no presuction treatment. Six patients had hypoxic levels below 60 mm Hg during suctioning. A significant fall in Po_2 was prevented by presuction oxygenation. Hyperinflation after suctioning rapidly returned the Po_2 to baseline.

Severe hypoxia can occur in children who have endotracheal suctioning and can be prevented by preoxygenation. Preoxygenation with an inspired oxygen fraction of 1 for 1 minute is recommended before suctioning. Intermittent hyperinflation with 100% oxygen during repeated suction passes will help to prevent hypoxia. These measures are especially important when the presuction Po_2 is low or borderline.

▶ This nicely done clinical study demonstrates that oxygenation with 100% oxygen before suctioning, followed by intermittent hyperinflation with 100% oxygen after suctioning, prevents any prolonged period of hypoxia from developing in ventilated neonates. The maneuvers are especially important in children with respiratory failure who already have low presuction Po_2.—G.W. Ostheimer, M.D.

Obstetrics—General

A Comparison of the Effect of Epidural, General, and No Anesthesia on Funic Acid-Base Values by Stage of Labor and Type of Delivery

Shyken JM, Smeltzer JS, Baxi LV, Blackemore KJ, Ambrose SE, Petrie RH (Washington Univ; Johns Hopkins Univ; Columbia Univ)
Am J Obstet Gynecol 163:802–807, 1990   6–40

The influence of type of anesthesia and of anesthesia itself on neonatal acid-base status was examined in 142 women who delivered infants at 36–42 weeks' gestation. Umbilical cord blood was sampled before, during, and after labor and elective section delivery. Vaginal deliveries were carried out without anesthesia and with epidural analgesia. Sections were performed with the use of general or epidural anesthesia.

The use of epidural analgesia for vaginal delivery was associated with longer labor, a lower umbilical artery pH, and higher arterial P_{CO_2} and bicarbonate values. In women having section delivery in the active phase of labor, epidural anesthesia was attended by lower arterial and venous values of partial pressure of oxygen compared with women who received general anesthesia. In contrast, epidural anesthesia for elective section delivery was associated with acid-base values similar to those of women given general anesthesia.

No advantage of epidural analgesia-anesthesia for the uncompromised term fetus, whether delivered vaginally or by cesarean section, was apparent. In vaginal deliveries the arterial pH is lower, presumably because a longer labor is associated with epidural analgesia.

▶ I have read the article by Shyken et al. (1) and feel there are several points regarding their methodology and results that deserve comment.

First, this retrospective review analyzed umbilical arterial and venous acid-base values, *when available* (italics ours). In most institutions, analysis of umbilical acid-base values is not done on a routine basis, especially following uncomplicated vaginal or cesarean delivery. What is the routine at Barnes Hospital? If indeed acid-base values are not done on all infants at this institution, some comments are necessary to sort out the possibility of selection bias. Although the authors attempted to exclude all patients with antenatal risk factors which may impact upon acid-base status, the unanswered question that remains is why were umbilical blood gas determinations obtained on these otherwise uncomplicated deliveries?

Second, the description of the anesthetic technique is incomplete. No mention is made of maternal inspired F_{IO_2} after induction of general anesthesia nor of the administration (or lack thereof) of supplemental oxygen to the mothers during epidural anesthesia. This information is critical to the interpretation of their results. The authors place considerable emphasis on their finding of significantly lower umbilical arterial and venous P_{O_2} values in the infants born during epidural anesthesia vs. general anesthesia for cesarean delivery. However, the emphasis here is misplaced. Rather than dwelling on the lower P_{O_2} values in the epidural group, the authors should have emphasized that the general anesthesia group had higher P_{O_2} values, a result easily explained by the fact that administration of general anesthesia usually includes 30% to 50% inspired F_{IO_2} (via endotracheal tube and positive pressure ventilation) after preoxygenation with 100% oxygen (2). It is unlikely that maternal F_{IO_2} (and thus maternal P_{O_2} —a parameter not mentioned by Shyken et al.) was comparable in the general vs. epidural group during cesarean delivery. Moreover, by what mechanism do the authors propose that epidural anesthesia can lower neonatal P_{O_2} values? Their statement, "Another reason for relative hypoxemia and hypercarbia associated with the use of epidural analgesia is hypotension as a result of sympathetic blockade" is made without reference. The article by Brizgys (3) (referred by the authors) only found a slightly lower pH (7.31 vs. 7.33) when hypotension occurred during cesarean delivery; P_{O_2} and P_{CO_2} values were unaffected.

Third, the acid-base values of the neonates born by vaginal delivery are claimed by the authors to be attributable to the longer labors of these women.

Considerable controversy exists regarding the acid-base sequelae of long labors (4). This retrospective study is subject to all the selection biases that flaw the numerous other retrospective studies correlating the length of labor with the use of epidural analgesia. One wonders if the results of Shyken et al. would have been different if all the patients in the vaginal delivery group had been randomized to receive either epidural or no analgesia during labor? As stated in a recent letter to this Journal (5), the time has come for a prospective, randomized trial of epidural analgesia vs. no epidural during labor (however, it would appear difficult to ethically design and execute such a study).

Finally, and most important, is that the study by Shyken et al. makes no mention of maternal risks of general vs. epidural anesthesia. A recent review discusses the inherent risks of general anesthesia for the parturient, in which all anesthetic-related deaths over a 40-year period in North Carolina were attributable to complications of general anesthesia (6). Another similar review in Massachusetts found that the vast majority of anesthetic-related deaths over a 30-year period were related to general anesthesia, and all such deaths over the last decade were a result of general anesthetic complications (7). At our institution, we perform over 2,500 cesarean deliveries per year and our rate of general anesthesia has been steadily declining over the last two decades, and currently is about 8%. We are proud of this accomplishment. Shyken concludes by stating that his results are "unlikely . . . to be clinically important for the term fetus with a normal electronic monitor pattern." We quite agree, and, therefore, other factors must be considered when choosing an anesthetic technique. If the data by Shyken et al. is ever used to discourage a woman from having epidural analgesia during labor, or, conversely, to encourage the use of general anesthesia for cesarean delivery, then a great disservice will have been done, not only to the obstetric and anesthetic communities, but especially to the women and infants who seek our expertise in obtaining safe and comfortable childbirth.—W.R. Camann, M.D.

References

1. Shyken JM, et al: *Am J Obstet Gynecol* 163:802, 1990.
2. Norris MC, Dewan DM: *Anesthesiology* 62:827, 1985.
3. Brizgys RV, et al: *Anesthesiology* 67:782, 1987.
4. Maresh M, et al: *Br J Obstet Gynaecol* 90:623, 1983.
5. Thorp JA, Parisi VM: *Am J Obstet Gynecol* 163:247, 1990.
6. May WJ, Greiss FC: *Am J Obstet Gynecol* 161:555, 1989.
7. Sachs BP, et al: *J Clin Anesth* 1:333, 1989.

Effect of Uterine Contractility and Maternal Hypotension on Prolonged Decelerations After Bupivacaine Epidural Anesthesia
Steiger RM, Nageotte MP (Univ of California, Irvine; Long Beach Mem Women's Hosp)
Am J Obstet Gynecol 163:808–812, 1990   6–41

Abnormal fetal heart rate patterns are reported more often when bupivacaine is used for epidural anesthesia, for reasons that are not clear. In a retrospective, case-control study, patients with prolonged decelerations after bupivacaine epidural anesthesia were matched with control patients for age, parity, and gestational age. The estimated frequency of prolonged decelerations after bupivacaine was 8.5%.

Prolonged decelerations did not correlate with the fall in mean arterial pressure after epidural anesthesia. Uterine hypertonus was noted in 82% of the study group and in 11% of the control group. Terbutaline was used in 30% of study cases and in no controls. Internal uterine pressure monitoring suggested that basal uterine tone was higher when decelerations occurred (Fig 6–8; see pp 192 and 193). There were no substantial differences in Apgar scores.

A rapid-acting tocolytic agent such as terbutaline may be indicated when prolonged decelerations occur after epidural anesthesia. The occurrence of prolonged decelerations after bupivacaine epidural anesthesia does, however, seem to have only a minimal, if any, effect on the immediate fetal outcome.

▶ Bupivacaine has been shown to produce uterine hypertonus in vivo and uterine artery vasoconstriction in vitro. The combination of these 2 pharmacologic responses appears to produce prolonged decelerations after bupivacaine epidural anesthesia on occasion. Interestingly, these actions can occur without alteration in maternal systolic pressure.

I have observed this phenomenon over many years and have clinically noted uterine hypertonus secondary to the unintentional intravascular injection of bupivacaine during epidural anesthesia. I have not believed that bupivacaine was present in high enough concentrations to produce uterine artery vasoconstriction. It would appear from this retrospective analysis that, in fact, uterine hypertonus and uterine artery vasoconstriction can occur without alteration in maternal systolic blood pressure and result in prolong accelerations. This information should be emphasized to obstetricians and nursing personnel, along with the fact that the occurrence of these prolonged decelerations does not have any effect on fetal outcome. Whether utilization of a tocolytic agent is necessary in these circumstances remains to be proven, in my opinion.—G.W. Ostheimer, M.D.

Effect of Adrenaline, Fentanyl, and Warming of Injectate on Shivering Following Extradural Analgesia in Labour
Shehabi Y, Gatt S, Buckman T, Isert P (Royal Hosp for Women, Paddington, NSW, Australia)
Anaesth Intens Care 18:31–37, 1990   6–42

Shivering occurs in 20% to 61% of parturients after extradural analgesia and in 23% of parturients without extradural analgesia. The etiology of shivering in parturients remains unclear. Local warming of the thermoreceptors in the spinal cord by warming the injectate may reduce the incidence of shivering. A prospective trial was carried out to determine

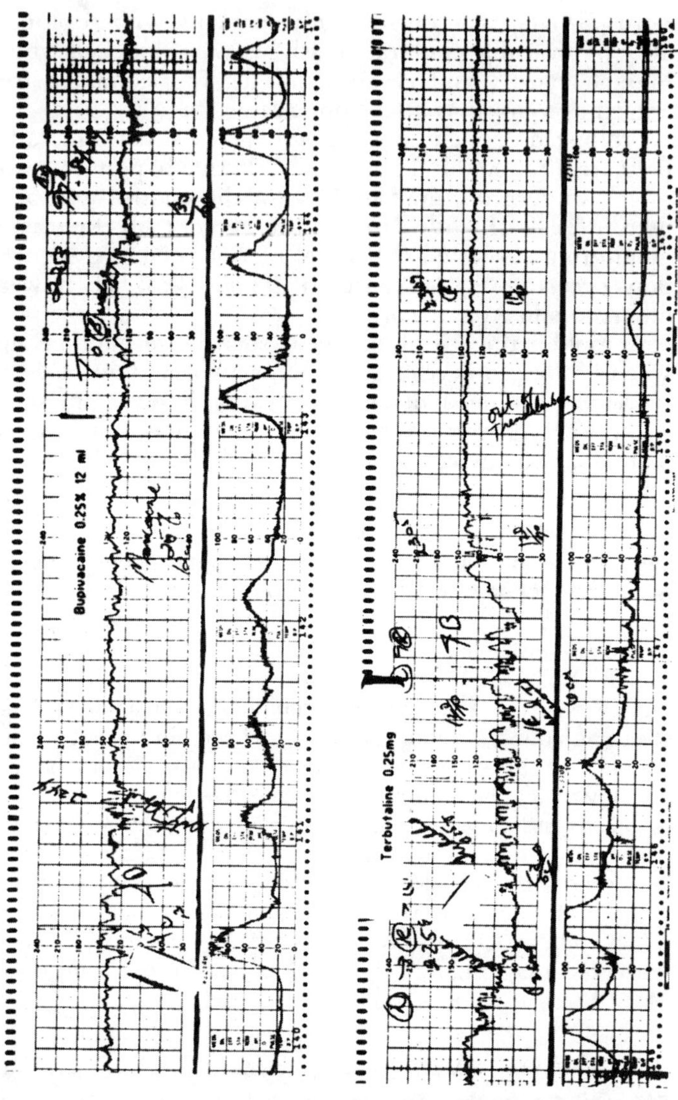

whether the addition of epinephrine or fentanyl to bupivacaine or warming the injectate has any effect on the incidence of shivering after extradural analgesia in laboring parturients.

Of 84 healthy, term, laboring women enrolled in the study, 20 received an extradural block with 10 mL of bupivacaine .5% plain at ambient temperature, 22 received 10 mL bupivacaine .5% that had been warmed to 38.5° or 39°C, 21 received an extradural block of 10 mL of bupivacaine .5% with 1:200,000 epinephrine at ambient temperature, and 21 received extradural 9 mL of bupivacaine .5% and 1 mL fentanyl (50 μg)

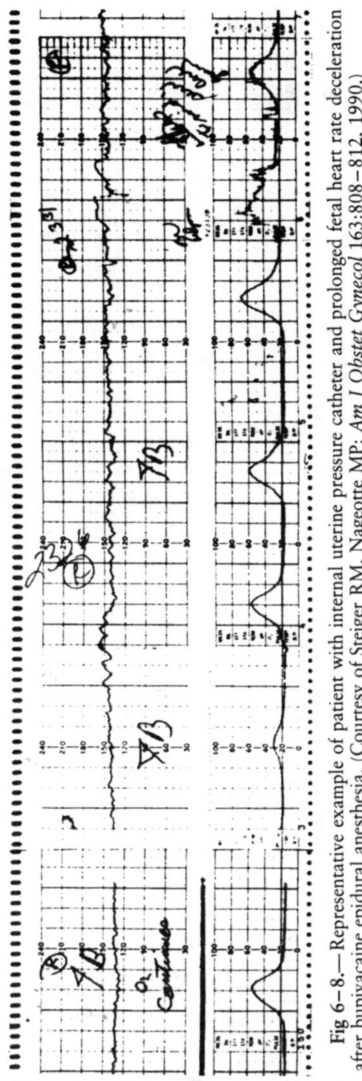

Fig 6–8.— Representative example of patient with internal uterine pressure catheter and prolonged fetal heart rate deceleration after bupivacaine epidural anesthesia. (Courtesy of Steiger RM, Nageotte MP: *Am J Obstet Gynecol* 163:808–812, 1990.)

at ambient temperature. The 4 groups were comparable for mean age, height, weight, gestational age, level of sensory block to pinprick, systemic blood pressure, pain and anxiety analogue scores, and mean baseline temperatures.

Sixteen patients (76.2%) in the epinephrine group shivered at some time during the 30-minute observation period. By contrast, only 27.3% of the patients who received warmed injectate and 33.3% of those who were given fentanyl shivered. The incidence of shivering among patients who received bupivacaine plain at ambient temperature was 55% (table).

Total Number of Patients Who Shivered During the Study Period (Including the Pre-Block Shiverers) (Patients in Group 1 Make Up the Control Group)

| | | | Number of Patients Shivering | | Chi-Square with Yates |
		Total	Yes	No	Correction
Group 1 (Control group)	10 ml bupivacaine, room temp 22.3°C	20	11	9	
Group 2	10 ml bupivacaine, warmed to 36.3°C	22	6	16	$P < 0.001$
Group 3	10 ml bupi + adrenaline, ambient temperature	21	16	5	$0.20 < P < 0.30$
Group 4	9 ml bupi + 50 μg fentanyl, ambient temperature	21	7	14	$0.02 < P < 0.05$

(Courtesy of Shehabi Y, Gatt S, Buckman T, et al: *Anaesth Intens Care* 18:31–37, 1990.)

Fentanyl was particularly effective in reducing shivering in patients who were already shivering before insertion of the extradural block. The increased incidence of shivering among epinephrine recipients did not reach statistical significance. Warming the injectate or adding fentanyl to local anesthetic solution markedly decreased the incidence of shivering among parturients with extradural analgesia.

▶ The addition of opioid to the epidural injectate has a significant effect on decreasing the incidence of shivering. Many years ago, meperidine was recommended to decrease shivering in the postoperative period, and then there was the utilization of the agonist/antagonist drugs such as butorphanol and, now, nalbuphine. It appears that opioids have a significant effect on the thermoregulatory center of the patient, whether pregnant or not, in decreasing the incidence of shivering. The issue of warming the epidural injectate is still controversial, based on a review of several studies.—G.W. Ostheimer, M.D.

Continuous Epidural Infusion of 0.0625% Bupivacaine-0.0002% Fentanyl During the Second Stage of Labor

Chestnut DH, Laszewski LJ, Pollack KL, Bates JN, Manago NK, Choi WW (Univ of Iowa)

Anesthesiology 72:613–618, 1990   6–43

The use of epidural analgesia during the second stage of labor remains controversial. In a previous study, continuous epidural infusion of .125% bupivacaine until delivery provided effective analgesia, but prolonged the second stage of labor and increased the incidence of instrumental delivery. In a subsequent study, continuous epidural infusion of .0625% bupivacaine—.0002% fentanyl produced first-stage analgesia similar to that produced by .125% bupivacaine alone, but epidural infusion was discontinued at full cervical dilation. A randomized, double-blind, placebo-controlled trial was conducted to determine whether continuing epidural infusion of bupivacaine-fentanyl until delivery provides effective second-stage analgesia without increasing the incidence of instrumental delivery or prolonging the second stage of labor.

The study included 63 nulliparous parturients who were all given identical epidural analgesia for the first stage of labor. Both groups had similar pain scores during the first stage of labor (Table 1). When the cervix was fully dilated, 29 women were given continuous epidural infusion of bupivacaine-fentanyl and 34 women were given saline placebo. Although pain scores during the second stage in the saline-treated group were significantly higher at each 30-minute interval 60–150 minutes after full cervical dilation, the difference in pain scores between the 2 groups was small but significant. One woman in the bupivacaine-fentanyl group underwent cesarean section during the second stage for apparent cephalopelvic disproportion. Surgical perineal anesthesia was adequate for vaginal delivery in 11 (39%) of 28 women in the bupivacaine-fentanyl group and 5 (15%) of 34 women in the placebo group. The median duration of the second stage was 53 minutes in the bupivacaine-fentanyl group and 63 minutes in the placebo group. Instrumental vaginal delivery was used in 6 (21%) women in the bupivacaine-fentanyl group and 5 (15%) in the placebo group (Table 2). These differences were statistically not significant.

Continuing epidural infusion of .0625% bupivacaine-.0002% fentanyl until delivery did not prolong the second stage, nor did it increase the incidence of instrumental delivery. Although patients in the bupivacaine-fentanyl group had somewhat better analgesia in the second stage than those in the placebo group, contrary to expectation, continuing epidural

TABLE 1.—Conduct of Labor

	Bupivacaine-Fentanyl (n = 29)	Saline-Placebo (n = 34)
Duration of active phase of first stage (min)*	316 ± 188	317 ± 199
Duration of known bupivacaine-fentanyl infusion (min)*	227 ± 159	215 ± 164
Bupivacaine dosage before start of study solution (mg)*	47 ± 30	44 ± 29
Bupivacaine dosage after start of study solution (mg)*	16 ± 13	0
Fentanyl dosage before start of study solution (μg)*	169 ± 80	161 ± 84
Fentanyl dosage after start of study solution (μg)*	50 ± 41	0
Duration of second stage (min)†	53 (5–283)	63 (16–181)
Position of vertex immediately before delivery		
Occiput anterior	27 (93%)	31 (91%)
Occiput posterior	1 (3%)	3 (9%)
Occiput transverse	1 (3%)	0 (0%)

Note: P was not significant.
*Mean ± SD.
†Mean (range) (excluding 1 woman in the bupivicaine-fentanyl group who underwent cesarean section after full cervical dilation).
(Courtesy of Chestnut DH, Laszewski LJ, Pollack KL, et al: *Anesthesiology* 72:613–618, 1990.)

infusion with the test solution until delivery did not consistently provide satisfactory second-stage analgesia.

▶ We are indebted to Dr. Chestnut for his series of studies relating to the effect of epidural anesthesia with or without narcotic on the progress of labor. However, I am afraid that .0625% bupivacaine with fentanyl is bordering on homeopathic doses. I know that there are readers who will argue with that state-

TABLE 2.—Method of Vaginal Delivery

	Bupivacaine-Fentanyl (n = 28)	Saline-Placebo (n = 34)
Spontaneous	22 (79%)	29 (85%)
Outlet forceps	0 (0%)	0 (0%)
Low forceps	2 (7%)	4 (12%)
Midforceps	2 (7%)	1 (3%)
Midvacuum followed by low forceps	2 (7%)	0 (0%)

Note: P was not significant.
(Courtesy of Chestnut DH, Laszewski LJ, Pollack KL, et al: *Anesthesiology* 72:613–618, 1990.)

ment, but I believe if we are asked to give continuous pain relief during labor and delivery that we should provide the patient with a appropriate anesthetic realizing that there may be some prolongation of the first and second stages of labor.

I am always asked what is the effect of epidural anesthesia on the progress of labor at various meetings around the country. I simply state that I believe epidural anesthesia prolongs the first and second stages of labor to varying degrees, but that a tremendous number of factors are interrelated. One must consider when the epidural was initiated and the reason for which it was initiated. Prolongation of the first stage of labor may be more pronounced in the primigravid patient and less so in the multiparous patient. Some obstetricians say that the second stage of labor is prolonged because the patients do not have perineal sensation and cannot adequately push. Well, folks, in more than 20 years of providing pain relief for labor and delivery, I have never had any patient say to me, "Please, Doctor, do not give me a top-up or continue my infusion (of local anesthetic with or without narcotic) because it will prolong my second stage of labor!"

I think this issue about the effect of epidural anesthesia on the progress of labor is concocted by some obstetricians or midwives who do not want to work with the anesthesiologist, labor nurse, and the parturient to provide a comfortable labor and delivery because it requires their attention to the labor and an understanding of epidural anesthesia. It is very easy for obstetricians and midwives to give parenteral medication, avoid continuous epidural anesthesia, and then just do the delivery without concern for the parturient's pain. I will not review the advantages of epidural anesthesia for the laboring patient, but suffice it to say that the well-managed obstetric anesthetic for labor and delivery provides a very satisfying and safe experience for both the mother and husband (or significant other). I have been privileged to work with obstetricians who understand and utilize epidural anesthesia for many years. I am not trying to sell "epidural anesthesia." It has sold itself over the years and does not need a front man.

The final point that I would like to make is that obstetric anesthesiologists are physicians who have devoted their professional careers to providing a safe course through labor and delivery for the parturient and the fetus about to be born. The denial of epidural anesthesia when it is available to the parturient or, even worse, to have an epidural anesthetic wear off so that the parturient can push "better" is barbaric. In fact, I know several instances when the parturient refused to push until she had appropriate epidural anesthesia! (I have reviewed the effects of labor and its pain on the mother and the fetus in several previous YEAR BOOKS so I will not repeat them.)

There are only a few instances in which the laboring patient will not benefit from a judiciously administered epidural anesthetic that provides pain relief for both labor and delivery. A slight prolongation of the first and second stages of labor is a small price to pay by a laboring parturient who will enjoy the outcome of her pregnancy in a comfortable and safe environment with her obstetrician, anesthesiologist, labor nurse, and support persons in attendance. It is time we stop apologizing and take pride in the fact that we are able to provide pain relief for the laboring patient and be of assistance to her during very trying and difficult circumstances.— G.W. Ostheimer, M.D.

Regional Epidural Analgesia for Labour Following Previous Caesarean Section: A 15 Year Review, 1972–1987
Meehan FP, Rafla NM, Burke G (Univ College Hosp, Galway, Ireland)
J Obstet Gynaecol 10:312–316, 1990   6–44

The use of regional anesthesia during labor has several advantages for women who have previously had a cesarean section. Some may require instrumental delivery or a repeat cesarean section. The epidural block may, however, mask the early signs of uterine scar rupture, although such ruptures are uncommon. At the study institution, regional epidural anesthesia has proved safe for mother and fetus in patients who had a previous cesarean section.

During a 15-year period, 345 of 1,350 patients undergoing labor after a previous cesarean section were delivered with the use of epidural analgesia. Vaginal delivery was achieved in 85% of the patients. Because stricter management of labor was instituted in 1982, the study was divided into 2 parts: 1972–1982 and 1982–1987. Oxytocin was given to induce or accelerate labor in 50% of the patients overall, but its use decreased from 57% in the first 10 years of the study to 44% in the last 5 years.

Nine of the 10 perinatal deaths occurred between 1972 and 1982. One of 5 neonatal deaths was associated with true rupture of the uterus and another followed prolonged labor and failed forceps. Between 1982 and 1987 there was 1 stillbirth before the onset of labor and no neonatal deaths (table). Although no maternal deaths occurred in the women who labored after previous cesarean section, there were 2 deaths among those who had elective repeat cesarean sections.

With regional anesthesia, women who have had a previous cesarean section may achieve vaginal delivery without added risk of true rupture or perinatal death. The complete relief of pain allows the patient to be ready for instrumental delivery or a cesarean section, if necessary.

▶ It's nice to see the Irish experience concur with what is rapidly becoming the American experience with vaginal birth after previous cesarean delivery utilizing regional anesthesia. Two points not covered by the above summary require mentioning. Of the 2 patients who died during surgery, death in both was caused by profuse hemorrhage and cardiac arrest, associated with placenta previa percreta invading the bladder. One patient was having her fourth cesarean section and the other was having her sixth cesarean section. This further substantiates the study of Clark et al. (1) who demonstrated that, as the incidence of cesarean delivery increases, so does the risk of placenta previa, and as the risk of placenta previa increases, so does the risk of placenta accreta and percreta.

Delivery After Previous Cesarean Section

| | 1972–1982 | | | | 1982–1987 | | | |
| | Excluding regional analgesia | | Regional analgesia | | Excluding regional analgesia | | Regional analgesia | |
	No.	(%)	No.	(%)	No.	(%)	No.	(%)
Total patients	1306		192		763		173	
Allowed to labour	657		187		348		158	
Induction rate	204	(31·0%)	84	(44·9%)	77	(22·1%)	50	(31·6%)
Successful vaginal delivery	538	(81·9%)	164	(87·7%)	266	(76·4%)	129	(81·6%)
Emergency caesarean section	119	(18·1%)	23	(12·3%)	82	(23·6%)	29	(18·3%)
True rupture	3	(0·5%)	2	(1·1%)	1	(0·3%)	0	(0·0%)
Bloodless dehiscence	5	(0·8%)	7	(3·7%)	2	(0·6%)	3	(1·9%)
Total babies	664		192		352		162	
Stillbirths	17	(2·6%)	4	(2·1%)	7	(2·0%)	1	(0·6%)
Neonatal deaths	9	(1·4%)	5	(2·6%)	0	(0·0%)	0	(0·0%)
Perinatal deaths	26	(3·9%)	9	(4·7%)	7	(2·0%)	1	(0·6%)

(Courtesy of Meehan FP, Rafla NM, Burke G: *J Obstet Gynaecol* 10:312–316, 1990.)

The other point is the overall cesarean delivery rate of approximately 11% in a tertiary referral center. At the Brigham and Women's Hospital, an American tertiary care referral center, the incidence of cesarean delivery has been in the 24% to 25% range in the past several years. I am at a lost to explain the difference in cesarean delivery rate between the Irish and the Americans centers with the exception of a more homogeneous population in the Irish centers, although they do get many high-risk referrals.—G.W. Ostheimer, M.D.

Reference

1. Clark SL, et al: *Obstet Gynecol* 66:89, 1985.

Distance From Skin to the Lumbar Epidural Space in an Obstetric Population
Meiklejohn BH (Leicester Royal Infirmary, Leicester, England)
Reg Anesth 15:134–136, 1990   6–45

The distance from the skin to the epidural space is quoted in standard textbooks as averaging 8 cm. However, surveys of obstetric populations show an average epidural space depth of 4.7 cm. The epidural space depth was measured in 163 women receiving epidural analgesia during labor. Other factors that may be related to epidural space depth (e.g., ethnic origin, height, weight, and the presence of edema) also were investigated.

The study population included 125 white women and 33 Asian women. The mean depth of the epidural space for all women was 4.78 cm and ranged from 3 cm to 8 cm. The distance from the skin to the epidural space was significantly greater in white women than in Asian women. There was no correlation between epidural space depth and age or height. However, the epidural space in women with clinically significant edema was significantly deeper than in those without edema. Thus there is no evidence to support an average epidural space depth of 8 cm, as still stated in standard textbooks.

▶ We are indebted to Dr. Meiklejohn for this very simple and straightforward study documenting the distance from the skin to the epidural space in the obstetric patient. I was surprised to learn that the depth of 8 cm is quoted in standard obstetric anesthesia textbooks. I guess I never thought very much about it.—G.W. Ostheimer, M.D.

Serious Non-Fatal Complications Associated With Extradural Block in Obstetric Practice
Scott DB, Hibbard BM (Royal Infirmary, Edinburgh; Univ of Wales, Cardiff)
Br J Anaesth 64:537–541, 1990   6–46

Extradural block is commonly used in obstetric practice in the United Kingdom. There, the mortality associated with extradural block is known, but accurate morbidity data are not available. A retrospective survey was done by mail to obtain data on serious nonfatal complications of extradural block occurring in obstetric practice in the United Kingdom. A questionnaire was mailed to all obstetric units in the United

TABLE 1.—Adverse Events Associated With
Extradural Block

Complication	No.	No. with permanent effects
Cardiac arrest	3	1 (brain damage)
Neuropathy involving spinal cord	1	1 (paraplegia)
Neuropathy involving a single spinal nerve	38	1 (quadriceps weakness)
Extradural abscess	1	? (still improving)
Extradural haematoma	1	? (still improving)
Urinary problems	6	0
Severe backache	5	0
Memory loss	1	0 (? from vasovagal faint)
Dural tap with:		
Prolonged headache	16	0
Cranial nerve palsy	5	0
Subdural haematoma	1	0
Acute toxicity (convulsions)	20	0
High or total spinal	8	0
Anaphylaxis	1	0
Total	108	5

(Courtesy of Scott DB, Hibbard BM: *Br J Anaesth* 64:537–541, 1990.)

Kingdom asking for data on the incidence and nature of serious adverse events that occurred during and after extradural block from 1982 through 1986.

Of 271 obstetric units contacted, 203 returned the requested information. The responding units delivered 516,000 infants yearly, representing 78% of all births reported annually in the United Kingdom. Of the 101,200 extradural blocks given annually, 84% were for pain relief and 16% for cesarean section. A total of 506,000 extradural blocks were administered during the 5-year survey period.

TABLE 2.—Other Reported Adverse Events Probably Not
Associated With Extradural Block

Complication	No.	Comment
Quadriplegia	1	Thrombosis of cervical haemangioma 10 days after delivery
Hypotension caused by cardiomyopathy	1	Heart transplant after delivery
Extradural abscess	1	Developed in diabetic 11 months after delivery
Facial weakness	1	?Multiple sclerosis

(Courtesy of Scott DB, Hibbard BM: *Br J Anaesth* 64:537–541, 1990.)

There were 108 serious adverse events associated with extradural block (Table 1). Thirty-eight women sustained damage to a single spinal nerve or nerve root that caused transient neuropathy. Two women had irreversible spinal cord lesions. Two others had postextradural spinal cord compression. Both were still recovering from their neurologic deficit at the time of the survey. Twenty-one women experienced acute toxicity with convulsions. All recovered, although 1 woman probably had transient cardiac arrest. There were 8 high or total spinal anesthetics after inadvertent subarachnoid injection of local anesthetic. All women recovered. Several miscellaneous complaints were probably not associated with extradural block (Table 2).

The incidence of serious nonfatal complications of extradural block is low in United Kingdom obstetric practices. Serious complications could be further reduced by meticulous technique.

▶ This retrospective study demonstrates that we cannot decrease our vigilance in obstetric anesthesia. Clearly, the message of how to treat unintentional intravascular injection and high or total spinal anesthesia has been received, because there were no fatalities in the women who experineced these adverse reactions. I agree with Drs. Scott and Hibbard that we need to undertake a major prospective study on the incidence of neurologic complications, particularly after epidural anesthesia. It is unfortunate that we are not able to gather such data in the United States, as has been possible over several years in the United Kingdom.—G.W. Ostheimer, M.D.

Patient Variables and the Subarachnoid Spread of Hyperbaric Bupivacaine in the Term Parturient
Norris MC (Thomas Jefferson Univ)
Anesthesiology 72:478–482, 1990 6–47

Several investigators have reported a correlation between height and the spread of hyperbaric bupivacaine in women undergoing cesarean section. However, a more recent study could not confirm this correlation. The effect of vertebral column length on the spread of sensory blockade after subarachnoid injection of hyperbaric bupivacaine was further examined in 52 term parturients, aged 20–42 years, undergoing cesarean section.

With the patient in the supine position, the distance from the sacral hiatus to the C7 vertebral prominence was measured immediately before subarachnoid injection of 15 mg of hyperbaric bupivacaine. Vertebral column length was recorded along with the patient's age, height, and weight. At 15 minutes after subarachnoid injection, the maximum cephalad extent of sensory analgesia and anesthesia was determined. Analgesia was defined as the loss of sensation of sharpness to pin prick, and anesthesia as the loss of perception of light touch.

There was a weak correlation between vertebral column length and patient height. However, age, height, weight, body mass index, and vertebral column length did not correlate with the spread of sensory analgesia or anesthesia. Thus the dose of injected hyperbaric bupivacaine need not be adjusted for any of the patient variables studied.

▶ I agree. After I began using hyperbaric bupivacaine for cesarean delivery I realized that the formula based on height did not uniformly give adequate anesthesia for the operative procedure. We religiously followed a formula based on height for hyperbaric tetracaine spinal anesthesia, and it served us well over many years. However, hyperbaric bupivacaine is different from hyperbaric tetracaine. I routinely use between 1.6 and 2 mL of hyperbaric .75% bupivacaine and add 10–25 μg of fentanyl for parturients undergoing cesarean delivery. I may decrease my dose in the very short patient (less than 5 ft) or increase my dose in the very tall patient (more than 6 ft).

Interestingly, a high thoracic or low cervical sensory level of anesthesia is not very distressing when the patient receives hyperbaric bupivacaine. In contrast, the patient who receives hyperbaric tetracaine becomes extremely uncomfortable and, even with no change in blood pressure, would have severe anxiety and the feeling of being unable to breath adequately.

My conclusion is that hyperbaric bupivacaine for surgical procedures and operative deliveries is outstanding. I believe that hyperbaric tetracaine should be reserved for surgical procedures in which a lower thoracic block provides adequate anesthesia for the surgery, such as lower abdominal and orthopedic procedures. Hyperbaric lidocaine behaves in a similar fashion to hyperbaric bupivacaine; however, the duration of the block is approximately 60–75 minutes and may not be adequate, even with subarachnoid opioid supplementation in this era of the slow surgeon.—G.W. Ostheimer, M.D.

Transient Maternal Hypotension Following Epidural Anesthesia
Philipson EH, Kuhnert BR, Pimental R, Amini SB (Case Western Reserve Univ; Cleveland Metropolitan Gen Hosp)
Anesth Analg 69:604–607, 1989   6–48

Maternal hypotension is a common complication of lumbar epidural anesthesia. Maternal hypotension can significantly lower umbilical cord pH values. Although there appear to be no clinical consequences to the neonate if the maternal hypotension is rapidly corrected, acidosis could increase placental transfer of local anesthetic agents as a result of ion trapping. The clinical and pharmacologic consequences of transient maternal hypotension after epidural anesthesia were assessed in 40 women with normal singleton term gestations undergoing elective cesarean delivery.

The women were given epidural anesthesia with .5% bupivacaine without epinephrine. Maternal blood pressure was measured every minute from the time of epidural anesthesia until delivery of the infant, and every 5 minutes thereafter until completion of the operation. If maternal hypotension occurred, it was corrected immediately with the intra-

Effect of Maternal Hypotension on Umbilical Cord Acid-Base
Status at Delivery

Umbilical cord	Normotensive group	Hypotensive group	Significance (P value)
Vein			
pH	7.34 ± 0.05*	7.30 ± 0.05	<0.05
P_{CO_2}	40.9 ± 4.9	39.9 ± 6.0	NS
P_{O_2}	32.1 ± 10.7	29.5 ± 5.2	NS
Artery			
pH	7.26 ± 0.06	7.22 ± 0.08	<0.05
P_{CO_2}	52.2 ± 6.7	55.2 ± 8.1	NS
P_{O_2}	15.9 ± 5.0	16.1 ± 3.8	NS

Abbreviation: NS, not significant.
*Values are mean ± 1 SD.
(Courtesy of Philipson EH, Kuhnert BR, Pimentel R, et al: *Anesth Analg* 69:604–607, 1989.)

venous administration of ephedrine. Maternal and umbilical cord blood samples were assayed for drug levels.

After epidural anesthesia, 13 of the 40 patients became hypotensive; this was corrected within 2.1 minutes. The other 27 patients remained normotensive. The mean pH of umbilical cord venous and arterial blood was significantly lower in hypotensive than in normotensive mothers (table). Whereas normotensive and hypotensive mothers had similar venous bupivacaine concentrations at delivery, neonates of hypotensive mothers had significantly lower bupivacaine concentrations in their umbilical cord vein than did neonates of normotensive mothers. The fetal/maternal ratio of bupivacaine levels was lower in the hypotensive group than in the normotensive group, but the difference did not reach statistical significance. Transient maternal hypotension does not lead to a greater placental transfer of bupivacaine because of ion trapping, even though the neonatal cord blood pH decreases.

▶ Dr. Kuhnert and her associates continue their evaluation of local anesthetics and the fetus and neonate in this excellent study. Our concern has been that an acidotic pH in the fetus would lead to increased trapping of an amide local anesthetic in the fetus with resultant adverse neurobehavioral effects. This study clearly demonstrates that transient maternal hypotension, even with a decrease in umbilical cord pH, does not lead to increased concentrations of bupivacaine presented to the fetus at the time of delivery.

A note of caution must be raised, however, to resist transferring this information to the parturient and fetus who demonstrate a pH of less than 7.2 during labor, which then necessitates emergency cesarean delivery. To my knowledge, this investigation has not been undertaken. However, in a clinical situation it would seem that the rapid administration of lidocaine (bupivacaine would be inappropriate in this context) should not significantly pass the placenta to the fetus because the operative delivery will be accomplished in a short period of time (less than 20 minutes). The current opinion is to utilize chloroprocaine as a top-up for emergency operative delivery in these circumstances. Although one cannot argue that pharmacologically it is the correct approach to use the ester local anesthetic instead of the amide local anesthetic to prevent placental transfer, are we raising a question that is more theoretical than real?

As the use of chloroprocaine continues to be assessed, and we have recent evidence of back pain persisting in the parturient after epidural administration, is it time that a reassessment, as started here by Kuhnert and her associates, be made of the utilization of the amide local anesthetics for emergency delivery? Certainly, the pH adjustment of 2% lidocaine, with or without epinephrine, to provide operative conditions for emergency cesarean delivery would then allow the administration of opioids for postoperative pain relief, which is negated by the use of chloroprocaine. I certainly would not put patient comfort ahead of fetal safety, but it is probably time to assess this pharmacologic dilemma. I hope that the study looking at the utilization of chloroprocaine versus lidocaine for emergency cesarean delivery can be undertaken because of this study by Kuhnert and her associates, which demonstrates that the transient development of an acidotic pH does not increase amide local anesthetic transfer to the fetus.—G.W. Ostheimer, M.D.

Aspiration Pneumonitis Prophylaxis in Obstetric Anaesthesia: Comparison of Effervescent Cimetidine-Sodium Citrate Mixture and Sodium Citrate

Ormezzano X, Francois TP, Viaud J-Y, Bukowski J-G, Bourgeonneau M-C, Cottron D, Ganansia M-F, Gregoire FM, Grinand MR, Wessel PE (Centre Hospitalier de Saint-Nazaire, Nantes, Cholet, d'Angers, and La Roche-sur-Yon, France)
Br J Anaesth 64:503–506, 1990   6–49

Aspiration of gastric contents into the lungs remains the major cause of anesthetic death among obstetric patients. Women with a gastric pH of less than 2.5 are particularly susceptible to aspiration pneumonitis. In a multicenter trial the efficacy of an effervescent cimetidine formulation, given before anesthesia induction to increase the gastric pH in women undergoing cesarean section, was assessed.

A total of 147 women undergoing elective or emergency cesarean section were randomly allocated to 3 groups. Twenty-eight patients received no premedication (group 1), 58 were given 15 mL of a solution containing 1.16 g of sodium citrate (group 2), and 61 received half a Tagamet 800 effervescent tablet containing 400 mg of cimetidine and .9 g of sodium citrate taken with 15 mL water (group 3). All medications were given 10–50 minutes before surgery. Gastric contents were sampled after tracheal intubation and immediately before extubation.

The mean pH immediately after tracheal intubation was 2.25 in the control group, 4.38 in the sodium citrate group, and 5.07 in the cimetidine-sodium citrate group. At extubation the mean pH was 2.83 in the control group, 4.57 in the sodium citrate group, and 5.37 in the cimeti-

The pH Values at Intubation (pH1) and Extubation (pH2), and
Number and Percentages of Patients With pH1 and pH2
Less Than 2.5 in Groups 1 (Control), 2 (Sodium Citrate), and 3
(Cimetidine With Sodium Citrate)

	Group 1 (n = 28)	Group 2 (n = 58)	Group 3 (n = 61)
pH1	2.25 (1.35)***	4.38 (1.44)††	5.07 (1.13)
pH2	2.83 (1.64)***	4.57 (1.51)††	5.37 (1.30)
Patients with			
pH1 $\leqslant$ 2.5	21 (75%)***	8 (13.8%)*	1 (1.6%)
pH2 $\leqslant$ 2.5	14 (50%)†††**	6 (10.3%)	1 (1.6%)

Note: Values are means ±1 SD. *** $P < .001$ compared with other groups at the time control was ended. †††$P < .001$ compared with group 3; **$P < .01$ compared with group 2; ††$P < .01$ compared with group 3; *$P < .05$ compared with group 3.

(Courtesy of Ormezzano X, Francois TP, Viaud J-Y, et al: *Br J Anaesth* 64:503–506, 1990.)

dine-sodium citrate group (table). After intubation, 75% of the controls had a pH of 2.5 or less, compared with 13.8% of patients given sodium citrate solution alone and 1.6% of patients given cimetidine with sodium citrate.

This effervescent cimetidine-sodium citrate combination preparation administered 10–50 minutes before anesthesia induction for planned or emergency cesarean section effectively increases the gastric pH at tracheal intubation and at extubation. It is more effective than sodium citrate solution alone in increasing gastric pH.

▶ Well, we have talked about using sodium citrate with or without cimetidine or another H_2 antagonist for years. Finally, we have evidence that a oral mixture of the 2 drugs does an excellent job in decreasing gastric acidity. I wonder when we will be able to utilize this mixture in the United States.—G.W. Ostheimer, M.D.

Gastro-Oesophageal Reflux in Pregnancy at Term and After Delivery

Vanner RG, Goodman NW (Southmead Hosp, Bristol, England)
Anaesthesia 44:808–811, 1989

6–50

Lower esophageal pH monitoring in pregnant women has shown an increased incidence of gastroesophageal reflux (GER) at term, even in asymptomatic patients. Because GER increases the risk of aspiration pneumonitis, pregnant women who require general anesthesia at term need to be protected against this risk. As it is not known for how long precautions need to be continued after delivery, the incidence of GER at term was compared with that on the second postpartum day.

Lower esophageal pH monitoring was carried out before and on the second day after delivery in 25 pregnant women, 22 of whom had symptoms of GER at term. An electrode mounted in a plastic catheter was in-

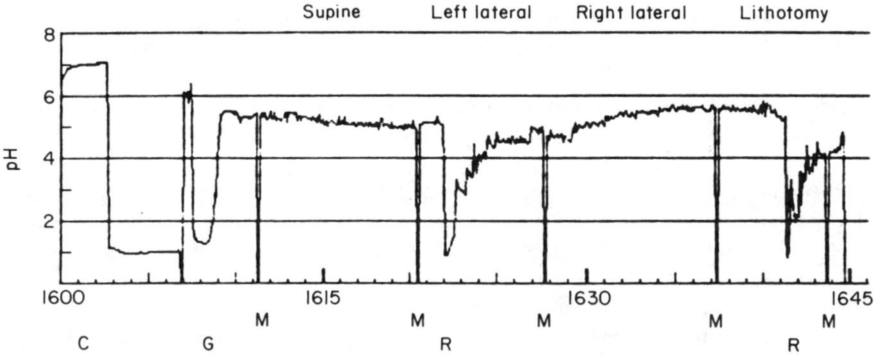

Fig 6–9.—Esophageal pH in a pregnant woman at term. *C,* calibration of the electrode at pH 7 and pH 1; *G,* gastric pH as the electrode is inserted into the stomach before withdrawal to the esophagus; *M,* a marker to indicate changes of position; *R,* clear episodes of GER, esophageal pH is the same as gastric pH. Each reflux episode lasted for about 2 minutes. (Courtesy of Vanner RG, Goodman NW: *Anaesthesia* 44:808–811, 1989.)

verted via an anesthetized nostril and swallowed with 200 mL of water. Reflux was defined as a decrease in pH to below 4. Patients were asked to perform a sequence of maneuvers designed to provoke reflux while in the supine, left lateral, right lateral, and lithotomy positions (Fig 6–9). Esophageal pH was plotted against time during the 45-minute test.

At term, 17 of the 25 women had reflux a total of 29 times. After delivery, 5 women had reflux, each on 1 occasion. The decrease in GER episodes was statistically significant. Three of the 29 reflux episodes at term and 3 of the 5 postpartum episodes lasted for less than 12 seconds, appearing as spikes on the graph (Fig 6–10). Both women who had reflux episodes lasting longer than 12 seconds after delivery had shown more than 1 reflux episode at term. Sixteen of the 29 episodes at term were spontaneous and 13 were provided.

The incidence of GER in pregnant women decreases by the second day after delivery. However, as other factors also contribute to the increased

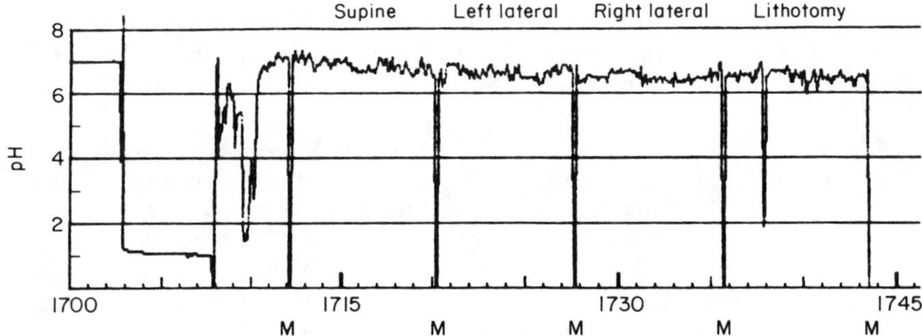

Fig 6–10.—Esophageal pH in a woman after delivery. The sequence of calibration, placement, and the reflux test is as in Fig. 6–9. *M,* a marker to indicate changes of position. A reflux episode occurred in the lithotomy position that lasted for 8 seconds and appears as a spike on the graph. (Courtesy of Vanner RG, Goodman NW: *Anaesthesia* 44:808–811, 1989.)

risk of aspiration pneumonitis, it is still not possible to state with certainty how long precautions should be continued after delivery.

▶ This nicely done study demonstrates that there is a significant decrease in GER by the second day after delivery. However, as the authors state, reflux is only one factor predisposing to regurgitation and aspiration, and it is still necessary to safeguard the recently delivered patient in the postpartum period. At the Brigham and Women's Hospital, we regard the recently delivered parturient to be at risk for regurgitation and aspiration throughout her postpartum stay, which averages approximately 3 days for vaginal delivery and 5–7 days for a patient who has undergone cesarean delivery. Precautions for these patients include the administration of metoclopramide and a clear nonparticulate antacid before induction of anesthesia. Some "at-risk" patients will also receive an H_2 antagonist before the induction of anesthesia, whether it be regional or general.— G.W. Ostheimer, M.D.

Denitrogenation in Pregnancy

Norris MC, Kirkland MR, Torjman MC, Goldberg ME (Thomas Jefferson Univ)
Can J Anaesth 36:523–525, 1989   6–51

A previous comparison of preoxygenation techniques in parturients undergoing rapid-sequence anesthesia induction for cesarean section reported that 3 minutes of tidal breathing of 100% oxygen or 4 deep breaths of 100% oxygen within 30 seconds provided similar increases in arterial oxygen concentration. Pregnancy produces significant changes in the respiratory system that affect the rate and degree of denitrogenation. To better understand how pregnancy affects denitrogenation with both breathing techniques, a Nitralyzer 505 gas meter and vacuum pump were used to continuously measure nitrogen concentrations during the experiments.

Using a circle anesthesia system and 8 L/min^{-1} fresh gas flow, 10 healthy parturients (mean age, 23 years) and 9 healthy nonpregnant women (mean age, 29 years) breathed 100% oxygen for 3 minutes and took 4 deep breaths of 100% oxygen within 30 seconds. The women breathed room air for at least 25 minutes between trials. Three of the parturients smoked cigarettes; none of the healthy controls was a smoker.

The parturient women achieved 95% denitrogenation significantly faster than the nonpregnant controls. Nonpregnant women required 110.8 seconds to reach 5% expired nitrogen, whereas parturients required only 54.5 seconds. In the parturients, tidal breathing for 3 minutes lowered the mean expired nitrogen concentration to 1%, whereas 4 deep breaths lowered it to 5%. This difference was statistically significant. However, the difference between the 2 techniques amounted to only a 56 mL increase in lung oxygen stores that provided only an extra 10–15 seconds of protection against hypoxemia. The difference was therefore not clinically significant. Both breathing techniques provide adequate denitrogenation and protection against apneic hypoxemia in normal parturients undergoing rapid sequence anesthesia induction before cesarean section.

▶ A number of studies in recent years have demonstrated that 3 minutes of tidal breathing of 100% oxygen or 4 deep breaths of 100% oxygen provide similar increases in Pao_2 before induction of general anesthesia in parturients. This study substantiates the previous findings. I am delighted that we are finally calling the technique exactly what it is; that is, we are not speaking of preoxygenation, which would mean *before* oxygenation, but of *denitrogenation,* which is the correct physiologic term. Let's hope that the correct terminology will now be used throughout the anesthetic literature.—G.W. Ostheimer, M.D.

Effects of Oral Caffeine on Postdural Puncture Headache: A Double-Blind, Placebo-Controlled Trial
Camann WR, Murray RS, Mushlin PS, Lambert DH (Brigham and Women's Hosp, Boston; Harvard Med School)
Anesth Analg 70:181–184, 1990   6–52

Previous studies have shown that intravenously administered caffeine effectively relieves postdural puncture headache (PDPH). In a double-blind, randomized study the use of orally administered caffeine was investigated in 40 women with postpartum PDPH. Twenty patients (mean age, 30 years) were given a capsule containing 300 mg of anhydrous caffeine powder USP and 20 women (mean age, 31 years) received a placebo capsule.

A visual analogue scale (VAS) was used to score headache severity at baseline and at 4 hours and 24 hours after ingestion of the capsule. If headaches failed to resolve within 4 hours, patients were instructed to rest, increase their fluid consumption, and take analgesics. An epidural blood patch was made available to patients with persistent PDPH.

At 4 hours after capsule ingestion 18 caffeine-treated patients and 12 placebo-treated patients had improved VAS scores. The mean VAS score at 4 hours was 33 in the caffeine-treated group and 49 in the placebo-treated group. Moreover, the magnitude of decrease in the VAS was more than 300% greater in the caffeine-treated group. At 24 hours there was no longer any difference in VAS scores between the groups. Thirty percent of the caffeine-treated patients had higher VAS scores at 24 hours than at 4 hours. Headache did not recur in 70% of the caffeine-treated patients. Although fewer epidural blood patches were required in the caffeine group, the difference did not reach statistical significance. One patient in each group complained of mild, transient flushing and jitteriness after taking the capsule.

Caffeine Content of Common Substances	
Substance	Caffeine content (mg)
Coffee*	
Freeze-dried	66
Percolator	107
Drip grind	142
Tea*	
Black	
1-min brew	28
5-min brew	47
Green	
1-min brew	15
5-min brew	32
Cocoa*	13
Coca-Cola †	65
Pepsi-Cola	43
Dr. Pepper	61
Mountain Dew	55
Jolt Cola	71
Chocolate candy bar (1.2 oz)	5
No Doz‡(Bristol-Myers)	100
Vivarin‡(Beecham)	200

*Coffee, tea, and cocoa measured as 5-oz (150 mL) cup.
†Cola beverages as 12-oz can.
‡Per tablet.
(Courtesy of Camann WR, Murray RS, Mushlin PS, et al: *Anesth Analg* 70:181–184, 1990.)

A single, oral dose of 300 mg of caffeine rapidly relieves PDPH. Although caffeine is widely available in many beverages and over-the-counter preparations (table), a pharmaceutical caffeine preparation provides a more exact caffeine dose in the treatment of PDPH.

▶ What would you rather do: Drink 3 cups of coffee, 5 cokes, or take 1 capsule to help relieve your PDPH? I guess I have always felt that I was rehydrating the postpartum patient as well as giving caffeine to help relieve her PDPH. It would be interesting to do a much larger study and see if the incidence of epidural blood patch was significantly reduced in patients with PDPH in a caffeine versus placebo group.

My therapy for PDPH is increased hydration, either intravenously or orally, as well as caffeine (usually in the oral form), a nonsteroidal anti-inflammatory drug, and reassurance. Ibuprofen is approved by the American Academy of Pediatrics as a postpartum analgesic in nursing mothers. After 24 hours of this conservative management and with little or no improvement, I will discuss the possibility of administering an epidural blood patch. Often, the postpartum patient prefers to wait and see what another 24 hours will bring while maintaining conservative therapy. If there is no further improvement at 48 hours after onset of the headache, I will administer an epidural blood patch unless the patient wants an additional trial of conservative therapy. I have no problem in sending the patient home and then having her return to do an epidural blood patch in an outpatient setting.— G.W. Ostheimer, M.D.

Effect of Epinephrine on Intrathecal Fentanyl Analgesia in Patients Undergoing Postpartum Tubal Ligation

Malinow AM, Mokriski BLK, Nomura MK, Kaufman MA, Snell JA, Sharp GD, Howard RA (Univ of Maryland; Univ of Maryland Hosp)
Anesthesiology 73:381–385, 1990   6–53

Eighty women who received spinal anesthesia for postpartum tubal ligation entered a double-blind study of the effects of epinephrine on postoperative analgesia induced by intrathecal fentanyl. In addition to 70 mg of hyperbaric lidocaine, patients received .2 mg of epinephrine or 10 μg of fentanyl, both epinephrine and fentanyl, or saline.

The peak rostral level of sensory anesthesia and the time to peak anesthesia were similar in all groups. Pain was delayed only in patients given both fentanyl and epinephrine (Fig 6–11). Three of these patients and 1 who was given saline requested no analgesia for 24 hours after surgery. Narcotic requirements over 24 hours did not differ among the various groups (table). Pruritus was more frequent in patients given fentanyl alone.

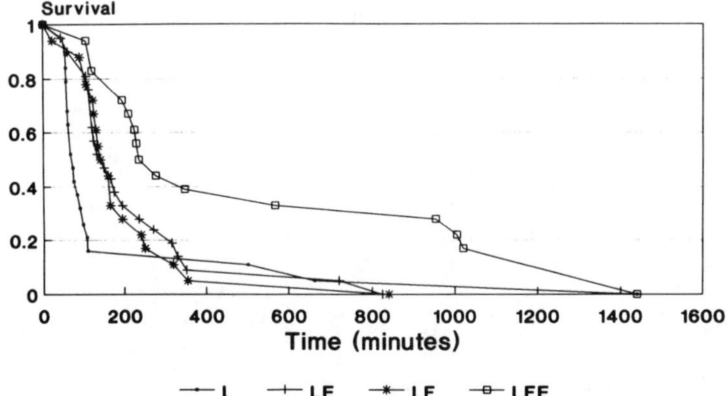

Fig 6–11.—Kaplan-Meier survival curves showing duration of effective analgesia for patients who received saline (L), epinephrine plus saline (LE), fentanyl plus saline (LF), or fentanyl plus epinephrine (LFE). Survival is proportion of each study group not yet requesting supplemental analgesia as function of time. Time zero is intrathecal injection of study drug. Time to first request for supplemental analgesia for LFE is different from other 3. (Courtesy of Malinow AM, Mokriski BLK, Nomura MK, et al: *Anesthesiology* 73:381–385, 1990.)

Characteristics of Analgesia

	L (n = 19)	LE (n = 21)	LF (n = 19)	LFE (n = 18)	Significance
Duration of pain score = 0 (min)	65 ± 36	76 ± 32	85 ± 44	137 ± 47*	$P < 0.0005$
Time to first request for supplemental analgesia (min)	198 ± 342	227 ± 201	203 ± 178	562 ± 504*	$P < 0.005$
Range	(48–1440)	(44–825)	(23–840)	(105–1440)	
Quantiles	(60, 73, 107)	(120, 150, 270)	(123, 150, 240)	(195, 255, 1005)	
24-h opioid requirements (mg morphine equiv.)	10 ± 8	8 ± 4	10 ± 7	8 ± 13	NS

Abbreviation: NS, no significant difference among patient groups.
*Different as compared to all other patient groups.
(Courtesy of Malinow AM, Mokriski BLK, Nomura MK, et al: *Anesthesiology* 73:381–385, 1990.)

Intrathecal administration of epinephrine plus fentanyl prolongs analgesia after postpartum tubal ligation in patients who receive subarachnoid anesthesia with hyperbaric lidocaine. Recovery of sensory and motor function is moderately prolonged. Epinephrine also makes pruritus less prevalent. The finding that the addition of 10 μg of fentanyl did not prolong postoperative analgesia raises the question of altered sensitivity of the parturient to subarachnoid opioids.

▶ The interesting finding from this investigation is that 10 μg of fentanyl without epinephrine did not prolong postoperative pain relief. The question that needs to be answered is whether there is altered sensitivity to subarachnoid opioids in the parturient that changes in the immediate postpartum period. A well-done dose response study should be able to provide the answer to that question.—G.W. Ostheimer, M.D.

Obstetrical Pulmonary Embolism Mortality, United States, 1970–85

Franks AL, Atrash HK, Lawson HW, Colberg KS (Ctrs for Disease Control, Atlanta)
Am J Public Health 80:720–722, 1990   6–54

It is not clear whether pulmonary embolism is becoming a more prominent cause of maternal deaths. Vital records data for 1970 to 1985 were reviewed, and it was found that for both whites and blacks the number of deaths from obstetric pulmonary embolism per 100,000 live births fell by 50% during this period (Fig 6–12). Black women remained at a greater than 2.5-fold higher risk, however, and black and white women aged 40 years and older had a tenfold higher risk of death from obstetric pulmonary embolism (Fig 6–13).

Although the risk of death from obstetric pulmonary embolism has declined overall, some groups remain at relatively high risk. It may be fea-

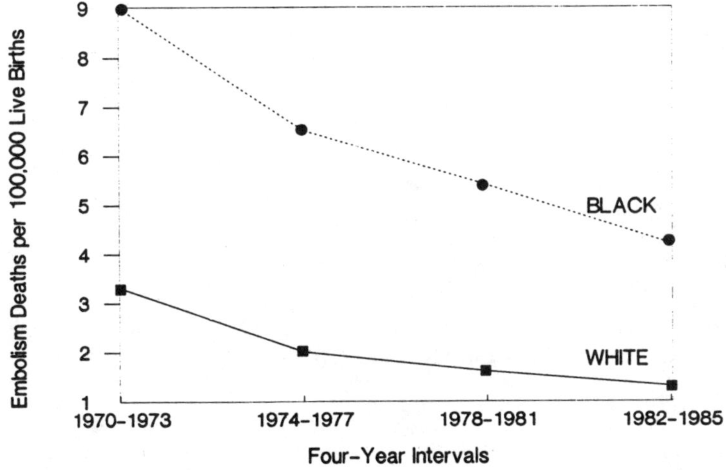

Fig 6–12.—Obstetric pulmonary embolism deaths per 100,000 live births, United States, 1970–1985, standardized to age distribution of live births to white women in this period. (Courtesy of Franks AL, Atrash HK, Lawson HW, et al: *Am J Public Health* 80:720–722, 1990.)

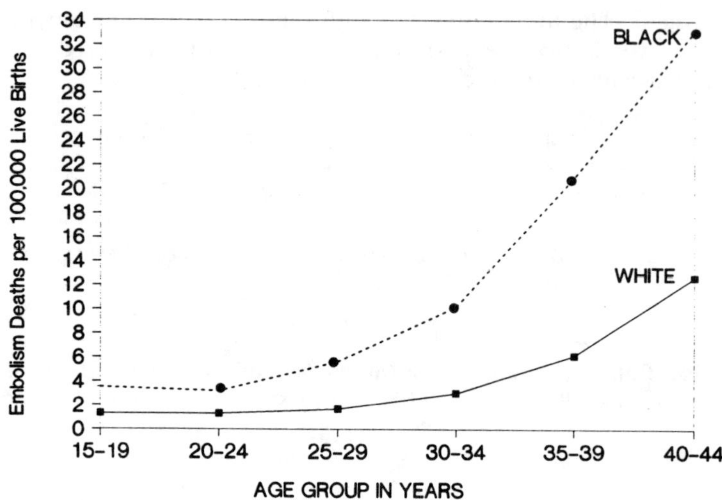

Fig 6–13.—Obstetric pulmonary embolism deaths by age and race, United States, 1970–1985. (Courtesy of Franks AL, Atrash HK, Lawson HW, et al: *Am J Public Health* 80:720–722, 1990.)

sible to implement and evaluate interventions such as the prophylactic use of pressure gradient stockings or anticoagulation in those at highest risk.

▶ Interesting observations.—G.W. Ostheimer, M.D.

Additional Reading

The following were presentations to a recent symposium on obstetric anesthesia.

Westmore MD: Epidural opioids in obstetrics: A review. *Anaesth Intensive Care* 18:292, 1990.

Brownridge P: Epidural medication after the initial dose: Reflections on current methods of administration during labour. *Anaesth Intensive Care* 18:300, 1990.

Crowhurst JA, Burgess RW, Derham RJ: Monitoring epidural analgesia in the parturient. *Anaeth Intensive Care* 18:308, 1990.

Paull JD: The place of caudal anaesthesia in obstetrics. *Anaesth Intensive Care* 18:313, 1990.

Sage DJ: Epidurals, spinals, and bleeding disorders in pregnancy: A review. *Anaesth Intensive Care* 18:319, 1990.

Lah F: Anaesthesia and the sick foetus. *Anaesth Intensive Care* 18:327, 1990.

Hewett E, Livingstone P: Management of failed endotracheal intubation at caesarean section. *Anaesth Intensive Care* 18:330, 1990.

Gatt S: Haematological disorders responsible for maternal bleeding in late pregnancy. *Anaesth Intensive Care* 18:335, 1990.

Roy RN, Betheras FR: The Melbourne chart: A logical guide to neonatal resuscitation. *Anaesth Intensive Care* 18:348, 1990.

Kliman L: Drug dependence and pregnancy, antenatal and intrapartum problems. *Anaesth Intensive Care* 18:358, 1990.

Obstetrics—Cesarean Section

The Effect on Uteroplacental Blood Flow of Epidural Anaesthesia Containing Adrenaline for Caesarean Section

Skjöldebrand A, Eklund J, Lunell N-O, Nylund L, Sarby B, Thornström S (Karolinska Inst at Huddinge Univ Hosp, Stockholm)
Acta Anaesthesiol Scand 34:85–89, 1990   6–55

Epinephrine is commonly added to anesthetic solutions used in epidural anesthesia (EDA). However, there is controversy over the safety of epinephrine in EDA for cesarean section because studies of the effect on uteroplacental blood flow (PBF) are inconclusive. Dynamic placental scintigraphy was used before and during EDA to examine the effect of epinephrine on PBF in 10 healthy women scheduled for elective cesarean section.

Scintigraphy was performed after intravenous injection of ^{113m}In. This radiopharmaceutical is bound to transferrin and does not cross the placental barrier. Preload infusion with a balanced electrolyte solution, 10 mL/kg, was initiated after injection of ^{113m}In. Bupivacaine, 5 mg/mL, with epinephrine, 2.5 µg/mL, was used in all 10 women. The total anesthetic dose ranged from 18 mL to 22 mL, adjusted for patient height. The mean blood pressure and pulse rate were determined every 5 minutes.

Nine of the 10 women had a decrease in PBF (table). The median decrease in total maternal PBF was 34%, which was statistically significant. The mean maternal blood pressure decreased by 3 mm Hg, also a statistically significant difference. The decrease in PBF was significantly negatively correlated with the decrease in mean blood pressure. The mean pulse rate increased significantly by 19 beats per minute. However, the change in pulse rate did not correlate with the change in PBF. The fetal heart rate was within normal range and was not affected by the EDA. Apgar scores at 1 minute and 5 minutes were normal. The median umbilical artery pH was 7.29. There was no correlation between the pH and blood flow index, or between the pH and the change in that index. Epinephrine, 2.5 µg/mL, in doses up to 45–55 µg, added to bupivacaine, 5 mg/mL, in EDA for cesarean section, when combined with a preload infusion of a balanced electrolyte solution, 10 mL/kg, reduces the total PBF.

Uteroplacental Blood Flow Measured by Placental Scintigraphy During Epidural Anaesthesia for Cesarean Section

Skjöldebrand A, Eklund J, Johansson H, Lunell N-O, Nylund L, Sarby B, Thornström S (Karolinska Inst at Huddinge Univ Hosp, Stockholm)
Acta Anaesthesiol Scand 34:79–84, 1990   6–56

Although epidural anesthesia (EDA) is commonly used in cesarean section, little is known about its effect on uteroplacental blood flow (PBF). A scintigraphic technique using intravenously injected ^{113m}In and a com-

Mean Blood Pressure, Pulse Rate, and Uteroplacental Blood Flow Indices of 10 Women Before and During Extradural Anesthesia (EDA) for Cesarean Section

Patient number	Mean blood pressure (mmHg) (kPa)			Maternal pulse rate (beats/min)			Uteroplacental blood flow index		
	Before EDA	During EDA	Change	Before EDA	During EDA	Change	Before EDA	During EDA	Change %
1	—	—	—	80	120	+40	93	63	−33
2	102 (13.6)	100 (13.3)	−2 (−0.3)	96	124	+28	100	63	−36
3	103 (13.7)	92 (12.3)	−11 (−1.5)	92	92	± 0	51	41	−19
4	100 (13.3)	87 (11.6)	−13 (−1.7)	78	88	+10	32	44	+39
5	103 (13.7)	100 (13.3)	−3 (−0.4)	70	104	+34	97	51	−48
6	93 (12.4)	87 (11.6)	−6 (−0.8)	80	90	+10	178	100	−44
7	103 (13.7)	85 (11.3)	−18 (−2.4)	80	90	+10	97	73	−25
8	77 (10.3)	74 (9.9)	−3 (−0.4)	84	74	−10	184	55	−70
9	98 (13.1)	103 (13.7)	+5 (+0.6)	76	120	+44	160	39	−76
10	93 (12.4)	92 (12.3)	−1 (−0.1)	90	120	+30	153	105	−31
Median	100 (13.3)	92 (12.3)	−3 (−0.4)	80	98	+19	98	59	−34
			($P < 0.05$)			($P < 0.05$)			($P < 0.01$)

Note: The statistical comparisons between the values before and during epidural anesthesia were performed with Wilcoxon's paired rank sum test. (Courtesy of Skjöldebrand A, Eklund J, Lunell N-O, et al: *Acta Anaesthesiol Scand* 34:85–89, 1990.)

puter-linked gamma camera was validated in animal experiments. Subsequently, the PBF was measured before and during EDA with the dynamic placental scintigraphy technique in 11 healthy women aged 24–39 years who were undergoing elective cesarean section. The women were given

Uteroplacental Blood Flow Indices and Mean Blood Pressures and Pulse Rates Before and During Epidural Anesthesia

Patient	Utero-placental blood flow index		Change of index (per cent)	Mean blood pressure (mmHg) (kPa)			Pulse rate (beats/min)		
	Before EDA	After EDA		Before EDA	After EDA	Change	Before EDA	After EDA	Change
1	96	50	−48	97 (12.9)	93 (12.4)	−4 (−0.5)	68	82	+14
2	81	40	−51	87 (11.6)	60 (8.0)	−27 (−3.6)	72	72	±0
3	88	68	−23	103 (13.7)	90 (12.0)	−13 (−1.7)	100	96	−4
4	88	54	−39	103 (13.7)	100 (13.3)	−3 (−0.4)	84	84	±0
5	267	119	−55	103 (13.7)	100 (13.3)	−3 (−0.4)	82	88	+6
6	125	164	+31	88 (11.7)	88 (11.7)	±0 (±0.0)	64	70	+6
7	96	89	−7	100 (13.3)	88 (11.7)	−12 (−1.6)	76	82	+6
8	55	87	+58	87 (11.6)	93 (12.4)	+7 (+0.8)	84	130	+46
9	39	51	+31	90 (12.0)	87 (11.6)	−3 (−0.4)	88	80	−8
10	119	94	−21	97 (12.9)	93 (12.4)	−4 (−0.5)	84	86	+2
11	65	54	−17	88 (11.7)	90 (12.0)	+2 (+0.3)	72	92	+20
Median	88	68	−21	97 (12.9)	90 (12.0)	−3 (−0.4)	82	84	+6

Note: The decrease in mean blood pressure was significant ($P < .05$).
(Courtesy of Skjöldebrand A, Eklund J, Johansson H, et al: *Acta Anaesthesiol Scand* 34:79–84, 1990.)

18–22 mL of bupivacaine .5% without epinephrine as the anesthetic, and all received a preload intravenous infusion of balanced electrolyte solution at a dose of 10 mL/kg.

Blood volume is a crucial factor when repeated dynamic scintigraphic blood flow measurements are compared. To determine to what extent rapid intravenous crystalloid infusion affects blood volume, hemoglobin concentrations were measured before and after the preload infusion in another 13 women who were similarly delivered by cesarean section during EDA.

Changes in PBF before and during EDA varied greatly. Uteroplacental blood flow decreased in 8 women and increased in 3 (table). The median decrease in PBF was 21%, but the difference was not statistically significant. The mean blood volume increased by 12% after preload crystalloid infusion. There was a small, but significant, decrease in the mean blood pressure but no significant change in pulse rate between first and second scintigraphic measurements. Uteroplacental blood flow did not correlate with mean blood pressure either before or after EDA. The level of anesthesia did not correlate with the change in PBF. Fetal heart rates before and after PBF measurements were normal. The effect of EDA on PBF in women undergoing cesarean section is unpredictable.

▶ Just when we thought we were beginning to understand PBF from a variety of studies, these 2 articles point out its unpredictability of after epidural anesthesia and demonstrate that there appears to be no correlation between maternal blood pressure and PBF. Clearly, this technique (Abstract 6–56) is different from the ^{133}Xe technique used by Rekonen et al. (1), which looked at a flow per unit volume over a small area of the placenta; the present study looks at total PBF flow. I, for one, am confused about which technique is more valid.

In the second study looking at PBF during epidural anesthesia using bupivacaine with epinephrine (Abstract 6–55), 9 of the 10 parturients investigated had a decrease in PBF. Again, the question is raised about the adverse effect of epinephrine on PBF. Even with this decrease in PBF, the fetal heart rate remained within normal ranges and the Apgar scores at 1 minute and 5 minutes were normal, as was the umbilical artery pH. The impression of the investigators that the addition of epinephrine seems to maintain maternal blood pressure at the expense of PBF is interesting.

It is increasingly evident that the addition of subarachnoid opioid to the local anesthetic mixture will intensify the anesthetic for the operative procedure. The next logical step in these studies would be to evaluate a solution of lidocaine plain vs. lidocaine plus opioid vs. lidocaine plus epinephrine. The results of this proposed study may have far-reaching effects on our practice of epidural anesthesia for cesarean delivery. I would also hope that the authors would expand their investigations to the utilization of spinal and general anesthesia.—G.W. Ostheimer, M.D.

Incidence of Electrocardiographic Changes During Cesarean Delivery Under Regional Anesthesia

Palmer CM, Norris MC, Giudici MC, Leighton BL, DeSimone CA (Thomas Jefferson Univ Hosp, Philadelphia)
Anesth Analg 70:36–43, 1990

6–57

Parturient women undergoing cesarean delivery under regional anesthesia often complain of chest pain and dyspnea. The cause of these symptoms has not been identified. Because of the similarity between these complaints and the classic symptoms of myocardial ischemia, a study was conducted to determine the incidence of ECG changes during nonemergent cesarean delivery.

Serial ECGs were obtained on 93 healthy ASA physical status I and II term parturient women aged 19–43 years who were undergoing nonemergent cesarean delivery under spinal or epidural anesthesia. Seven leads were recorded at predetermined intervals, including after anesthesia induction, skin incision, hysterotomy, delivery, 4 minutes after delivery, 8 minutes after delivery, and skin closure. Baseline preoperative 12-lead ECGs had been obtained as part of the routine preoperative laboratory evaluation and were therefore not repeated. Complaints by patients were recorded concurrently. All tracings were interpreted by a cardiologist.

Electrocardiographic changes occurred in 44 of the 93 women. In 35 of these women the changes were interpreted as characteristic or suggestive of myocardial ischemia (Fig 6–14). Fifteen women complained of chest pain, pressure, and dyspnea concurrent with the ECG changes. None of the women without ECG changes reported symptoms of chest pain, pressure, or dyspnea. The association between symptoms and ECG changes was statistically significant. Electrocardiographic changes and symptoms were transient, as symptoms resolved and ECGs returned to baseline by the end of the delivery in all patients. Women with ECG changes were likely to have slightly higher heart rates and lower systolic and diastolic arterial pressures than those without ECG changes. Although the differences were slight, they reached statistical significance.

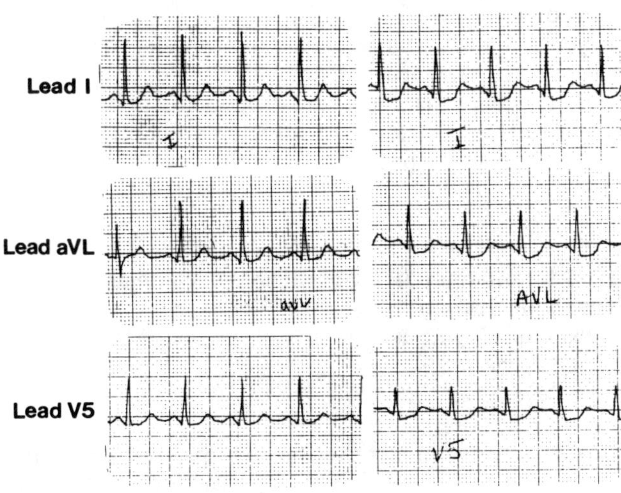

post–induction　　　　**4 min. post–delivery**

Fig 6–14.—Representative examples of the type of ECG changes observed. Patient 2 had ST-T elevation in leads I, aV_L, and V_5 after delivery; patients 12, 46, and 60 had ST-T depression of varying degrees in leads I, aV_L, and V_5 after delivery. (Courtesy of Palmer CM, Norris MC, Giudici MC, et al: *Anesth Analg* 70:36–43, 1990.)

These findings suggest that myocardial ischemia is a likely cause of the ECG changes and symptoms of chest pain and dyspnea that sometimes occur in parturient women undergoing cesarean delivery under regional anesthesia.

▶ The authors speculate that myocardial ischemia is a likely cause of both the ECG changes seen in the patients described and those symptoms of chest pain and dyspnea that patients sometimes experience during cesarean delivery. I respect the investigators observations and their opinions, but I think the overwhelming weight of evidence is that the signs of chest pain and dyspnea appear to be related to various emboli (air, most likely) that can occur during cesarean delivery. I have personally seen ST depression associated with a rapid heart rate (more than 140 beats per minute) secondary to persistent hypotension and aggressive management with intravenous ephedrine. I suspect that the ephedrine has "flogged" the heart sufficiently to produce myocardial ischemia.

It is unfortunate that the investigators did not correlate the ECG changes with Doppler findings, because I suspect that most of their findings would occur coincident with Doppler changes signifying various types of emboli, but the most probable would be air emboli. The investigators were not able to correlate the administration of ephedrine with subsequent ST changes to see if there is a causal relationship between the administration of ephedrine and myocardial ischemia with ST segment depression when the heart is stimulated to its maximum. This occurrence may give added impetus to reconsider the status of phenylephrine to treat acute hypotension during regional anesthesia for cesarean delivery. The prevailing evidence to date suggests that aggressive management during hypotension with phenylephrine until the baby's delivery does not cause any adverse effects on the newborn. However, one is reminded that long-term administration may have a significant effect on uteroplacental perfusion, and caution in that regard is advised. I wonder how many readers have noted ST depression with a very rapid heart rate during cesarean delivery occurring either spontaneously or in response to intravenous ephedrine.—G.W. Ostheimer, M.D.

A Double-Blind Comparison of Epidural Bupivacaine and Bupivacaine-Fentanyl for Caesarean Section

Paech MJ, Westmore MD, Speirs HM (King Edward Mem Hosp for Women, Perth, Western Australia)
Anaesth Intens Care 18:22–30, 1990

6–58

The quality of sensory anesthesia during epidural cesarean section using lidocaine 2% with epinephrine, or bupivacaine .5%, with or without epinephrine, is enhanced by the addition of fentanyl. However, studies of the effect of fentanyl addition on other characteristics of the epidural block and on maternal side effects have been inconclusive. Furthermore, the neonatal effect of fentanyl has not been determined. A randomized, double-blind, controlled study was done to assess the quality of intraop-

Characteristics of Epidural Anesthesia

	Fentanyl (n = 27)	Saline (n = 27)
Maximum intraoperative pain (0-100)	*6 (9)	21 (24)
Range	0-38	0-74
Zero pain score (no.)	12 (44%)	8 (30%)
Onset of sensory anaesthesia (min)	31 (15)	31 (7)
Duration of sensory anaesthesia (min)	314 (71)	319 (122)
Sensory anaesthesia at S_1		
— partial (no.)	19 (70%)	16 (59%)
— complete (no.)	8 (30%)	11 (41%)
Duration of motor block (min)	238 (83)	269 (124)

*$P = .004$.
†Standard deviation or percentage in parentheses.
(Courtesy of Paech MJ, Westmore MD, Speirs HM: *Anaesth Intens Care* 18:22–30, 1990.)

erative analgesia, the effect on all characteristics of the epidural block, and the effect on neonatal outcome when fentanyl was added to bupivacaine .5%.

Of 54 healthy women undergoing elective cesarean section, 27 were given 20 mL of bupivacaine .5% with 2 mL solution containing 100 μg of fentanyl, and 27 received 20 mL of bupivacaine .5% with 2 mL saline solution. All women received similar preoperative doses of ranitidine, sodium citrate, metoclopramide, and warmed crystalloid solution. The quality of intraoperative analgesia was assessed by the anesthetist and the patient. Patient characteristics were similar for both groups.

Onset of epidural sensory anesthesia and its subsequent duration were similar in both groups. However, 81% of the patients in the fentanyl-treated group had excellent intraoperative analgesia compared with 48% of the controls (table). The difference was statistically significant. The incidence and severity of maternal side effects were similar for both groups, and there was no significant difference for any specific side effect. Other characteristics of epidural anesthesia were unaltered by the addition of fentanyl, nor was neonatal outcome affected. The addition of 100 μg of fentanyl to .5% bupivacaine for epidural cesarean section is a valuable clinical maneuver because it significantly improves the quality and reliability of intraoperative analgesia without producing significant maternal side effects or causing adverse neonatal effects.

▶ This study demonstrates that the addition of fentanyl, 100 μg, to .5% bupivacaine for epidural anesthesia for cesarean delivery improves the quality and reliability of intraoperative pain relief without producing adverse maternal or neonatal side effects and should be an impetus to the investigators mentioned previously to evaluate uteroplacental blood flow using this technique.

When .75% bupivacaine was no longer recommended for cesarean delivery, we used .5% bupivacaine in doses similar to those of .75% bupivacaine that had been used. This would equate 30 mL of .5% bupivacaine with 20 mL of .75% bupivacaine. Our patients for cesarean deliveries and our anesthesiologists were unimpressed by the analgesia/anesthesia provided by .5% bupivacaine even though the amount of drug used was similar to that of .75% bupivacaine. After a trial we discontinued the use of .5% bupivacaine in our institution because it was inadequate for cesarean delivery. Now there are a number of reasons why the pain stimulus may be different in our patient population, including exteriorization of the uterus after delivery for surgical closure. Otherwise, I wonder if there is a difference in pain perception between other individuals and parturients in the United States in whom .5% bupivacaine alone is not looked upon as adequate for cesarean delivery. Clearly, in this study, 81% of the patients who received bupivacaine-fentanyl had an excellent intraoperative course compared to 48% of the patients in the control groups. Is it possible that we have been giving patients inadequate intraoperative anesthesia because of the unavailability of appropriate solutions? Certainly, 2% lidocaine with and without epinephrine should be available worldwide for operative procedures. Perhaps the place of epidural fentanyl is in intensifying the intraoperative anesthesia for cesarean delivery and not for postoperative analgesia.

Finally, studies evaluating uteroplacental blood flow with bupivacaine and fentanyl must be done and compared with 2% lidocaine, with and without fentanyl and with and without epinephrine.—G.W. Ostheimer, M.D.

Does Ephedrine Influence Newborn Neurobehavioral Responses and Spectral EEG When Used to Prevent Maternal Hypotension During Caesarean Section?

Kangas-Saarela T, Hollmén AI, Tolonen U, Eskelinen P, Alahuhta S, Jouppila R, Kivelä A, Huttunen P (Univ of Oulu, Finland)
Acta Anaesthesiol Scand 34:8–16, 1990   6–59

Maternal hypotension is a frequent complication of spinal anesthesia for cesarean section. Ephedrine is commonly used to prevent or treat maternal hypotension. Maternal ephedrine administration stimulates the neonatal CNS. Whether small doses of ephedrine given to the mother affect the neonatal spectral electroencephalogram (EEG), and whether such EEG changes are reflected in neurobehavioral testing, were determined in 16 infants delivered by elective cesarean section with spinal anesthesia.

Eight women were given intravenous ephedrine in 10-mg increments as soon as any fall in systolic blood pressure from baseline was noted. In the other 8 women hypotension was prevented with a large preload of Ringer's solution at a dose of 20 mL/kg. Scanlon's neurobehavioral tests were performed on all neonates at ages 3 hours and 1, 2, and 4–5 days. Electroencephalographic signals were recorded from age 30 minutes to 150 minutes, and again 24 hours later.

All infants were healthy and free from gross abnormalities. Neurobehavioral testing showed no differences between infants of either group. The spectral EEG showed significant differences between the 2 groups, but only during the first 2 hours after delivery. At age 24 hours none of the recorded spectral EEG parameters showed any significant differences between the groups.

When used to prevent maternal hypotension during spinal anesthesia for cesarean section, ephedrine did not affect neurobehavioral testing in neonates. The spectral EEG did show evidence of significant subclinical differences, but only within the first few hours after delivery.

▶ I am not sure what the difference in the spectral EEG at 2 hours after delivery in the ephedrine-treated group means. However, I am sure that there will be increasing investigations using a variety of CNS evaluations in all phases of obstetric anesthesia in the future.—G.W. Ostheimer, M.D.

Are Doppler-Detected Venous Emboli During Cesarean Section Air Emboli?

Fong J, Gadalla F, Pierri MK, Druzin M (New York Hosp:Cornell Univ Med Ctr; Mem Sloan Kettering Inst, New York)
Anesth Analg 71:254–257, 1990   6–60

It has been assumed that the venous emboli detected by precordial ultrasonic Doppler monitoring during section delivery are air emboli, but amniotic fluid embolism is also a possibility, as is thromboembolism. Intraoperative Doppler monitoring and precordial 2-dimensional echocardiography were performed in 50 parturients in ASA physical status I or II who were having cesarean section under lumbar epidural or general anesthesia.

In the 49 evaluable patients there was excellent correlation between embolic events detected by Doppler monitoring and those detected by echocardiography. Venous emboli occurred in 26% of patients (11 of 42) during epidural anesthesia and 42% of patients (3 of 7) during general anesthesia. Embolism sometimes occurred more than once during surgery. It did not correlate with chest pain, dyspnea, oxygen desaturation, or premature ventricular contractions. Embolism was not more frequent when the placenta was manually removed or when the uterus was exteriorized for hysterotomy repair. Doppler-detected venous emboli in women having cesarean section appear to be air emboli, based on their echocardiographic appearance.

▶ My compliments to the authors for confirming what our group has believed for several years.—G.W. Ostheimer, M.D.

The Effect of Continuous Epidural Analgesia on Cesarean Section for Dystocia in Nulliparous Women

Thorp JA, Parisi VM, Boylan PC, Johnston DA (Univ of Texas, Houston; MD Anderson Cancer Ctr, Houston)
Am J Obstet Gynecol 161:670–675, 1989   6–61

The rate of cesarean section for dystocia in nulliparous women can be considered epidemic. Because only few women will deliver vaginally after cesarean section, the increase in cesarean section for dystocia in nulliparous women is the single most important factor responsible for the current cesarean epidemic. The use of epidural labor analgesia has increased similarly in recent years. However, the effects of epidural analgesia on cesarean section rates have not been well studied. To assess the effects of epidural labor analgesia on the incidence of cesarean section for dystocia in nulliparous women, 711 nulliparous women with cephalic fetal presentations, singleton gestations, and spontaneous onset of labor were studied.

Of the women, 142 were given no analgesia in labor, 122 were given narcotic analgesia only, 378 had epidural analgesia only, and 69 had epidural plus narcotic analgesia. Thus 447 women received only epidural or epidural plus narcotic analgesia and 264 women received either no analgesia or narcotic analgesia only. The 2 groups had similar ages, gestational weeks, and racial backgrounds.

Cesarean section for dystocia was performed in 3.5% of the women who had no analgesia, 4% of those who had narcotic analgesia only, 10% who had epidural analgesia, and 10% who had epidural plus narcotic analgesia (table). After controlling for potentially confounding variables, the incidence of cesarean section for dystocia was 10% in the epidural group and almost 4% in the nonepidural group. This difference was statistically significant. Both groups had similar frequencies of cesarean section for fetal distress, similar cord arterial and venous blood gas parameters, and similar proportions of low 5-minute Apgar scores and low cord pH values. Although the role of selection bias cannot be excluded from this nonrandomized study, these data strongly suggest that epidural analgesia in labor increases the incidence of cesarean section for dystocia in nulliparous women.

▶ I included this study by obstetricians concerning the effect of continuous epidural analgesia on cesarean section for dystocia in nulliparous women for the benefit of anesthesiologists who do not frequently read the obstetric literature. As the authors state in their discussion, the role of selection bias cannot be excluded from this nonrandomized study. Also, there is no anesthesiologist involved in the group of investigators to analyze the data from the standpoint of an anesthesiologist. Currently, there are studies of randomized patients that may give us a little more insight into whether continuous epidural analgesia actually does increase the cesarean delivery rate in nulliparous women.—G.W. Ostheimer, M.D.

Comparison of Analgesia Subgroups

	No analgesia	*Narcotic analgesia*	*Epidural analgesia*	*Epidural and narcotic analgesia*
Cesarean section for dystocia*	3.5% (5/142)	4.1% (5/122)	10.3% (39/378)	10.1% (7/69)
Cesarean section for dystocia,† birth weight < 4000 gm	3.0% (4/135)	2.6% (3/117)	9.4% (32/342)	6.7% (4/60)
Birth weight‡ (gm)	3272 ± 450	3237 ± 464	3392 ± 465	3448 ± 472

Note: All values are expressed as proportions or mean ± SD.

*A χ^2 analysis demonstrates a significant difference between the following subgroups: no analgesia vs. epidural; no analgesia vs. epidural and narcotic; narcotic vs. epidural; narcotic vs. epidural and narcotic ($P < .05$).

†A χ^2 analysis demonstrates a significant difference between the following subgroups: no analgesia vs. epidural narcotic vs. epidural ($P < .05$).

‡Analysis of variance and Scheffé test show a significant difference in birth weight between the following subgroups: narcotic vs. epidural ($P = .03$); narcotic vs. epidural and narcotic ($P = .02$). No difference in birth weight was noted between the no analgesia vs. the epidural subgroups, yet there was a significant increase in cesarean section for dystocia between these subgroups ($P < .01$).

(Courtesy of Thorp JA, Parisi VM, Boylan PC, et al: *Am J Obstet Gynecol* 161:670–675, 1989.)

Intravenous Propofol During Cesarean Section: Placental Transfer, Concentrations in Breast Milk, and Neonatal Effects: A Preliminary Study

Dailland P, Cockshott ID, Lirzin JD, Jacquinot P, Jorrot JC, Devery J, Harmey J-L, Conseiller C (Hôp Cochin; Univ Paris; ICI Pharma, Cergy, France; ICI Pharmaceuticals, Cheshire, England)

Anesthesiology 71:827–834, 1989

An open, noncomparative study was done to investigate the placental transfer of propofol, the transfer of propofol into breast milk and colostrum, and the neonatal assessments used when propofol was administered to 21 women for induction of anesthesia or induction and maintenance of anesthesia during elective cesarean section.

In both phases of the study, anesthesia was induced with an intravenous bolus of propofol, 2.5 mg/kg. In phase 1, anesthesia was maintained in 10 women with 50% nitrous oxide in oxygen and halothane. In phase 2, involving 11 women, a continuous infusion of propofol was initiated in 11 women after the induction dose at a rate of 5 mg · kg^{-1}· h^{-1}. Maternal venous and umbilical cord arterial and venous samples were taken at delivery. Propofol crossed the placenta, as shown by concentrations in umbilical venous blood in phases 1 and 2. The ratio of drug concentration in umbilical venous blood to that in maternal blood at delivery was .70 in phase 1 and .76 in phase 2. The ratio of the propofol concentration in the umbilical artery to that in the umbilical vein was 1.09 and .70, respectively. The mean drug concentration in samples taken by a heel prick 2 hours after brith in 8 neonates in phase 2 was low, representing about 10% of the corresponding umbilical cord artery concentration at delivery. Propofol concentrations were low in milk/colostrum, although these data were very limited. Propofol cleared rapidly from the neonatal circulation, so neonatal exposure through breast milk/colostrum would be negligible compared with placental transfer. The drug seemed to have little effect on the healthy newborns in both study phases.

These findings justify the performance of additional research on propofol administration during anesthesia for cesarean section. Studies are especially needed to compare propofol with thiopental and to assess the effect of this drug on high-risk fetuses.

▶ The incidence of maternal awareness after propofol induction was 40% in phase 1 and 9% in phase 2. I am very concerned about this high incidence of awareness with propofol. Obviously, increasing the induction dose may significantly decrease the incidence of awareness, but then one must consider an anesthetic-related effect in the fetus/neonate because there is very rapid placental transfer of this agent. I have personal knowledge of several instances of recall from an ineffective induction dose of propofol in pregnant and nonpregnant patients. Therefore, I believe the jury is still out on propofol as an agent for induction for cesarean delivery and look forward to additional studies comparing it with thiopental. Further in-depth assessment of this drug on normal and high-risk fetuses/newborn must also be undertaken.—G.W. Ostheimer, M.D.

Isoflurane With Either 100% Oxygen or 50% Nitrous Oxide in Oxygen for Caesarean Section

Piggott SE, Bogod DG, Rosen M, Rees GAD, Harmer M (Univ Hosp of Wales, Cardiff)

Br J Anaesth 65:325–329, 1990

Women undergoing general anesthesia for cesarean section usually receive 50% oxygen and nitrous oxide, supplemented with a volatile agent. To confirm earlier findings that the use of 100% oxygen significantly improved fetal oxygenation during cesarean section, the 2 types of anesthesia were compared.

The patients underwent either elective or emergency cesarean section. By random allocation, 103 received isoflurane in 100% oxygen (group 100) and 97 received isoflurane in 50% nitrous oxide in oxygen (group 50). Concentrations of isoflurane were calculated to deliver 1.5 of the maximum allowable concentration (MAC) for the first 5 minutes after induction and 1 MAC thereafter. Umbilical venous and arterial blood samples were taken at delivery. At 24 hours and 48 hours after delivery, the hemoglobin concentration and packed cell volume were measured to estimate operative blood loss.

Arterial Blood-Gas Data

	Elective surgery		Emergency surgery	
	Group 50	Group 100	Group 50	Group 100
Umbilical vein				
pH	7.33 (0.03)	7.33 (0.03)	7.26 (0.11)	7.29 (0.06)
P_{CO_2} (kPa)	6.02 (0.64)	6.04 (0.71)	6.77 (1.66)	6.28 (1.06)
P_{O_2} (kPa)	4.89 (0.99)	5.84 (1.81)	4.00 (1.2)	5.01† (1.79)
Base deficit (mmol litre^{-1})	2.03 (1.35)	2.14 (1.87)	4.76 (4.88)	3.71 (2.65)
Umbilical artery				
pH	7.18 (0.04)	7.30 (0.06)	7.23 (0.12)	7.27 (0.08)
P_{CO_2} (kPa)	7.02 (7.59)	7.00 (0.73)	7.56 (1.52)	7.05 (1.09)
P_{O_2} (kPa)	3.12 (0.76)	3.06 (0.90)	3.06 (0.90)	2.73 (1.22)
Base deficit (mmol litre^{-1})	2.04 (0.97)	2.14 (2.14)	5.4 (5.89)	4.3 (4.19)
Arteriovenous difference (kPa)	1.67 (0.87)	2.83† (1.55)	1.29 (1.2)	2.11* (1.73)

Note: Values are means ±1 SD.
*P < .05 between groups within same surgical category.
†P < .01.
(Courtesy of Piggott SE, Bogod DG, Rosen M, et al: *Br J Anaesth* 65:325–329, 1990.)

Blood loss did not differ significantly between groups. The infants born to mothers in group 100 required less resuscitation and tended to have higher Apgar scores at 1 minute than those born to mothers in group 50. Two women in group 100 and 3 in group 50 reported dreaming, but there were no instances of awareness with either anesthetic regimen. No significant differences in arterial blood-gas data were noted between groups, (table) nor were there significant differences in time to first breath and sustained ventilation. The requirement for intubation did not differ between groups.

Increasing the maternal inspired oxygen concentration to 100%, particularly in emergency cesarean sections, achieves a greater umbilical venous partial pressure of oxygen. This improvement in fetal oxygenation results in a lower incidence of neonatal resuscitation.

▶ This study demonstrates that 100% oxygen plus a volatile agent can significantly improve fetal oxygen and, at the same time, prevent maternal awareness. There is no excuse for inadequate maternal anesthesia during emergency cesarean delivery. On the rare occasion when very little volatile agent can be used, predelivery supplementation with ketamine or postdelivery supplementation with diazepam or midazolam and narcotic should significantly reduce the incidence of maternal recall.—G.W. Ostheimer, M.D.

A Randomized Double-Blind Comparison of Epidural Versus Intravenous Fentanyl Infusion for Analgesia After Cesarean Section

Ellis DJ, Millar WL, Reisner LS (Univ of California, San Diego)
Anesthesiology 72:981–986, 1990   6–64

There is no clinical advantage to epidural infusion over intravenous infusion of fentanyl for analgesia after cesarean section because the doses required epidurally may be similar to those for intravenous administration. A prospective, randomized, double-blind clinical trial was designed to compare plasma fentanyl concentrations and the severity of side effects at comparable levels of analgesia with intravenous and epidural fentanyl administration in women undergoing elective cesarean section.

Of 28 women scheduled to undergo elective cesarean section, 12 were randomly allocated to receive fentanyl intravenously for postoperative analgesia and 16 to epidural fentanyl analgesia. Epidural patients were given fentanyl epidurally and saline intravenously, and intravenous patients received fentanyl intravenously and saline epidurally. Fentanyl and saline infusion rates were adjusted until the patient was comfortable. Sedation was evaluated by an observer. Each patient was monitored for respiratory depression. Patients rated nausea, pain, and pruritus on unmarked visual analogue scales. Plasma fentanyl concentrations were measured at 12 hours and 24 hours after the final adjustment of fentanyl infusion rates.

Three patients in the intravenous group were excluded from the study because of inadequate pain relief despite having received the maximum allowable infusion rate of fentanyl. Similar infusion rates of fentanyl were required to produce similar levels of analgesia at 12 hours and 24 hours in the remaining 25 patients. Patients who received intravenous fentanyl had significantly greater plasma fentanyl concentrations at 12 hours, but both groups had similar plasma fentanyl levels at 24 hours. There was no significant difference in the severity of nausea, pruritus, or sedation between the 2 groups. None of the patients had evidence of respiratory depression. Patient satisfaction with pain control, evaluated at the end of 24 hours, was also similar for both groups. Epidural fentanyl infusion offers no clinical advantage over intravenous fentanyl infusion for analgesia after cesarean section.

▶ The study has finally been done to confirm the suspicions of a number of investigators and pharmacologists that the highly lipid-soluble opioids produce their effect not only on the spinal cord but also in the supraspinal area from vascular uptake. I am sure we will now see a number of studies looking at the other opioids that are administered epidurally to provide postoperative pain relief. I am curious what this will do to our postoperative pain programs in which fentanyl has been used primarily in the postoperative period. The search continues for the optimal opioid to use in epidural infusion to achieve postoperative analgesia.

It will be interesting to assess the concentrations of opioid in the blood in comparison to the CSF, at least in animal preparations, because it would appear that the subarachnoid administration of the opioid does produce its effect directly on the spinal cord.—G.W. Ostheimer, M.D.

Epidural Morphine for Analgesia After Caesarean Section: A Report of 4,880 Patients

Fuller JG, McMorland GH, Douglas MJ, Palmer L (Univ of British Columbia; Grace Hosp, Vancouver)
Can J Anaesth 37:636–640, 1990   6–65

TABLE 1.—Effectiveness of Epidural Morphine

Dose (mg)	No. of patients	Duration of analgesia ($\pm SD$) (hr)	No. of patients receiving no analgesic in first 48 hr
2	8	19.3 ± 11.2	0
2.5	7	17.4 ± 8.7	0
3	210	19.6 ± 10.3	17 (8.1%)
3.5	60	22.7 ± 11.3	9 (15%)
4.0	313	22.7 ± 10.2	25 (8.0%)
4.5	66	24.0 ± 10.5	5 (7.6)
5	4216	23.0 ± 10.0	485 (11.2%)
Total	4880	22.9 ± 10.1	545 (11.2%)

Note: Correlation coefficient between dose and duration of analgesia = .066.
(Courtesy of Fuller JG, McMorland GH, Douglas MJ, et al: *Can J Anaesth* 37:636–640, 1990.)

Although epidural morphine is effective in controlling postoperative pain, undesirable side effects may occur. The side effects of epidural morphine were reviewed in a group of 4,880 women who underwent cesarean section with epidural anesthesia. It was thought that the most serious

TABLE 2.—Patients With Respiratory Rate Less Than 10 per Minute

	Age (yr)	Height (cm)	Weight (kg)	Epidural morphine dose (mg)	Resp. depression		Naloxone (mg)	Intraop supplemental medications	Postop medications
					Rate	Time after morphine (hr)			
1	38	162	73	5	9	1		Fentanyl 50 μg	
2	30	172	73	5	8	11		Fentanyl 50 μg	Diphenhydramine 50 mg
3	30	150	62	5	6	1		Fentanyl 150 μg	
4	32	160	70	5	7	2.5		Fentanyl 100 μg	
5	31	151	66	5	9	6			Diphenhydramine 50 mg
					9	7			
6	32	156	69	5	9	5	0.15	Droperidol 0.5 mg	
					7	8			
					8	9			
					8	12			
7	33	165	63	5	8	6	0.4		Demerol 50 mg
8	35	175	89	5	9	2			
					9	3			
9	39	165	81	5	8	6			Dimenhydrinate 50 mg
10	27	160	75	5	8	12	0.1		Dimenhydrinate 50 mg
11	32	152	55	4	9	2			
12	32	152	60	5	8	1		Fentanyl 50 μg	

(Courtesy of Fuller JG, McMorland GH, Douglas MJ, et al: *Can J Anaesth* 37:636–640, 1990.)

side effect of the analgesia, respiratory depression, would be uncommon in healthy obstetric patients.

The cesarean sections were done between July 1, 1983, and June 30, 1986. The duration of the analgesic effect varied widely from patient to patient (Table 1) and was not related to the dose of morphine. Eleven percent of the patients needed no additional analgesics during the first 48 hours after surgery. Only 12 patients had respiratory depression, defined as a respiratory rate of less than 10 breaths per minute (Table 2), and 3 of these required naloxone injection. Perioperative medication was not related to respiratory depression (Table 3).

Side effects included nausea and vomiting (40%), pruritus (58%), and dizziness (9.8%) (Table 4). The dose of epidural morphine was related only to the occurrence of pruritus. The postpartum nurses believed that

TABLE 3.—Perioperative Medications and Respiratory Depression

No. of patients receiving:

	No. of patients	*Intraop fentanyl*	*Postop parenteral narcotic*	*Postop gravol*	*Postop benadryl*
RR <10	12	5 (41.7%)	1 (8.3%)	2 (16.7)	2 (16.7)
RR ≥10	4868	2143 (43.9%)	627 (12.8%)	923 (18.9)	926 (19.0)

(Courtesy of Fuller JG, McMorland GH, Douglas MJ, et al: *Can J Anaesth* 37:636–640, 1990.)

TABLE 4.—Common Side Effects of Epidural Morphine vs. Dose

Dose (mg)	No. of patients	Nausea & vomiting	Pruritus	Herpes simplex	Urinary retention
2	8	3	2		1
2.5	7	2	2		
3	210	80	101	6	10
3.5	60	17	31	3	2
4	313	108	170	6	15
4.5	66	30	39	3	4
5	4216	1707	2500	153	170
Total	4880	1947 (39.9%)	2845 (58.3%)	171 (3.5%)	202 (4.1%)
P-	NS	<0.05	NS	NS	

(Courtesy of Fuller JG, McMorland GH, Douglas MJ, et al: *Can J Anaesth* 37:636–640, 1990.)

dizziness was more frequent and more profound in these women than in patients who had not received epidural morphine.

Overall, the review confirms the effectiveness of epidural morphine for the control of pain after cesarean section. The optimal dose of the drug is 3 mg. Because of the potential for respiratory distress, postoperative respiratory monitoring is essential.

▶ We are indebted to the obstetric anesthesia group at the Grace Maternity Hospital in Vancouver for this excellent clinical report on the efficacy and safety of epidural morphine. It is hoped that an oral preparation will be available in the near future to administer to postoperative patients to prevent the occurrence of respiratory depression and diminish the other troublesome side effects of epidural opiate administration. It is interesting to find that 3 mg of morphine appears to be the optimal dose, rather than the 5- to 10-mg dose advocated previously.—G.W. Ostheimer, M.D.

Orthopedics

Coagulation and Fibrinolytic Parameters in Patients Undergoing Total Hip Replacement: Influence of the Anesthesia Technique
Donadoni R, Baele G, Devulder J, Rolly G (Univ Hosp, Ghent, Belgium)
Acta Anaesthesiol Scand 33:588–592, 1989   6–66

Anesthesia may contribute to coagulation changes during and after surgery and thereby to the pathogenesis of thromboembolism. Findings were compared in 29 patients having total hip replacement under general anesthesia, 29 others given epidural anesthesia, and 22 given both epidural and general anesthesia but with a lower concentration of isoflurane.

Antithrombin III levels were depressed just after surgery in all groups but recovered significantly more rapidly in the epidural group. The activated partial thromboplastin time was significantly prolonged only in the general anesthesia group. Prothrombin times did not change significantly. Changes in the protein C level were similar in all groups. Tissue plasminogen activator activity did not change significantly. Plasminogen levels were higher in patients given epidural analgesia. The comparatively benign changes in antithrombin III and plasminogen associated with epidural blockade may partly explain why this technique helps to prevent thromboembolic complications after hip replacement surgery.

▶ This study was an attempt to explain why epidural anesthesia is associated with less immediate postoperative deep vein thromboses and pulmonary emboli than is general anesthesia. Although the authors think that it might be related to antithrombin III's quicker return to normal, the data seem "iffy" at best and the changes seem only marginal, that is, 92% vs. 104% of control (as seen by my unaided eye). Thus I don't make as much of the data as they do, although it is a very well-done study.—M.F. Roizen, M.D.

Blood-Gas and Circulatory Changes During Total Knee Replacement: Role of the Intramedullary Alignment Rod
Fahmy NR, Chandler HP, Danylchuk K, Matta EB, Sunder N, Siliski JM (Massachusetts Gen Hosp, Boston)
J Bone Joint Surg 72-A:19–26, 1990   6–67

Routine hemodynamic changes were observed in patients undergoing total knee replacement arthroplasty in which cemented components were used, whereas such changes did not occur in those who received uncemented knee prostheses. A later study found serious hypotension and a marked decrease in oxygen saturation of arterial blood immediately after insertion of an intramedullary alignment rod in a patient undergoing uncemented total knee replacement. Because intramedullary alignment rods are being used increasingly with most modern cementless total knee replacement systems, a prospective study was initiated to measure the intramedullary pressures and the changes in circulatory and blood gas values associated with insertion of different intramedullary alignment rods.

The study population consisted of 21 women and 14 men aged 48–84 years (mean, 70 years) having total knee replacement with noncemented prostheses. None had evidence of active cardiac or pulmonary disorders. Patients were divided into 5 groups on the basis of type of alignment rod used. Examined were the effects of the use of an 8-mm solid alignment rod with and without venting, an 8-mm fluted alignment rod with venting, and an 8-mm fluted or solid alignment rod inserted through a 12.7-mm drill hole but without other venting.

There was a statistically significant reduction in oxygen saturation, arterial oxygen tension, and end-tidal carbon dioxide tension after insertion of both solid and fluted 8-mm alignment rods through an 8-mm hole in both vented and unvented femoral canals, resulting in a significant increase in intramedullary pressure. Bone marrow contents and fat were retrieved from blood samples obtained from the right atrium, indicating that embolization of marrow contents had occurred during insertion of the alignment rod. However, these changes did not develop in any of the patients in whom a 12.7-mm drill hole was made at the entry site for the 8-mm fluted alignment rod. Insertion of an intramedullary alignment rod in the femur causes embolization of marrow contents that can be prevented by making a drill hole at the entry site of a fluted alignment rod at least 4.7 mm larger than the diameter of the rod.

▶ These data demonstrate the importance of a surgical maneuver that prevents increases in intramedullary pressure during insertion of the alignment rod. If this maneuver does not alter the success of the operation, it would seem to be a reasonable step to include.— R.K. Stoelting, M.D.

Airway

Local Anesthesia for Fibreoptic Bronchoscopy: Transcricoid Injection or the "Spray As You Go" Technique?
Webb AR, Fernando SSD, Dalton HR, Arrowsmith JE, Woodhead MA, Cummin ARC (St George's Hosp, London)
Thorax 45:474–477, 1990   6–68

Local anesthesia for fiberoptic bronchoscopy can be administered by a single transcricoid injection of lidocaine or by using a "spray-as-you-go" technique. The single injection method generally requires a lower dose of local anesthetic than the spray technique. To compare the safety, patient comfort, and convenience to the bronchoscopist of the single transcricoid lidocaine injection and the lidocaine spray technique, studies were made in 62 patients scheduled for outpatient fiberoptic bronchoscopy. Of the patients, 32 were randomly allocated to receive lidocaine, 240 mg, instilled through the bronchoscope under direct vision, and 30 to receive lidocaine, 100 mg, by a single cricothyroid puncture. Additional doses of lidocaine were given to both groups as needed.

The mean total dose of lidocaine administered by spray was 451 mg, compared with 322 mg in the group given transcricoid injection. Despite the lower dose of local anesthetic administered, the cough rate in the latter patients was lower than in the spray-treated group. Neither technique was perceived as more or less unpleasant by the patient. The transcricoid injection was not associated with any complications. Because the primary reason for topical anesthesia of the respiratory mucosa in bronchoscopy is to reduce cough, the transcricoid injection technique with its reduced cough rate, produced with a lower dosage of local anesthetic, offers a clear advantage over the "spray-as-you-go" technique.

▶ After the initial doses (100 mg and 240 mg) were given, the average amount of additional lidocaine required in the 2 groups was 211 mg and 122 mg. Although this difference may be significant (statistically), was it different from a clinical standpoint (no complications occurred in either group).— R.R. Kirby, M.D.

Transcarinal Aspiration of a Mediastinal Cyst to Facilitate Anesthetic Management
McDougall JC, Fromme GA (Mayo Clinic and Found, Rochester, Minn)
Chest 97:1490–1492, 1990   6–69

Major airway obstruction that can complicate the perioperative management of patients with mediastinal masses may be fatal. Severe obstruction, which occurred during anesthesia secondary to a large mediastinal cyst, was deflated endoscopically during surgery.

Woman, 35, a smoker, had a 4.5-cm subcarinal mass and a productive cough, as well as wheezing of recent onset. The mass had enlarged in the preceding 2 weeks and compressed both the bronchus intermedius and the midesophagus. Ventilation proved difficult; chest films obtained after anesthetic induction showed left lower lobe collapse and marked compression at the carinal level. Bronchoscopy showed compression of both mainstem bronchi and partial occlusion of the left bronchial tree by thick secretions, which were aspirated. The cyst was decompressed by a needle passed through the bronchoscope. Ventilation improved markedly as a result, and a benign cyst was removed. The left lower lobe was totally reexpanded at the end of surgery.

Although most of these obstructions involve solid tumors, cystic mediastinal masses can compress major airways to a significant degree. The cystic nature of the mass in this patient provided an opportunity for transcarinal decompression. Endoscopic deflation of the cyst allowed more effective ventilation and made removal of the lesion easier and safer.

▶ Interesting solution to a difficult and potentially lethal problem.—R.R. Kirby, M.D.

What Is the Safest Endotracheal Tube for Nd-YAG Laser Surgery? A Comparative Study
Sosis MB (Indiana Univ, Indianapolis)
Anesth Analg 69:802–804, 1989   6–70

The neodymium-yttrium-aluminum-garnet (Nd-YAG) laser is increasingly being used in airway surgery, particularly in the treatment of tracheobronchial tumors for which this laser is very effective. However, life-threatening airway burns from Nd-YAG laser-induced combustion of polyvinylchloride endotracheal tubes and fiberoptic bronchoscopes have been reported. The safest endotracheal tube for use with the Nd-YAG laser under stringent conditions sought.
A combined carbon dioxide/Nd-YAG laser was used for the experiments. The laser's output was set at 50 W in the continuous mode of operation. Laser emission was continued for 1 minute or until combustion occurred. The Nd-YAG laser was directed at 6 different commercially

available endotracheal tubes, with 5 liters of oxygen per minute flowing through them.

The Nd-YAG laser ignited and perforated 4 of the 6 endotracheal tubes within 12 seconds, namely, the plain Rusch red rubber endotracheal tube, the Bivona Fome-cuff laser endotracheal tube, the stainless steel Mallinckrodt Laser-Flex endotracheal tube, and the Xomed Laser-shield endotracheal tube. Only plain red rubber endotracheal tubes that had been wrapped with 3M no. 425 tape or with Venture copper foil tape were unaffected by 1 mixture of exposure to the laser beam, and they are therefore recommended for clinical use. Because of the flammable nature of the adhesive on the Venture copper foil, the 3M tape is preferred. Wrapped red rubber endotracheal tubes are still subject to indirect combustion from sparks or from a high temperature near the tube.

▶ The potential for airway fires is a well-recognized hazard during anesthesia for laser surgery. In this report, the endotracheal tubes were tested under extreme conditions—high power level from the laser and oxygen flowing through the endotracheal tube. We would hope that, during use of the laser in the operating room, it would be possible to avoid these extreme conditions.—R.K. Stoelting, M.D.

Liver Transplantation

Mortality During Intensive Care After Orthotopic Liver Transplantation
Park GR, Gomez-Arnau J, Lindop MJ, Klinck JR, Williams R, Calne RY (Addenbroke's Hosp, Cambridge, England; Kings College Hosp, London)
Anaesthesia 44:959–963, 1989   6–71

The current indications for orthotopic liver transplantation (OLT) are end-stage liver disease, acute hepatic failure, inborn errors of metabolism, and certain liver tumors. To determine the incidence of OLT patients who died in the intensive care unit (ICU), and the major causes of postoperative death in the ICU, data were reviewed retrospectively on 335 adults who underwent OLT in 1968–1987. The procedure was performed on 41 patients in 1968–1975, 60 in 1976–1980, 45 in 1981–1983, 27 in 1984, 45 in 1985, 57 in 1986, and 60 in 1987. Of the 335 patients who underwent OLT, 195 died, 86 (44%) in the ICU. Intensive care unit mortality peaked in 1984 (48%), but decreased to 11% in 1987.

The main causes of death in the ICU were infection (55%) and hemorrhage (19%). Multisystem failure and renal failure accounted for 60% of all contributory causes of death. Although many factors influence survival after OLT, the development of renal failure in these critically ill patients is associated with high mortality. The period in which the maximum incidence of renal failure occurred coincided with the introduction of cyclosporine A, which was then administered immediately after OLT. The high incidence of renal failure led to a change in policy whereby ini-

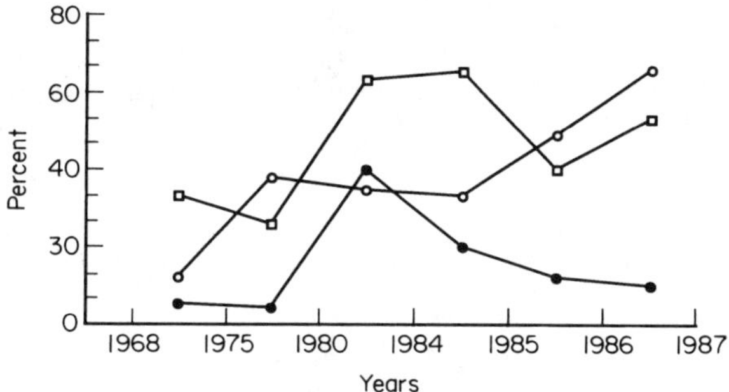

Fig 6–15.—Incidence of renal failure during the period of intensive care in patients who had undergone liver transplantation in 1968–1987. Mortality (as a percentage of all deaths) and 1-year survival for the same period are also shown. *Open circles* indicate 1-year survival; *closed circles,* renal failure; *squares,* ICU deaths. (Courtesy of Park GR, Gomez-Arnau J, Lindop MJ, et al: *Anaesthesia* 44:959–963, 1989.)

tiation of cyclosporine therapy is delayed for 48 hours after the end of operation until the patient is hemodynamically stable and has adequate renal function.

Whereas renal failure occurred in 45% of patients who died in the ICU in 1981–1983, the incidence of renal failure gradually decreased over time, to a 10% incidence in 1986 (Fig 6–15). The reduction in incidence of renal failure has resulted in a decrease in ICU mortality and an increase in 1-year survival. There were no deaths in the ICU attributed primarily to rejection, pulmonary embolism, or biliary problems. Other factors that appeared closely related to ICU mortality were the volume of blood transfused intraoperatively, longer duration of tracheal intubation, and more days spent in the ICU. The current 1-year survival rate at this institution is 66%.

Postoperative infection and hemorrhage after OLT continue to be the primary causes of death in the ICU. The high incidence of postoperative infection is attributable to the severity of preexisting illness, the magnitude of the operation, and the need for immunosuppression. The high incidence of postoperative hemorrhage may represent a complication of surgery, a derangement in the coagulation mechanism as a result of preexisting poor synthetic liver function, or failure of synthetic function of the new liver.

▶ This study says essentially that if patients don't do well intraoperatively or postoperatively, they die, and that the major cause of death is renal failure. Over the years since 1968, a major reduction in mortality has been related to the major reduction in the incidence of renal failure. But once renal failure develops in a patient with liver failure, a high mortality results. A second comment is brought forth by this study: Lichtor et al. (1) showed that preoperative ICU requirements, preoperative encephalopathy, and preoperative coagulation disturbances predispose patients to not do well; such patients required more transfusions intraoperatively, and they had a higher death rate. This study's findings are consonant with those findings, as patients who had more blood loss did not do well and had a much higher mortality than other groups.—M.F. Roizen, M.D.

Reference

1. Lichtor L, et al: *Anesthesiology* 68:607, 1988.

7 Monitoring

Pulse Oximetry and Capnography

Pulse Oximetry for Hypoxemia: A Warning to Users and Manufacturers

Fanconi S (Univ of Zurich, Switzerland)
Intensive Care Med 15:540–542, 1989   7–1

Although pulse oximetry is a major advance in patient monitoring, it is most accurate at 80% to 100% saturation. Measurements made at 70% to 80% oxygen saturation have significant limitations. Although some manufacturers and users claim that it is not important to have great accuracy at lower saturations as long as an attempt is made to maintain an oxygen saturation level above 90%, some patients with profound hypoxemia require monitoring, and accurate readings are needed to prevent brain damage. Some manufacturers have made changes in their instruments and now claim improved correlations at low saturation levels.

Conflicting findings are reported in studies comparing ear probes with finger probes. Errors at low saturation may be explained in part by multiple light scattering or by lack of suitable calibration data. Nevertheless, there is substantial variability in pulse oximeter responses within subjects. No technical explanations for the divergent findings are at hand.

Invasive measurements of arterial saturation are warranted in patients whose pulse oximetry values are below 75% to 80% oxygen saturation. Manufacturers probably should avoid modifying their instruments until further studies are available.

▶ I don't think this report detracts from the use of pulse oximetry, but it does prove that the technique is not infallible. So long as one recognizes its limitations, the shortcomings can be dealt with.—R.R. Kirby, M.D.

Delayed Detection of Hypoxic Events by Pulse Oximeters: Computer Simulations

Verhoeff F, Sykes MK (Radcliffe Infirmary, Oxford, England)
Anaesthesia 45:103–109, 1990   7–2

Although the pulse oximeter is an essential monitor during anesthesia, the accuracy of the device may be affected in a number of ways. The alarm limit on the pulse oximeter is usually set at an oxygen saturation of 90%. But if there is a measurement delay of longer than 60 seconds between the decrease in alveolar oxygen concentration and the pulse oximeter response, the arterial saturation may have decreased far below 90% before the alarm sounds. In a series of simulations on the MacPuf computer model, the rate of decrease of arterial oxygen tension (PaO_2) and

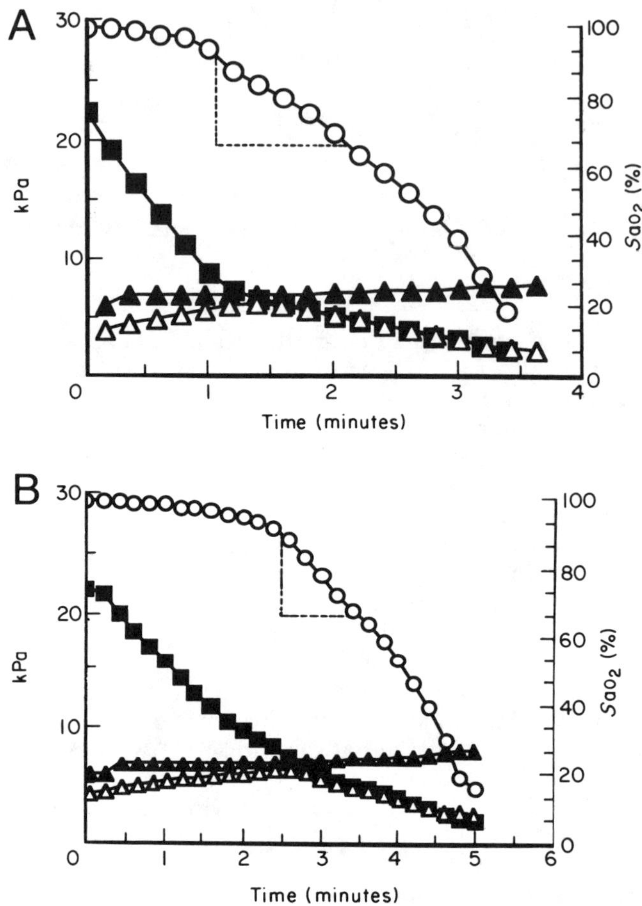

Fig 7–1.—Changes in Sa_{O_2} *(circles)*, arterial P_{CO_2} *(Pa_{CO_2}; closed triangles)*, alveolar P_{O_2} *(PA_{O_2}; squares)* and brain P_{O_2} *(Pb_{O_2}; open triangles)* in response to apnea. Inspired oxygen concentration 30%. **A,** functional residual capacity 1.5 L; **B,** functional residual capacity 3L. The *vertical dotted line* represents the time at which 90% saturation occurs and the *horizontal line* shows the saturation 1 minute later. (Courtesy of Verhoeff F, Sykes MK: *Anaesthesia* 45:103–109, 1990.)

saturation (Sa_{O_2}) that result from various causes of oxygen supply failure were assessed.

In the simulation, the standard MacPuf 70-kg subject with an oxygen consumption of 250 mL/min and a carbon dioxide output of 200 mL/min was ventilated mechanically with a tidal volume of 500 mL and a frequency of 12 breaths per minute. The clinical situations examined included disconnection of a paralyzed patient from the ventilator during controlled mechanical ventilation (CMV) (Figs 7–1 and 7–2); oxygen supply failure and continued CMV with a gas that contained no oxygen in a nonbreathing system (Fig 7–3); and a sudden decrease of the fresh gas flow to zero with a Mapleson D system and with a circle carbon dioxide absorption system (Fig 7–4).

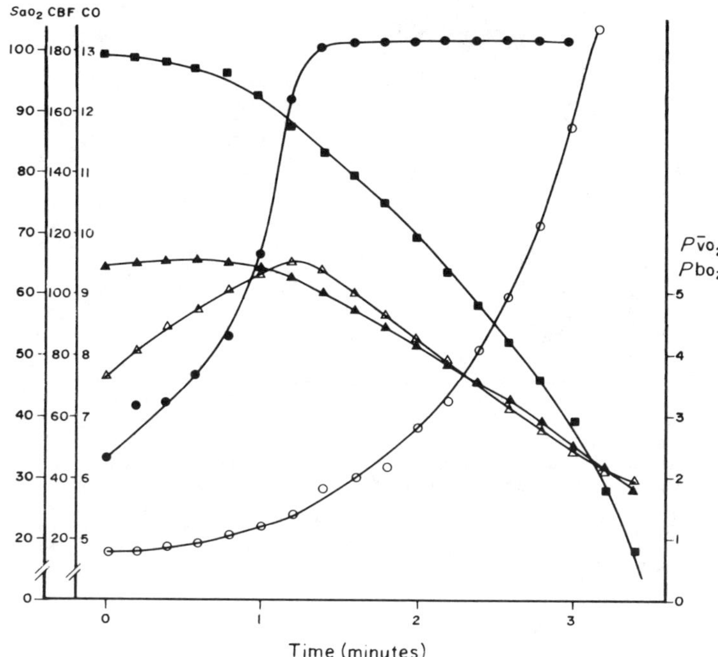

Fig 7–2.—Changes in Sao$_2$, cerebral blood flow *(CBF)*, cardiac output *(CO)*, brain Po$_2$ *(Pbo$_2$)*, and mixed venous Po$_2$ *(P$\bar{v}$o$_2$)* after disconnection from the ventilator with functional residual capacity of 1.5 L. arterial Paco$_2$ increased to 6.7 kPa at 3 minutes. *Open circles* indicate CO litres per minute; *closed circles*, CBF milliliters per minute per 100 g of tissue; *squares*, Sao$_2$ percent; *closed triangles*, P$\bar{v}$o$_2$ kPa; *open triangles*, Pbo$_2$ kPa. (Courtesy of Verhoeff F, Sykes MK: *Anaesthesia* 45:103–109, 1990.)

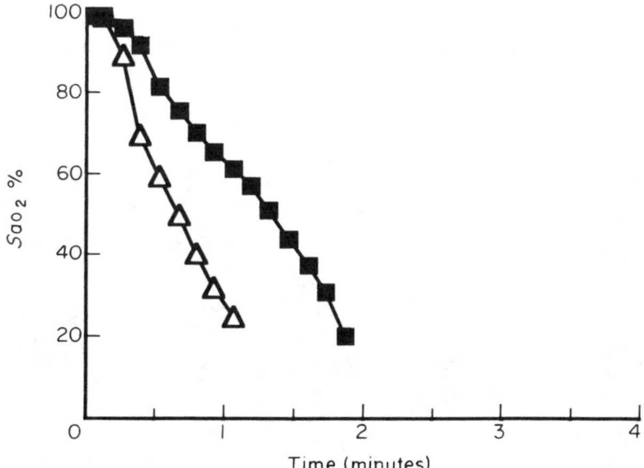

Fig 7–3.—Changes in Sao$_2$ after oxygen supply failure with continued ventilation with hypoxic gas mixture in a nonrebreathing system functional residual capacity 1.5 L, *triangles;* and 3 L, *squares.* (Courtesy of Verhoeff F, Sykes MK: *Anaesthesia* 45:103–109, 1990.)

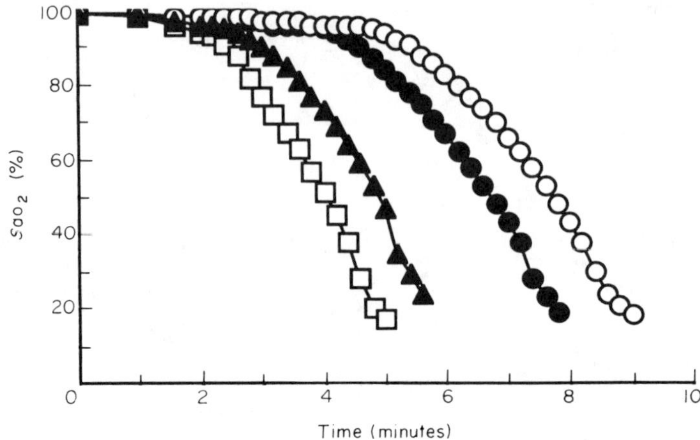

Fig 7–4.—Changes in SaO_2 resulting from simulated disconnection of the fresh gas flow into a Mapleson D system (functional residual capacity 1.5 L, system volume 2 L, *squares*) and circle CO_2 absorption system of 5 L volume with functional residual capacity of 1.5 L *(closed circles)* and 3.0 L *(open circles)*. The functional residual capacity 1.5 L, system volume 5 L *(triangles)* simulation was also performed with an increased oxygen consumption produced by the patient temperature to 40C. (Courtesy of Verhoeff F, Sykes MK: *Anaesthesia* 45:103–109, 1990.)

Marked differences were noted between the rate of arterial desaturation that resulted from each of the clinical situations involving oxygen supply failure. In the first simulation, SaO_2 could have decreased to 65% before the pulse oximeter alarmed at a reading of 90%, with the patient sustaining severe hypoxic damage. Continued ventilation with a hypoxic gas mixture in a nonrebreathing system may result in a decrease of SaO_2 to 30% to 40% within 1 minute.

Oxygen supply monitors must be able to detect a decrease in oxygen supply pressure or concentration and disconnection of the breathing system from either the fresh gas supply or the patient. Before a pulse oximeter alarm is activated, arterial oxygen saturation may reach dangerous levels.

▶ An interesting topic, the importance of which is well quantitated here. Perhaps the message is not that pulse oximetry is not as valuable as we have thought but, rather, that ventilatory catastrophes are best evaluated and detected by end-tidal CO_2 monitoring.—R.R. Kirby, M.D.

Reliability of Pulse Oximetry in Titrating Supplemental Oxygen Therapy in Ventilator-Dependent Patients

Jubran A, Tobin MJ (Univ of Texas, Houston)
Chest 97:1420–1425, 1990

7–3

Although pulse oximetry is widely used in critical care, few studies have assessed its utility in clinical decision making. Pulse oximetry may be useful in the titration of the fractional inspired oxygen concentration

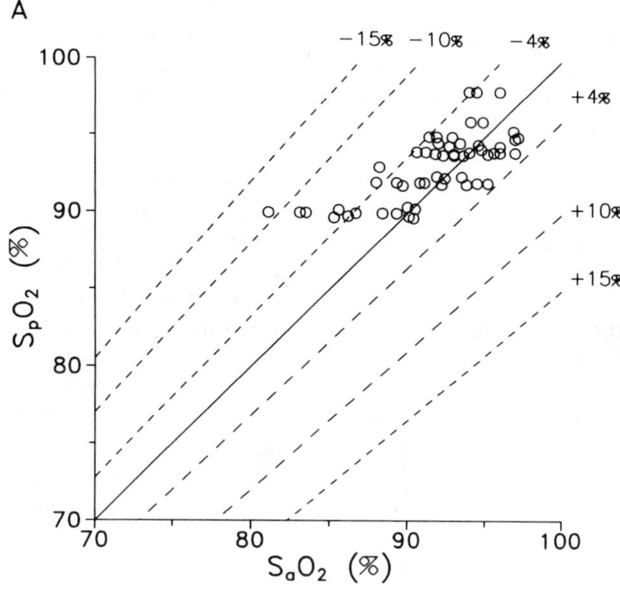

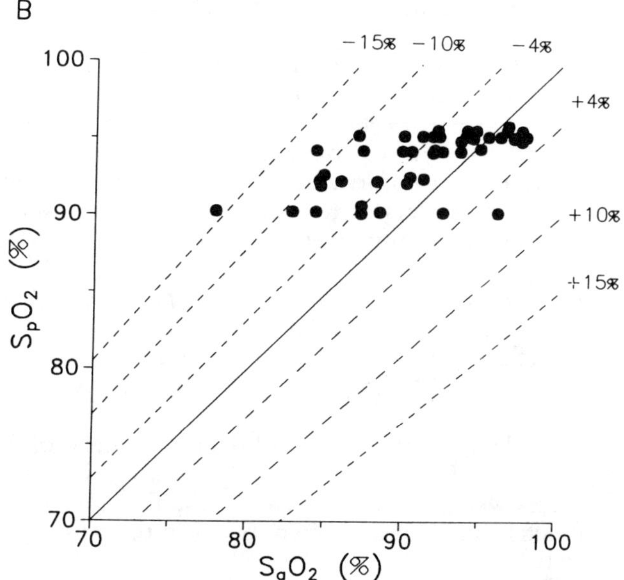

Fig 7–5.—The arterial O_2 saturation (Sao_2) vs. the pulse oximeter O_2 saturation values (Spo_2) for the 55 measurements obtained in white patients (grid **A**), and for the 43 measurements obtained in black patients (grid **B**). The *solid line* is the line of identity and the *dashed lines* are isopleths of different levels of bias. Pulse oximetry was less accurate in the black patients, and frequently overestimated the true Sao_2. (Courtesy of Jubran A, Tobin MJ: *Chest* 97:1420–1425, 1990.)

(FIO$_2$) in ventilator-dependent patients. However, guidelines for this use do not exist. A recent survey indicated that directors of intensive care units used a wide range of target O$_2$ saturation (SpO$_2$) values. To determine if SpO$_2$ could be reliably substituted for measures of arterial O$_2$ tension when adjusting FIO$_2$ in ventilator-dependent patients, 54 critically ill patients were studied. A number of SpO$_2$ target values were examined, aiming for arterial O$_2$ tension of 60 mm Hg or greater while minimizing the risk of O$_2$ toxicity. An SpO$_2$ target of 92% was reliable in white patients for predicting a satisfactory level of oxygenation. In black patients, however, this SpO$_2$ reading was commonly associated with significant hypoxemia. An SpO$_2$ target of 95% was required for this population. Inaccurate oximetry readings were also more common in black (27%) than in white (11%) persons (Fig 7–5).

▶ The problem is, what establishes the criteria that a PaO$_2$ of 60 mm Hg and an SpO$_2$ of 92% or 95%, or whatever, are really critical or even important? We go to great lengths in terms of ventilator support, fluid therapy, inotropic administration, and the like to obtain these values, but do we know that 60 mm Hg is really superior to 50 mm Hg? I know of no data to support such a conclusion. Thus the limits chosen are at best arbitrary.—R.R. Kirby, M.D.

Agreement Between Noninvasive Oximetric Values for Oxygen Saturation
Cahan C, Decker MJ, Hoekje PL, Strohl KP (Case Western Reserve Univ)
Chest 97:814–819, 1990   7–4

The Hewlett-Packard (HP) ear oximeter is an accurate means of monitoring oxygen saturation; unfortunately, however, it is no longer manufactured. Five pulse oximeters were evaluated for their ability to replace the HP ear oximeter in noninvasively estimating arterial oxygen saturation (SaO$_2$).

Studies were performed in 22 white and 6 black subjects during progressive isocapnic hypoxia over an SaO$_2$ range of 99% to 70%. The instruments used included the Criticare Model 501+, Nellcor N100, Nellcor N200, Ohmeda 3700, and Physiocontrol Lifestat 1600. All are equipped with a finger sensor.

Pulse oximetric data differed from HP data by a mean of 2.6% in the entire group. The mean difference was 1.9% in whites and 5.1% in blacks. Differences were greater below 80% than above 85% saturation. The 95% confidence limits of agreement between the pulse oximeters and the HP were ±10%.

Pulse oximeters yield consistently higher values for SaO$_2$ than the HP ear oximeter. Pulse oximetric values may be higher in black than in white persons. Agreement between these types of instrument worsens as the oxygen saturation declines. It cannot be assumed that pulse oximeters will provide the same clinical values as the HP.

Comparison of Four Pulse Oximeters: Effects of Venous Occlusion and Cold-Induced Peripheral Vasoconstriction
Langton JA, Lassey D, Hanning CD (Leicester Gen Hosp, Leicester, England)
Br J Anaesth 65:245–247, 1990
7–5

Different pulse oximeters have varying abilities to function under adverse conditions, particularly with motion or impaired peripheral perfusion. The ability of 4 pulse oximeters (the Ohmeda 3700, Nellcor N100 and N200, and Datex Oscar) to detect hypoxemia in the presence of venous obstruction or cold-induced peripheral vasoconstriction was evaluated.

The study included 20 healthy persons, who breathed 10% oxygen in nitrogen for periods of 2 minutes or until the reference oxyhemoglobin saturation (SaO_2) decreased to less than 75%. Venous occlusion was produced by inflating an arm cuff to 40 mm Hg, and vasoconstriction was achieved using a plastic wrap filled with cold water, cold bags, or a blood warmer with ice cold water circulating through it.

Detection times increased with both venous obstruction and peripheral vasoconstriction. Hypoxemia was detected within similar times by all of the instruments, but lower values of SaO_2 sometimes were recorded with the Ohmeda 3700. It is important to use consistent methods of producing vasoconstriction and to avoid venous congestion when recording SaO_2 with a pulse oximeter.

▶ There is increasing awareness that certain events may influence the overall accuracy of oxygen saturation readings displayed by pulse oximeters. Nevertheless, the clinical usefulness of these devices is rarely influenced by ±10% accuracy.—R.K. Stoelting, M.D.

Editorial: An International Consensus on Monitoring?
Winter A, Spence AA
Br J Anaesth 64:263–266, 1990
7–6

Guidelines on minimal standards of monitoring, originated at Harvard Medical School, have been adopted by the American Society of Anesthesiologists (ASA), a forum of Australian anesthetists, and the Association of Anaesthetists of Great Britain and Ireland (AAGBI). All groups' guidelines require the continuous presence of an appropriately qualified anesthetist, continuous monitoring of cardiopulmonary function, observation of reservoir bag and chest excursion, a ventilator disconnect alarm, and an oxygen analyzer of inspired gas. An oxygen supply failure alarm is also required by the AAGBI and Australian guidelines, but not by the Harvard or ASA guidelines.

Spirometry is optional according to the Harvard guidelines, recommended by ASA and AAGBI, and recommended when it is indicated by the Australian group. Noninvasive arterial pressure monitoring is required at appropriate intervals by all groups. Electrocardiography is required by all but the Australian guidelines, but not by the Harvard or ASA guidelines.

Spirometry is optional according to the Harvard guidelines, recommended by ASA and AAGBI, and recommended when it is indicated by the Australian group. Noninvasive arterial pressure monitoring is required at appropriate intervals by all groups. Electrocardiography is required by all but the Australian guidelines, which stipulate only that ECG be available. Pulse osimeters are recommended by the ASA, strongly recommended by the AABGI, and required when needed by the Harvard group. According to the Australian guidelines, pulse oximeters were to be required by 1990.

End-tidal carbon dioxide monitoring was either recommended, strongly recommended, or required when needed. Temperature was required when needed. All guidelines stipulate the use of invasive hemodynamic monitoring when indicated. The Harvard and AAGBI guidelines require that methods to monitor neuromuscular block be available. The Australian guidelines stipulate neuromuscular block monitoring when indicated. It is not included in the ASA guidelines.

Minimum monitoring criteria change as technology improves. A reasonable standard of care is also subject to current pressures for efficient use of finances. In each case the anesthesiologist must decide the level of monitoring required for the surgery at the initial preoperative assessment. Electromedical and other monitors should be included in the checks before a procedure is begun.

▶ Critics have argued that the routine use of certain monitors, as dictated by Standards, will distract the anesthesiologist's attention from the patient. With respect to pulse oximetry and capnography, I would take strong exception to this concern. These monitors greatly enhance the vigilance of the anesthesiologist and have clearly contributed to increased patient safety during the perioperative period.—R.K. Stoelting, M.D.

A Comparative Study of Methods of Detection of Esophageal Intubation
Sum-Ping ST, Mehta MP, Anderton JM (Univ of Iowa; Manchester Royal Infirmary, England)
Anesth Analg 69:627–632, 1989   7–7

Observance of the end-expired carbon dioxide (CO_2) waveform is the most reliable and popular method of confirming correct placement of the tracheal tube. However, normal-appearing CO_2 waveforms have been observed during inadvertent esophageal ventilation. To determine whether measurement of volume and temperature of expired gas would complement CO_2 waveforms in assessing the correct placement of tra-

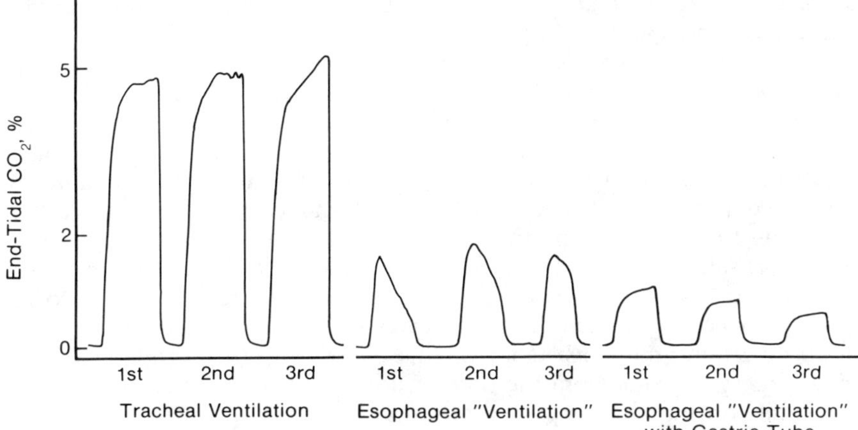

Fig 7–6.—Carbon dioxide waveforms of expired gas with tracheal and esophageal ventilation. Rate of decrease in CO_2 level from esophageal tube, before insertion of gastric tube, does not follow normal washout pattern. (Courtesy of Sum-Ping ST, Mehta MP, Anderton JM: *Anesth Analg* 69:627–632, 1989.)

cheal tubes, the trachea and esophagus of 21 patients were intubated simultaneously and ventilated in succession with the same inspiratory volume of 621 mL. Levels of CO_2 and volumes and temperatures of expired gas were measured.

End-expired CO_2 levels of gas from the trachea averaged 4.9%. In 7 patients CO_2 waveforms were recorded from the esophageal tube similar to that obtained with tracheal intubation, but the mean level of end-expired CO_2 was significantly lower (.6%) (Fig 7–6). Volumes expired from the tracheal tube were significantly higher than those expired from the esophageal tube. Furthermore, peak temperatures of expired gas recorded from the tracheal tube were significantly higher than those from the esophageal tube. The temperature waveforms obtained from the tracheal tubes were similar in shape and peak with each ventilation, whereas temperature waveforms were dissimilar with each esophageal ventilation.

The occasional detection of CO_2 waveforms from an esophageal tube may lead to incorrect assessment of tube placement. This limitation of the CO_2 analyzer can be offset by measuring the volume and temperature of expired gas.

▶ Insistence upon 3 consecutive end-expired CO_2 waveforms of more than 30 mm Hg is, in my opinion, undeniable evidence that the tube is placed in the trachea. It is difficult for me to accept the argument that 3 consecutive CO_2 waveforms of less than 5 mmHg could be confused with tracheal placement of the tube. It is my belief that the incidence of unrecognized esophageal intubation should approach zero if every tracheal tube placement was verified by "ETco₂ × 3 > 30 mm Hg."—R.K. Stoelting, M.D.

Stability of Arterial to End-Tidal Carbon Dioxide Gradients During Postoperative Cardiorespiratory Support
Russell GB, Graybeal JM, Strout JC (Pennsylvania State Univ, Hershey)
Can J Anaesth 37:560–566, 1990   7–8

Continuous measurement of end-tidal carbon dioxide ($ETCO_2$) by mass spectrometry or infrared capnometry is routinely used in mechanically ventilated patients as an indication of arterial carbon dioxide ($PaCO_2$) levels, as this policy helps to decrease the expense of frequent arterial blood gas sampling. However, the use of the $ETCO_2$ as a reflection of respiratory acid-base status is reliable only as long as there is a close correlation between $PaCO_2$ and $ETCO_2$, expressed as the $P(a-ET)CO_2$.

To determine the consistency of this correlation in postoperative cardiac surgery patients from the time of admission to the intensive cardiac care unit, during changing cardiorespiratory support, up to the time of tracheal extubation, 46 men and 13 women (mean age, 63 years) who had undergone a variety of cardiac operations, mostly coronary artery bypass grafting, were monitored postoperatively. None had obstructive lung disease. Individual factors evaluated for their effects on $P(a-ET)CO_2$ included rate of mechanical ventilation, infusion of vasoactive agents, and associated changes in hemodynamic pathophysiology.

A total of 382 comparisons of $PaCO_2$ and $ETCO_2$ were obtained during widely varying conditions of cardiorespiratory support. In the study population overall, the $ETCO_2$ and $PaCO_2$ measurements maintained a significant correlation throughout the study period. However, the $P(a-ET)CO_2$ did vary from patient to patient, and in many individual patients there was no statistically significant correlation between $PaCO_2$ and $ETCO_2$ measurements. Although the variation was typical of a normal population distribution, the lack of a positive correlation for individual patients limits the clinical relevance of this finding. Because of the individual variations in $P(a-ET)CO_2$ observed in this study, it is recommended that postoperative cardiac surgery patients undergo periodic arterial blood gas analysis until the time of extubation.

▶ The problems mentioned here are magnified greatly when patients with postoperative or posttraumatic respiratory insufficiency are followed with $ETCO_2$ monitoring. In the acute phase of such illness, our experinece has been most disappointing. Differences of the $P(a-ET)CO_2$ as high as 30 mm Hg have been noted frequently when high-pressure, large tidal volume ventilation is employed. In such cases there is no substitute for arterial blood gas analysis.—R.R. Kirby, M.D.

Neuromuscular

The Effect of Local Surface and Central Cooling on Adductor Pollicis Twitch Tension During Nitrous Oxide/Isoflurane and Nitrous Oxide/ Fentanyl Anesthesia in Humans

Heier T, Caldwell JE, Sessler DI, Miller RD (Univ of California, San Francisco)
Anesthesiology 72:807–811, 1990   7–9

A previous study during nitrous oxide/isoflurane anesthesia showed a direct relationship between the adductor pollicis muscle temperature and twitch response when the temperature in the muscle was reduced secondary to central (total body) cooling. The twitch response was studied in 20 unpremedicated patients to determine whether the method of cooling the hand (either central or local surface, hand only) influences the relationship between adductor pollicis temperature and twitch tension under isoflurane anesthesia, and whether the decreased evoked twitch response during central cooling results from reduced muscle temperature and/or the anesthetic drug used.

During isoflurane anesthesia in 15 patients, adductor pollicis temperature and twitch tension decreased significantly in a linear manner during local surface cooling, central body temperature was not allowed to decrease (Fig 7–7). The mean reduction in twitch tension per reduction in muscle temperature was 6% per degree C, which was only 43% of that observed during central cooling in a previous study under similar experimental conditions.

Because isoflurane can contribute to the reduction in twitch tension, the effect of central cooling on adductor pollicis twitch tension during nitrous oxide/fentanyl anesthesia was studied in 5 patients. Adductor pollicis twitch tension decreased significantly when muscle temperatures were less than 35.2° C. There was a significant linear relationship between central and adductor pollicis temperatures and adductor pollicis twitch tension, with a mean reduction in twitch tension of 16.4% per degree C. These findings were similar to those obtained in a previous study of patients anesthetized with nitrous oxide/isoflurane.

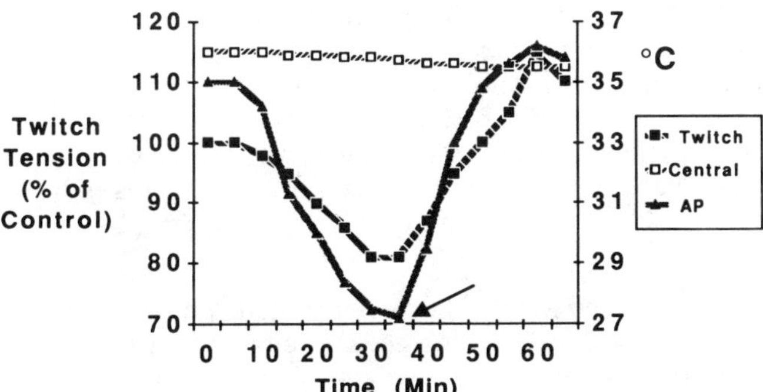

Fig 7–7.—Changes in central and adductor pollicis *(AP)* temperatures and adductor pollicis twitch tension in 1 patient undergoing local cooling and rewarming of the thenar eminence during isoflurane anesthesia. *Arrow* indicates when rewarming started. There was a significant linear relationship between twitch tension and muscle temperature during cooling and rewarming. Twitch tension decreased 19% when adductor pollicis temperature decreased from 35° to 27° C. Central temperature did not change significantly during the cooling period. (Courtesy of Heier T, Caldwell JE, Sessler DI, et al: *Anesthesiology* 72:807–811, 1990.)

Both central cooling and local surface cooling of the adductor pollicis muscle reduce twitch tension. These findings indicate that the decrease in adductor pollicis twitch tension caused primarily by the decreased temperature and is independent of the anesthetic technique used, whether nitrous oxide/isoflurane or nitrous oxide/fentanyl anesthesia.

▶ This study emphasizes that modest decreases in body and or peripheral temperature can significantly reduce the strength of hand muscle response to peripheral nerve stimulation. This should be taken into account when using a peripheral nerve stimulator clinically.— R.D. Miller, M.D.

Local Anaesthetic Block Protects Against Electrically-Induced Damage in Peripheral Nerve
Agnew WF, McCreery DB, Yuen TGH, Bullara LA (Huntington Med Research Insts, Pasadena, Calif)
J Biomed Eng 12:301–308, 1990   7–10

Little is known about the effects of prolonged electrical stimulation of nerves. If neuronal hyperactivity underlies neural injury by electrical stimulation, blocking the action potentials should reduce or abolish injury. Local anesthetic was infused onto nerves at the site of a stimulating electrode. High-frequency stimulation of the cat's peroneal nerve has been shown to cause irreversible neural damage in the form of axonal degeneration of large myelinated nerve fibers.

The application of 10% procaine or 2% lidocaine nearly prevented axonal degeneration from stimulation at 50 Hz. It was not necessary to block the action potential in all large myelinated axons to protect virtually all of the axons from stimulation-related damage. It proved possible to protect myelinated axons using a protocol that blocked action potentials, chiefly in the smaller axons.

It appears that neural damage from electrical stimulation does not result primarily from electrochemical processes associated with passage of current across the metal-tissue interface but, rather, from some physiologic process that is suppressed by local anesthetic. This may be depletion of a vital substrate or generation of a toxic product.

▶ This is an interesting article. I wonder whether it has any clinical significance? Should we use a local anesthesia before utilizing a peripheral nerve stimulator? Does the local anesthetic actually attenuate damage for needles when performing a nerve block?—R.D. Miller, M.D.

Correlation Between Integrated Evoked EMG and Respiratory Function Following Atracurium Administration in Unanesthetized Humans
Sharpe MD, Lam AM, Nicholas JF, Chung DC, Merchant R, Alyafi W,

Beauchamp R (St Joseph's Hosp; Univ of Western Ontario, London; Univ of Washington)
Can J Anaesth 37:307–312, 1990   7–11

Residual paralysis from the use of neuromuscular blocking agents during anesthesia may lead to hypoventilation or upper airway obstruction, or both. Integrated evoked electromyography (IEEMG) provides an accurate and quantitative assessment of neuromuscular blockade. In 6 healthy unanesthetized volunteers, IEEMG was used to correlate response to ulnar nerve stimulation with respiratory function during steady-state infusion of subparalytic doses of atracurium. The IEEMG findings were recorded in response to ulnar nerve stimulation at train-of-four $T_4/T_1 = .2$ and $T_4/T_1 = .6$.

At the level of maximum depression, when $T_4/T_1 = .2$, all subjects had difficulty with swallowing and phonation, none was able to sustain head lift, and hand grip was reduced to 26% to control. However, the tidal volume remained normal in all subjects, and although maximum negative inspiratory pressure (NIP) was 50% of control, forced vital capacity and forced expiratory volume in 1 second were 80% and 82% of control, respectively (Fig 7–8). At the lesser $T_4/T_1 = .6$, all assessments of peripheral strength were normal, and except for NIP (which was 73% of control) none of the respiratory variables differed significantly from control.

In unanesthetized subjects an IEEMG T_4/T_1 of .6 is consistent with near normal respiratory function after administration of atracurium. The

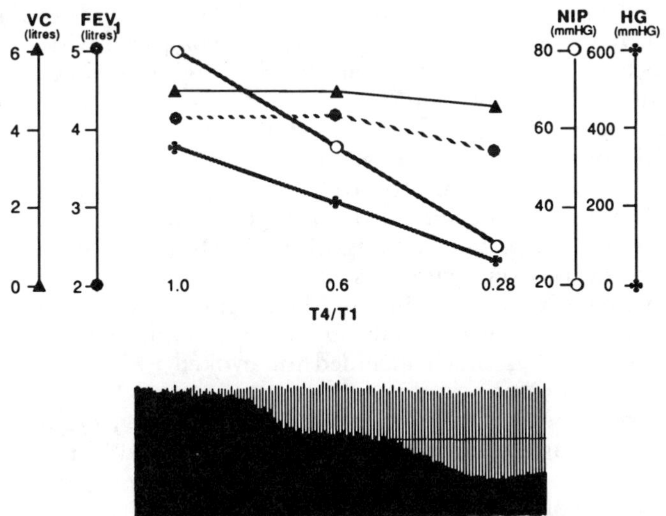

Fig 7–8.—Correlation of respiratory function and hand grip with IEEMG in 1 subject. Assessment of vital capacity (VC), forced expiratory volume in 1 second (FEV$_1$), NIP, and hand grip (HG) are summarized at top while corresponding IEEMG tracing is displayed below. Tracing depicts both T_1 and T_4 EMG (analogous to twitch height). Before administration of atracurium there is no fade and T_4 is identical and superimposed on T_1, creating dark shade in beginning. With onset of neuromuscular blockade, T_4 gradually declines, thus creating dark shade (T_4) and light shade (T_1). (Courtesy of Sharpe MD, Lam AM, Nicholas JF, et al: *Can J Anaesth* 37:307–312, 1990.)

reduced NIP at $T_4/T_1 = .6$ may be caused by weakness of pharyngeal muscles or vocal cord paresis, or both, which leads to a partial airway obstruction during maximal forced inspiration.

▶ This study has several similarities to the Pavlin et al. study with D-tubocurarine (1). Clearly, the train-of-four ratio appears to reflect adequacy in respiratory function. However, it does not appear to be sensitive enough to detect a weakness in the pharyngeal musculature necessary for maintaining patent airway. It also must be recognized that this study was conducted in human volunteers. The inclusion of a residual anesthetic creates problems in addition to the muscle relaxant in maintaining adequate ventilation and a patent airway.—R.D. Miller, M.D.

Reference

1. Pavlin EG, et al: *Anesthesiology* 70:381, 1989.

Clinical, Electrical and Mechanical Correlations During Recovery From Neuromuscular Blockade With Vecuronium
Dupuis JY, Martin R, Tétrault JP (Univ of Sherbrooke, Sherbrooke, PQ)
Can J Anaesth 37:192–196, 1990   7–12

Electromyographic (EMG) and mecanomyographic (MMG) responses are both used to monitor recovery from nondepolarizing neuromuscular blockade during and after anesthesia. The MMG responses of the adductor pollicis have been studied extensively and compared with clinical criteria of recovery from neuromuscular blockade with the long-acting muscle relaxant tubocurarine. An MMG train-of-four (T_4/T_1) value of .7 after using tubocurarine correlates with full recovery of respiratory function and is currently applied to other nondepolarizing muscle relaxants. However, there have been no controlled studies to determine whether the same T_4/T_1 value is valid for other nondepolarizing muscle relaxants.

To determine correlations among EMG, MMG, and clinical criteria of adequate recovery from neuromuscular blockade with the intermediate-acting muscle relaxant vecuronium, 7 healthy, conscious volunteers aged 24–34 years were given subparalyzing doses of vecuronium under neuromuscular monitoring, which included the evoked EMG response of the adductor digiti minimi and the simultaneous evoked MMG response of the adductor pollicis on the same side. Vital capacity, negative inspiratory pressure, peak expiratory flow rate, and 5-second head lift were assessed during recovery from the blockade.

Six of the 7 volunteers reported a pleasant sedative effect that began before evidence of onset of neuromuscular blockade and lasted for 30–60 minutes after complete recovery. Respiratory rate, tidal volume, end-tidal carbon dioxide, and oxygen saturation remained unchanged for the duration of the equipment.

Six volunteers could sustain head lift for 5 seconds at EMG T_4/T_1 of

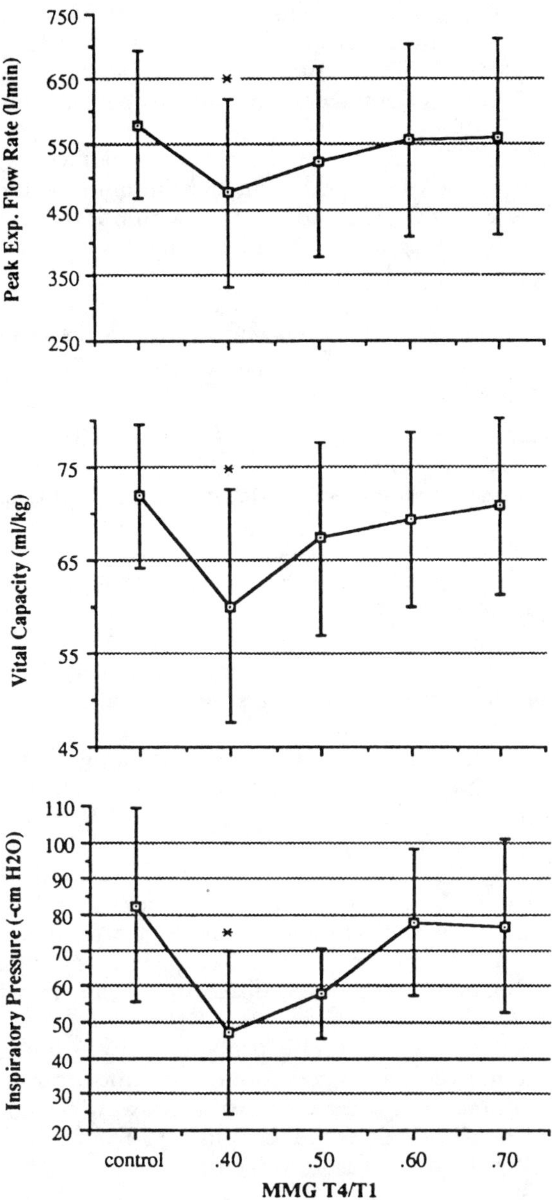

Fig 7–9.—Changes from control in mean ± standard deviation of peak expiratory flow rate, vital capacity, and inspiratory pressure at different evoked MMG train-of-4-responses of adductor policis. *P < .005 when compared with control. (Courtesy of Dupuis JY, Martin R, Tétrault JP: *Can J Anaesth* 37:192–196, 1990.)

.5, and all 7 maintained head lift for 5 seconds at EMG T_4/T_1 of .7. All volunteers achieved normal respiratory function at EMG T_4/T_1 of .9. However, the MMG T_4/T_1 required to perform normal respiratory tests was .5, at which time 6 volunteers were able to perform the head lift test adequately (Fig 7–9).

The evoked MMG response of the adductor pollicis lags behind the evoked EMG response of the adductor digiti minimi by about 20%. The reason for a lower MMG T_4/T_1 correlation with normal respiratory function when vecuronium is used instead of tubocurarine is not clear and should be further explored.

▶ One of the interesting results of this study is the suggestion that correlation of tests with respiration and peripheral nerve stimulation may be different with different neuromuscular blocking drugs.— R.D. Miller, M.D.

Cardiovascular

Transesophageal Echocardiography and Its Potential for Esophageal Damage
Urbanowicz JH, Kernoff RS, Oppenheim G, Parnagian E, Billingham ME, Popp RL (Stanford Univ; Hewlett-Packard Corp, Andover, Mass)
Anesthesiology 72:40–43, 1990   7–13

An animal study and a clinical study were undertaken to determine whether prolonged contact between a transesophageal echocardiography (TEE) probe and the esophageal wall can cause damage. Contact pressure was measured with a modified water-filled balloon designed to attach firmly to the tip of a TEE probe. High pressures against the esophageal wall were not produced in dogs. In all but 1 of 126 measurements in 3 animals the esophageal probe contact pressure was less than 7.7 mm Hg; autopsy studies failed to demonstrate mucosal or muscular damage.

Six patients having a range of operations under general anesthesia were studied using the same Silastic balloon. Contact pressures were less than 17 mm Hg in 5 of the 6 patients but in 1 case were as high as 60 mm Hg. The exceptional patient had a descending thoracic aneurysm. No complications were noted.

Contact pressures between a TEE probe and the esophageal wall generally are low, and even prolonged contact has not produced esophageal damage. High contact pressures are possible, however, in exceptional patients who may be at risk of esophageal injury. The probe should not be fixed in a flexed position for a prolonged period.

▶ This is an interesting article in the search for potential damage from TEE. It seems that just the epidemiology of it and its successful use in humans have not allowed the authors to conclude that it is safe for this purpose. The authors did this study with the Hewlett-Packard probe. Whether or not different probe designs result in different risks was not evaluated.

The authors leave us with more questions than they answer. For instance, if the pressure on the esophagus does go over 60 mm Hg, will this lead to esophageal damage? How long will it take at 60 mm Hg for esophageal damage to occur? Is the risk of changing positions and the friction rubbing up and down the esophagus and causing trauma in the esophagus and throat greater than the rare risk of it at 60 mm Hg? I don't have answers to those questions, but I do know that, in my experience with approximately 2,500 applications of TEE, we have yet to have a complication in a patient who did not have esophageal varices (which we knew about beforehand, were aware of the risk, and had informed the patients of it, as this is part of an experimental protocol dealing with myocardial function in liver transplantation).

Thus I am left thinking that this is a very nice laboratory finding, and the study is well done, but I wonder what it all means. Will I change my practice on the basis of this paper and move the probe up and down and avoid angulation and square-edged probes? No, because I think the risk to the patient from moving it up and down is probably greater than the rare chance of increased pressure occurring. I have fewer data to support my view than the authors have to support theirs, but perhaps more data will be accumulated in the next 10 years to answer these questions.—M.F. Roizen, M.D.

Noninvasive Measurement of Cardiac Output During Surgery Using a New Continuous-Wave Doppler Esophageal Probe

Kumar A, Minagoe S, Thangathurai D, Mikhail M, Novia D, Viljoen JF, Rahimtoola SH, Chandraratna PAN (Univ of Southern California, Los Angeles)
Am J Cardiol 64:793–798, 1989   7–14

A noninvasive, transcutaneous, continuous-wave Doppler technique to measure cardiac output by placing the Doppler transducer in the suprasternal notch correlates well with thermodilution cardiac output measurements. Because the transducer has to be hand held, an esophageal stethoscope was modified to serve as an esophageal Doppler probe. To evaluate the accuracy and utility of the new esophageal Doppler transducer for measuring cardiac output during surgery, 14 patients (average age, 61 years) underwent prolonged elective surgical procedures under general anesthesia.

All patients required continuous intraoperative hemodynamic monitoring because of underlying cardiopulmonary disease. A balloon-tipped pulmonary artery catheter to measure thermodilution cardiac output was inserted before anesthesia induction. The Doppler computer was calibrated for the aortic root diameter obtained from echocardiographic data. Descending aortic blood flow velocity signals were recorded via the esophageal probe and cardiac output was computed by the Doppler computer. A total of 246 paired Doppler and thermodilution cardiac output measurements were obtained in the 14 study patients.

The average thermodilution cardiac output was 5.90 L/min, and the average Doppler cardiac output was 6.21 L/min. There was good correlation between cardiac output measurements obtained by the 2 techniques. Reproducible measurements of Doppler cardiac output also were obtained during intraobserver and interobserver studies. The esophageal probe was easy to insert, and the Doppler computer operation was simple. This instrument can be used for hemodynamic monitoring during general anesthesia in selected patients with cardiopulmonary disease.

▶ It is possible to do things in the operating room today that weren't possible even in a cardiac catheterization laboratory 10 or 15 years ago. However, such technology comes at a high cost and has not been shown always to improve outcome. Although it is hard to envision that an anesthesiologist would not be helped by such sophisticated monitoring, I wonder if we aren't reaching a point of information overload. Is it possible that Doppler cardiac output transesophageal echocardiography, evoked potential monitoring, and compressed spectral array electroencephalography, together with the more commonly employed measurement of vital signs, SpO_2, $Petco_2$, and the like, will be too much for an anesthesiologist to integrate and, at the same time, conduct the anesthetic.—R.R. Kirby, M.D.

Effect of Pulmonary Artery Catheterization on Outcome in Patients Undergoing Coronary Artery Surgery

Tuman KJ, McCarthy RJ, Spiess BD, DaValle M, Hompland SJ, Dabir R, Ivankovich AD (Rush-Presbyterian-St Luke's Med Ctr, Chicago)
Anesthesiology 70:199–206, 1989   7–15

Prospective data are lacking on whether pulmonary artery catheterization (PAC) improves the outcome of cardiac surgery in higher-risk patients compared with central venous pressure (CVP) monitoring alone. It seems logical that prompt recognition of hemodynamic abnormalities should better the outcome. The benefit from PAC was assessed in relation to risk level in a prospective series of 1,094 patients having coronary surgery, of whom 537 had elective PAC.

No outcome variables differed significantly in relation to the use of PAC, even in higher-risk patients. There also was no substantial difference in outcome among some 40 patients assigned to CVP monitoring but who later had a clinical need for PAC because of serious hemodynamic occurrence. In the higher-risk group, the duration of stay in the intensive care unit was longer in patients having PAC.

Previous studies showing that PAC confers benefit have used historical controls or examined only a small number of patients. The present study indicates that PAC does not have a major influence on the outcome after coronary artery surgery, and that even high-risk patients can be managed safely without its routine use. If PAC is reserved until a clinical need arises, safety is maintained and there is considerable cost savings. Incorrect interpretation of routine PAC data could lead to inferior treatment planning and negate any positive effects on the outcome.

▶ Nowhere in this article can I find what was done once the PAC was in place. It isn't the PAC that should change outcome, but the management of the patient utilizing the data it supplies. Because that isn't specified, one can't tell whether anything was done to optimize patient care once the monitor was inserted, or how long the patient stayed in the intensive care unit and had hemodynamics normalized the way Rao et al. described in their 1983 article (1). Thus, one can't tell whether or not this test of PAC versus CVP is worth anything. One wishes that the editors of *Anesthesiology* had insisted on more data so that one could analyze the importance of this study, but alas we can only guess what the authors did. As written, I'm not sure that this article will help me in deciding whether or not to use a PAC. I wouldn't ever consider using a PAC catheter if I wasn't going to do anything with the data derived therefrom, and one can't tell if that was in fact the situation—was the catheter inserted and supposed to help the patient all by itself.—M.F. Roizen, M.D.

Reference

1. Rao TLK, et al: *Anesthesiology* 59:499, 1983.

Hyperkalemia-Like ECG Changes Simulating Acute Myocardial Infarction in a Patient With Hypokalemia Undergoing Potassium Replacement

Madias JE, Madias NE (City Univ of New York, New York; Tufts Univ, Boston, Mass)

J Electrocardiol 22:93–97, 1989   7–16

Elevation of the ST segment (+ST) in association with hyperkalemia has never been documented. Only a few cases of transient +ST and Q waves simulating acute myocardial infarction (MI) in association with hypokalemia have been reported. However, pseudoinfarctional ECG changes in patients with hyperkalemia have been described. A patient with severe hypokalemia experienced transient, marked +ST in the course of potassium (K^+) replacement while she was still hypokalemic.

Woman, 65, was evaluated for weakness, weight loss, and symptoms suggested of urinary tract infection of 2 months' duration. Physical and laboratory examination yielded a diagnosis of Hodgkin's disease stage 4B and urinary infection. She was given blood transfusions. Central hyperalimentation was initiated on day 8 and chemotherapy on day 9. Serial ECGs were unchanged from baseline. On day 14, laboratory testing revealed severe hypokalemia and hyperglycemia. The patient was given 40 mmol of potassium chloride (KCl) by mouth, the glucose-containing hyperalimentation solution was discontinued, and infusion with half-normal saline containing 60 mmol KCl per liter was started. Ten minutes after administration of a second oral dose of 40 mmol KCl, an ECG revealed marked +ST in leads V_1–V_4 consistent with acute anterior MI. The K^+ level obtained at that time was 3 mEq/L. An ECG obtained 15 minutes later showed further widening of the QRS complexes and essentially unchanged +ST segments and T waves. However, the patient was clinically stable and did not complain. An acute MI was ruled out on the basis of the absence of any clinical signs or evolutionary ECG changes and negative enzymatic screening. The ECG changes gradually returned to normal.

This unusual ECG feature may reflect a reduction of the intracellular/ extracellular K^+ ratio in a patient with a decreased level of intracellular serum K^+ who was undergoing rapid K^+ repletion.

▶ There are many dangers of potassium replacement in a patient with hypokalemia, including a 1 in 200 chance of dying, if you believe the data from the Boston Collaborative Drug Group. The data in this article show that, in fact, you can simulate an acute MI-like picture on ECG, probably related to a reduction in the intracellular to extracellular potassium ratio, by administering potassium to patients with decreased intracellular potassium. It is interesting to note that this patient had received about 130 mEq of potassium—80 mEq orally and 50 mEq intravenously—or roughly 3.3 mEq/kg over a period of 8 hours. There may not be any value to this rapid replacement of potassium, and it clearly is hazardous, not only in laboratory test abnormalities, but in actually causing electrophysiologic abnormalities resulting in severe dysrhythmias.—M.F. Roizen, M.D.

Miscellaneous

A Second Time-Study of the Anaesthetist's Intraoperative Period
McDonald JS, Dzwonczyk R, Gupta B, Dahl M (Ohio State Univ)
Br J Anaesth 64:582–585, 1990   7–17

The extent to which recent technological advances have raised the level of anesthetic vigilance was studied in a single operating room during 30 surgical procedures involving 10 resident anesthetists and 3 certified registered nurse anesthetists. The patients underwent general, gynecologic, or ear-nose-throat procedures lasting for a mean of 1.4 hours.

The anesthetists knew that they were the study subjects; activities were videotaped and analyzed independently by 3 reviewers. At the time of study, automatic noninvasive arterial pressure monitors were in use, as were automatic ventilators and patient breathing circuit disconnect alarms.

The greatest amount of intraoperative time was spent monitoring the patient directly (45%) or indirectly (14%). Overall monitoring time was longer than in a previous study. Anesthetists still spent about 10% to 12% of their time completing patient records (table), which may sometimes take place at the expense of direct monitoring.

▶ This is an exciting article because it says that automatic monitors may help us to have more time for direct patient monitoring. The percent of time the faculty have used for direct patient monitoring since the advent of more respiratory monitoring gadgets and the automated blood pressure went from 16.8% to more than 40%. Unfortunately, the authors don't define direct patient monitoring, how they determined it, or what it really means. Nor do they say that the definitions were the same this year as in 1980. The authors also state that 11.1% or so of our time could be spent on more direct patient monitoring if we eliminated record keeping and perhaps we all should have automated record keepers.

Percentage of Time Spent on 11 Activities: 1980 and 1985

Activity	1980 Study [5]	1985 (Present study)		
		Senior Faculty Anaesthetist	Junior Faculty Anaesthetist	Non-clinical Staff
Direct patient monitoring	16.8 (11.2)	53.5 (14.5)	38.7 (11.5)	42.1 (13.6)
Indirect patient monitoring	8.5 (7.7)	12.8 (6.1)	16.8 (7.6)	13.2 (5.4)
Record-keeping	12.1 (3.8)	10.3 (5.7)	11.4 (4.2)	11.1 (5.9)
Anaesthesia machine	4.8 (3.0)	4.5 (3.0)	4.7 (4.2)	4.8 (3.0)
I.v. cannulae	5.6 (3.1)	4.9 (4.6)	4.1 (4.3)	7.0 (5.6)
Breathing system	25.1 (14.0)	0.8 (0.7)	1.0 (0.9)	3.5 (2.8)
Surgical table	1.9 (1.3)	1.0 (1.3)	1.3 (1.6)	0.7 (1.4)
Drug-related activities	5.1 (2.7)	5.1 (4.8)	7.1 (6.3)	7.1 (10.2)
Communication	8.7 (5.1)	3.5 (5.5)	13.2 (12.7)	6.8 (8.3)
Idle time	4.4 (7.1)	0.0 (0.0)	0.4 (1.9)	0.3 (0.9)
Unclassified time	7.0 (3.5)	3.6 (4.3)	1.3 (2.7)	3.4 (4.3)

The data are presented as the mean (SD) of the numbers of procedures reviewed.
(Courtesy of McDonald JS, Dzwonczyk R, Gupta B, et al: *Br J Anaesth* 64:582–585, 1990.)

I gather valuable trend data by writing out a record myself and, although I believe that there are other ways of getting that same input and effect into my brain, I learn by writing things down; consequently, I'm not sure that 11.1% of my time could be spent more profitably in any other way. Some of us learn by writing, some by hearing, some by reading, and perhaps our learning style needs to be evaluated for our practice environment to be most conducive to favorable patient outcome. This article is provocative and stimulating.—M.F. Roizen, M.D.

8 Special Patient Groups

Obesity

Influence of Extreme Obesity on the Body Disposition and Neuromuscular Blocking Effect of Atracurium
Varin F, Ducharme J, Théorêt Y, Besner J-G, Began DR, Donati F (Univ of Montreal; McGill Univ, Quebec)
Clin Pharmacol Ther 48:18–25, 1990   8–1

Because atracurium is disposed of independently of hepatic or renal function, it should be useful in studying the relationship between obesity

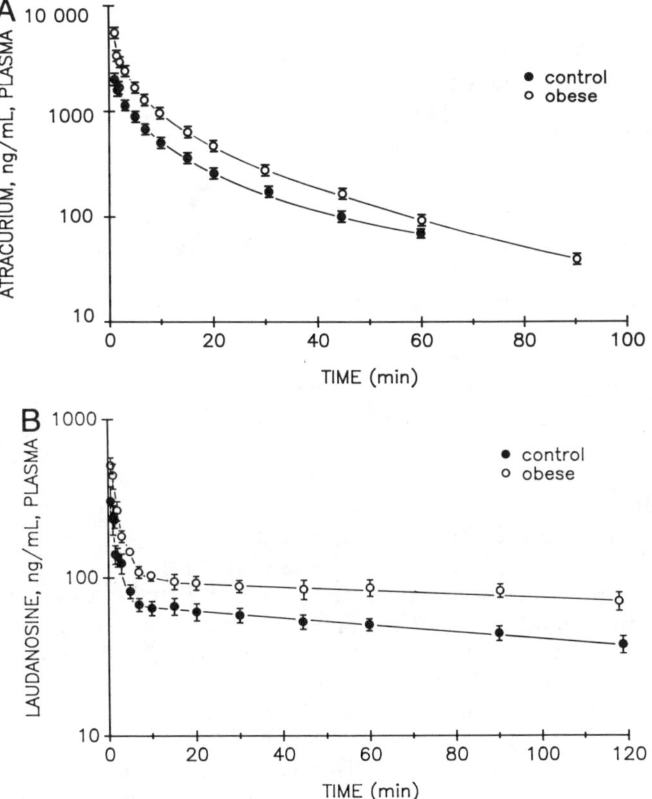

Fig 8–1.—Pharmacokinetic profiles of atracurium and laudanosine in obese patients and nonobese (control) patients. Mean arterial plasma concentrations (± standard error of mean) of atracurium (**A**) and laudanosine (**B**) are represented over time after intravenous bolus of atracurium besylate, .2 mg/kg. (Courtesy of Varin F, Ducharme J, Théorêt Y, et al: *Chin Pharmacol Ther* 48:18–25, 1990.)

and the curarizing effect of nondepolarizing neuromuscular blocking drugs. The disposition and pharmacodynamics of atracurium were compared in 9 morbidly obese patients at least 45 kg above ideal body weight who were scheduled for gastroplasty and 9 patients with normal body habitus. After succinylcholine, atracurium besylate was given intravenously in a dose of .2 mg/kg.

Plasma levels of atracurium were significantly higher in obese patients at all times, and the area under the plasma concentration curve was nearly twice as great as in the controls. The pattern of laudanosine concentration was similar (Fig 8–1). Half-lives and the mean residence time of atracurium did not differ significantly. The absolute mean plasma clearance was comparable in the 2 groups. The time to peak neuromuscular blockade also did not differ, and blockade was not prolonged in obese patients.

Because obese patients require a higher plasma level of atracurium to experience comparable neuromuscular blockade, the dose should be calculated on a total body weight basis. It is not clear whether this can be attributed to altered protein binding or to changes in acetylcholine receptors.

► This is an excellent study. Why obese patients would require a higher concentration of atracurium for neuromuscular blockade is puzzling. I wonder whether this conclusion applies to all neuromuscular blocking drugs.—R.D. Miller, M.D.

Hepatic Cirrhosis

"Endogenous" Benzodiazepine Activity in Body Fluids of Patients With Hepatic Encephalopathy
Mullen KD, Szauter KM, Kaminsky-Russ K (Case Western Reserve Univ)
Lancet 336:81–83, 1990   8–2

It has been hypothesized that an endogenous benzodiazepine-like substance is involved in hepatic encephalopathy. Benzodiazepine activity was examined in the body fluids of 30 patients with hepatic encephalopathy and in 18 controls. None of those involved in the study had taken synthetic benzodiazepines for at least 3 months.

Benzodiazepine receptor binding was significantly higher in the CSF of patients with hepatic encephalopathy than in controls. The severity of encephalopathy was significantly correlated with benzodiazepine activity by radioreceptor assay and radioimmunoassay in urine and plasma. Benzodiazepine activity equivalent to 900 ng/mL could be detected in patients with advanced encephalopathy.

Hepatic encephalopathy is associated with elevated levels of a substance having benzodiazepine activity. The identity, source, and effects of this substance have yet to be determined. It may have a role in the pathogenesis of the neural inhibition seen in hepatic encephalopathy.

► Hepatic encephalopathy is a very serious problem. We may encounter this type of patient in the liver or critical care unit. The mechanism has been illusive, although this paper is intriguing in that it suggests that a benzodiazepine-like substance may be contributing to the encephalopathy.—R.D. Miller, M.D.

Chronic Alcohol Intake Does Not Change Thiopental Anesthetic Requirement, Pharmacokinetics, or Pharmacodynamics

Swerdlow BN, Holley FO, Maitre PO, Stanski DR (Stanford Univ; VA Med Ctr, Palo Alto)
Anesthesiology 72:455–461, 1990   8–3

It is commonly believed that chronic alcoholic patients require larger than normal doses of thiopental for satisfactory induction of general anesthesia. However, the cross-tolerance to barbiturates in an alcoholic population has not been adequately characterized. Using an electroencephalographic (EEG) measure of thiopental's drug effect on the CNS and pharmacodynamic modeling to relate the thiopental serum concentration to drug effects, the thiopental anesthetic requirements, pharmacokinetics, and pharmacodynamics in 11 patients with a history of excessive alcohol intake, chosen from an inpatient alcohol rehabilitation program, were compared with those of 9 control patients or volunteers who were social drinkers. Five alcoholic subjects were restudied after 1 month of abstinence from alcohol consumption.

The alcoholic subjects had their last drink 9–17 days before the study and none had evidence of acute alcoholic intoxication or withdrawal at the time of study. The thiopental dose required to achieve EEG burst suppression (1–3 seconds of isoelectric signal) did not differ significantly between the alcoholic (mean dose, 823 mg) and control (mean dose, 733 mg) groups (Fig 8–2). Similarly, the rate of equilibration between the thiopental serum concentration and pharmacologic effect, the brain's

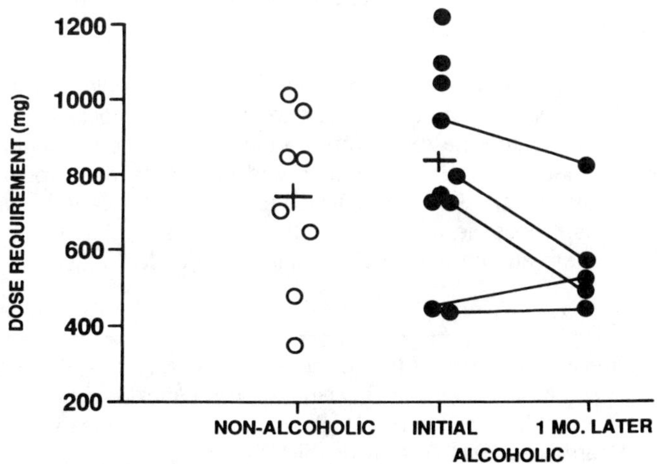

Fig 8–2.—The thiopental dose needed to achieve burst suppression with 3 seconds of isoelectric EEG during a constant infusion of 100 mg/min. The mean value is indicated with a *plus sign*. The individual alcoholic subjects who were studied a second time are indicated with a *connecting line*. (Courtesy of Swerdlow BN, Holley FO, Maitre PO, et al: *Anesthesiology* 72:455–461, 1990.)

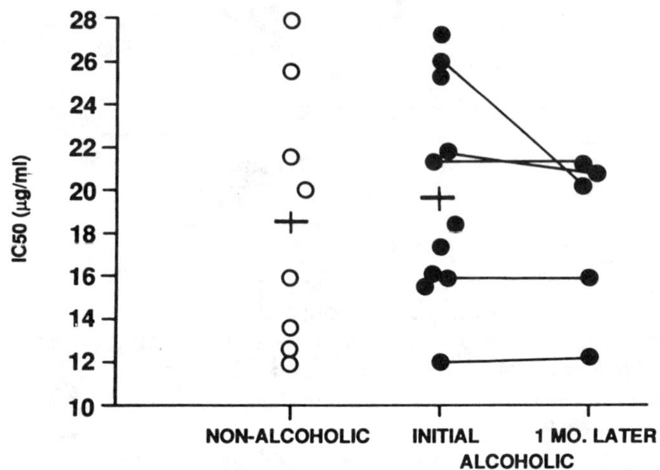

Fig 8–3.—The thiopental serum concentration needed to achieve one half of the maximal decrease of the spectral edge (IC_{50}). The mean value is indicated with a *plus sign*. The individual alcoholic patients who were studied a second time are indicated with a *connecting line*. (Courtesy of Swerdlow BN, Holley FO, Maitre PO, et al: *Anesthesiology* 72:455–461, 1990.)

maximal EEG response to thiopental, and the steady-state plasma concentration needed to cause half of the maximal EEG slowing (Fig 8–3) were not different between groups. Nor was there a significant difference in elimination clearance or elimination half-life between groups. There were no appreciable changes in thiopental dose requirement, pharmacokinetics, or pharmacodynamics among the 5 alcoholic subjects who were studied after 1 month of abstinence.

Apparently, thiopental induction doses should not be routinely increased in chronic alcoholic patients. Rather, they should be based on factors known to alter initial drug distribution and standard hemodynamic considerations.

▶ The results of this study are contrary to the commonly held clinical view that you need more thiopental to induce anesthesia in an alcoholic. This study was extremely well done and the results are certainly valid. The only concern that I would have is that the alcoholic subjects had not had a drink for 9–17 days before the study. I suspect that most alcoholics do not wait that long before taking a drink. Is it possible that the anesthetic biases are based on alcoholics who are both acute and chronic in their intake?—R.D. Miller, M.D.

Pharmacokinetics of Propofol Infusions in Patients With Cirrhosis

Servin F, Cockshott ID, Farinotti R, Haberer JP, Winckler C, Desmonts J-M (Hôp Bichat, Paris; Hôp de Brabois, Vandoeouvre; Hôp Charles Nicolle, Rouen, France; ICI Pharmaceuticals Dvsn, Cheshire, England)
Br J Anaesth 65:177–183, 1990   8–4

Propofol is used to maintain anesthesia by continuous infusion. The pharmacokinetics of infused propofol were examined in 10 patients with cirrhosis and 10 others with normal hepatic and renal function, all of whom were undergoing elective surgery. All of the patients with cirrhosis had previous clinical decompensation, but none had ascites or encephalopathy at the time of study. Propofol was infused at a rate of 21 mg/kg/hr for 5 minutes; 12 mg/kg/hr for 10 minutes; and 6 mg/kg/hr for the rest of the procedure, which lasted for at least 2 hours.

Patients with cirrhosis took longer to recover when the infusion ceased, but both groups had similar blood drug levels at the time of eye opening. Total body clearance was not significantly lower in the cirrhotic patients. The distribution volume at steady state was significantly greater in these patients, but the terminal elimination half-life did not change as a result.

Moderately severe cirrhosis does not substantially alter the pharmacokinetics of propofol when it is infused to maintain general anesthesia. It is important to titrate the infusion rate according to the individual's clinical response.

▶ These data are consistent with many similar studies evaluating the impact of cirrhosis on hepatic clearance of drugs other than propofol. The common observation is that hepatic dysfunction must be severe (ascites, encephalopathy, hypoalbuminemia) before clearance of drugs is likely to be significantly altered.—R.K. Stoelting, M.D.

The Perioperative Changes in Glomerular Filtration and Renal Blood Flow in Patients With Obstructive Jaundice
Thompson JN, Carolan G, Myers MJ, Blumgart LH (Royal Postgrad Med School, London)
Acta Chir Scand 155:465–470, 1989   8–5

Postoperative renal impairment is not uncommon in patients with obstructive jaundice. The pathophysiologic mechanism of this increased renal sensitivity to injury is not known. To assess alterations in renal blood flow and glomerular filtration rate in patients with obstructive jaundice, technetium-99m-diethylenetriaminepentaacetic acid renal scintigraphy was performed before and 8 weeks after elective hepatobiliary surgery in 6 patients with obstructive jaundice and 6 nonjaundiced controls.

Glomerular filtration rates were lower before the operation in the jaundiced patients. The filtration rates increased in the jaundiced patients postoperatively but decreased in the control patients (Fig 8–4). Renal blood flow was reduced postoperatively in the controls but not in the jaundiced patients.

Altered renal hemodynamics and reversible impairment of glomerular filtration were observed in 6 patients with obstructive jaundice. The alter-

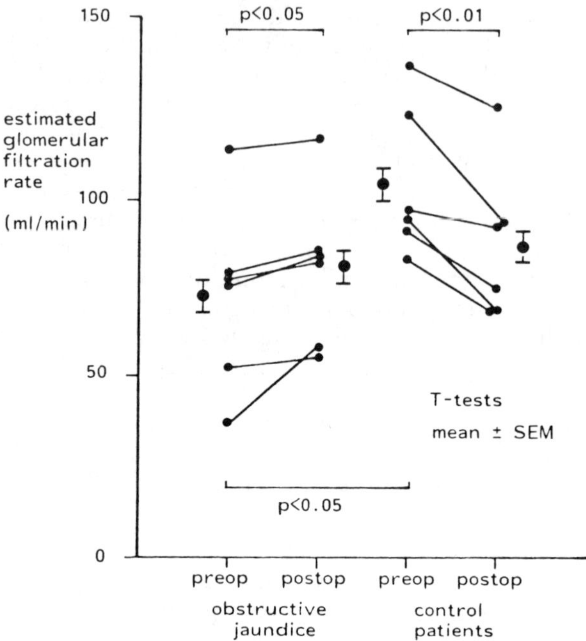

Fig 8–4.—Estimated glomerular filtration rates before and after surgery in patient with obstructive jaundice and nonjaundiced controls. (Courtesy of Thompson JN, Carolan G, Myers MJ, et al: *Acta Chir Scand* 155:465–470, 1989.)

ations in renal blood flow may provide a mechanism for the increased renal sensitivity to injury noted in obstructive jaundice.

▶ Several issues brought up by this article on perioperative changes in glomerular filtration and renal flow in patients with obstructive jaundice need to be dealt with before I accept its conclusions: (1) What was the renal function of these patients to begin with? Were they at risk of renal failure? That is, how high was their creatinine clearance before the start of surgery? Although that in the control group was roughly the same, it's not clear that the creatinine clearance was in fact equivalent between groups. (2) The 2 groups don't appear equal in a number of aspects. For example, only 1 of 5 patients with obstructive jaundice was female, but there were 5 females in the control group. (3) The group with obstructive jaundice received 4 times as many blood products as did the control patients, roughly 4 units compared to 1 unit. I think this presents a major difference for risk of operation. How the authors judged adequate hydration was not stated. They simply said that the patients were adequately hydrated. (4) I take issue with one statement in the paper: "Obstructive jaundice predisposes to the development of systemic hypotension, and if associated with an impaired renovascular response to stress might be expected to predispose to ischaemic renal failure." I would think quite the contrary. If you blunt the sympathorenal reflexes, I think renal blood flow is better and, in fact, may prevent the adverse effects of hypotension. That is, the protective mechanism of the sympathetic nervous system in this case protects the heart and brain but does not protect the kidney.

Like most good articles, this paper stimulates more questions than it answers, and we are left unsure as to the true effect of changes in glomerular filtration and renal blood flow in patients with obstructive jaundice compared to a group matched for surgical severity and gender.—M.F. Roizen, M.D.

Elderly

Population Pharmacokinetics and Pharmacodynamics of Thiopental: The Effect of Age Revisited

Stanski DR, Maitre PO (Stanford Univ; Univ of Bern, Switzerland)
Anesthesiology 72:412–422, 1990   8–6

The thiopental dose required for anesthesia induction decreases by 50% to 67% between the ages of 20 and 80 years. This decrease has been attributed to a decrease in the initial distribution volume for thiopental. The pharmacokinetics and electroencephalographic (EEG) pharmacodynamics of thiopental relative to age were reexamined. A 3-compartment model was used to analyze the bolus and rapid intravenous infusion thiopental serum concentration vs. time data obtained from 64 patients during an 8-year period.

Sixteen patients received an intravenous thiopental bolus and 48 were given a rapid intravenous infusion of thiopental for anesthesia induction. Using the EEG again as a measure of CNS drug effect, the data reconfirmed that age does not affect the brain's sensitivity to thiopental because thiopental EEG pharmacodynamics were not altered with increasing age. When thiopental was administered as a rapid intravenous bolus, the thiopental distribution phenomenon could not be characterized accurately. When thiopental was given as a rapid intravenous infusion, increasing age was associated with a decrease in thiopental rapid intercompartment clearance. Thus the decreased thiopental requirement in elderly persons can be attributed to a decreased rapid intercompartment clearance. The initial distribution volume of thiopental does not change with age.

The Relationship of Age to the Pharmacokinetics of Early Drug Distribution: The Concurrent Disposition of Thiopental and Indocyanine Green

Avram MJ, Krejcie TC, Henthorn TK (Northwestern Univ)
Anesthiology 72:403–411, 1990   8–7

The optimal dose of thiopental depends on its initial distribution kinetics and its pharmacodynamics. Older patients sometimes require lower doses of thiopental than younger patients. To determine the pharmacokinetic basis of this increased reactivity of the elderly to thiopental, 21 healthy men aged 20–80 years were simultaneously given thiopental and indocyanine green (ICG), a marker of intravascular space. Frequent early arterial blood samples were taken and the distribution of the 2 compounds was modeled.

The distribution of ICG could be considered as 2-compartment, whereas the distribution of thiopental was 4-compartment. Both models have in common a central volume (V1), the central blood pool. The ICG distributes from V1 by intravascular mixing to a peripheral blood volume that is a subset of a rapidly equilibrating peripheral thiopental compartment. Elimination of both drugs occurred from the peripheral compartments. The central volume did not decrease with increasing age. The intercompartmental clearance from V1 to the peripheral compartments decreased by 35% between the ages of 20 and 80 years.

Age cannot be used alone to adjust the dosage of thiopental in elderly patients. Appropriate doses of thiopental must be selected on the basis of physiologic factors that may affect the pharmacokinetics or pharmacodynamics of the drug.

How Far Can We Go With Compartmental Models?
Hull CJ (Royal Victoria Infirmary, Newcastle Upon Tyne, England)
Anesthesiology 72:399–402, 1990

8–8

Studies of drug disposition yield concentration-time data that must be simplified mathematically. Models that simulate what actually happens in the body produce the best approach. Such a model may consist of a number of perfusion-limited compartments, each defined by volume, blood flow, and apparent tissue-blood partition coefficient. Such models can account for hemodynamic changes but numerical values must be assigned to their many parameters.

Alternatively, drug disposition can be represented by simple compartmental models whose volumes are "apparent." In a parametric model the function that will govern the concentration-effect relationship is determined in advance.

Henthorn et al. proposed that early disposition of thiopental might be defined by considering the concurrent disposition of an intravascular marker such as indocyanine green (ICG), which follows 2-compartment kinetics. Thiopental, however, partitions into lung tissue and ICG does not; therefore, it cannot be assumed that they share identical central distribution volumes.

With respect to the early distribution period, the assumptions underlying the simple compartmental model make it inappropriate as an investigative tool. The model of Henthorn's group does not adequately account for the complexities of early distribution and does not attempt to represent the dynamics of pharmacologic effect. It is possible that this model could be developed to account for pulmonary uptake and real values of cardiac output if serial estimates of both arterial and mixed venous concentrations of thiopental are available. Such a model may be able to demonstrate the influence of age on thiopental kinetics in proper physiologic terms.

▶ What I take from these 2 articles (Abstracts 8–6 and 8–7) and the editorial (Abstract 8–8) is that, no matter what model is used, there is a reduced thiopental dose requirement in the elderly that is not related to sensitivity of the brain to thiopental or, as it is called, pharmacodynamics, but is caused by a pharmacokinetic mechanism of reduced distribution from the central compartment to peripheral compartments. Obviously, these compartments are theoretical constructs and do not actually exist, but this distribution from the central to the peripheral compartments appears to decrease by about 5% per decade. Thus the anesthetic requirement decreases between 50% and 70% from age 20 to age of 80, using EEG as a measure; almost all of this difference can be accounted for by the fact that thiopental stays in the central compartment and is distributed to the brain in a higher concentration in the aged.—M.F. Roizen, M.D.

Outcomes of Surgery in Patients 90 Years of Age and Older

Hosking MP, Warner MA, Lobdell CM, Offord KP, Melton LJ III (Mayo Clinic and Found, Rochester, Minn)
JAMA 261:1909–1915, 1989   8–9

The question was raised of how well the elderly withstand surgery. Data were reviewed on 795 patients aged 90 or more who underwent surgery at the Mayo Clinic from 1975 to 1985. Most of the patients were aged 90–94 years, but 14% were aged 95–99 years and 2% were at least 100 years. A substantial number of patients had chronic disorders, usually hypertension. Nearly 20% had sustained a myocardial infarction. Eighty percent of the group were in ASA class III or worse.

Nearly 10% of the patients had serious morbidity within 48 hours of surgery; the mortality rate was 1.6%. Short-term morbidity and short- and long-term mortality correlated closely with ASA physical status. Emergency surgery was associated with the highest risk. Preoperative renal, liver, and CNS disease predicted a poorer outlook, as did male gender and surgery on the mouth, nose, or pharynx.

Patients aged 90 or more years tolerate surgery relatively well. About half of the present operations involved general anesthesia, but this did not heighten short- or long-term mortality compared with regional anesthesia. Both increased rates of operation in the very elderly and improved survival may significantly influence health care costs in the future.

▶ Once again, the ASA physical status classification proved predictive of the risk of surgery. Added to the ASA physical status classification, the emergency nature of the procedure seems to be the best predictor of risk in operative procedures. In our own studies, these 2 risk factors were clearly superior to those used by Medicare for risk adjustment, or even those used by Medis groups, by a factor of more than 100%. The Medicare risk adjustments got you 30% of the way toward the correct risk assessment, and the Medis groups, 39%; using the ASA status plus emergency nature of the surgery and the known mortality of the procedure got you 89% of the way there.

This study shows that even in patients 90 years of age and older, of whom there will be an estimated 2 million in the United States by the year 2000, surgery can be attempted with relatively low mortality and overall serious morbidity rates—in this series, 1.6% mortality and 9.4% serious morbidity rates in a group already at high risk. Eye surgery on 91 patients carried absolutely no morbidity and mortality, whereas non-eye surgery was associated with progressively increasing mortality as age increased. Non-eye surgery done on an emergency basis resulted in a mortality rate of 7.9%, ranging from 1.7% in ASA physical status class III to 80% in ASA physical status class V patients. The Mayo Group that published this study is to be congratulated for their outstanding use of a large database to enlighten the rest of us concerning the risks of anesthesia and surgery in specific high-risk populations.—M.F. Roizen, M.D.

Hemodynamic Effect of Epidurally Administered Epinephrine in Middle-Aged and Elderly Patients

Tomoda MK, Ueda W, Hirakawa M (Kochi Med School, Kochi, Japan)
Acta Anaesthesiol Scand 33:647–651, 1989   8–10

Epinephrine is commonly added to local anesthetic solutions to decrease the rate of vascular absorption and prolong the duration of epidural analgesia. The hemodynamic effects of epidural epinephrine have been well studied but only in relatively young patients. The hemodynamic effects of epidural epinephrine were compared in 14 middle-aged men aged 52–65 years and 18 elderly men aged 75–82 years who underwent elective transurethral resection of the prostate under epidural anesthesia.

Seven middle-aged patients and 9 elderly patients were injected with 10 mL of 1.5% lidocaine solution into the epidural space. The remaining patients were given 10 mL of 1.5% lidocaine solution with 1:200,000 epinephrine added. Bupivacaine was used to provide supplemental analgesia as needed. Arterial blood samples to measure the plasma epinephrine concentration were obtained before epidural injection, and 5, 10, and 20 minutes after completion of the initial injection.

There was no significant difference in the plasma epinephrine concentration and level of analgesia at 20 minutes between the 2 age groups. Eight middle-aged patients and 4 elderly patients required supplemental bupivacaine injection to restore an adequate quality of surgical analgesia. Of these 12 patients, 9 had been given lidocaine and 3 had received lidocaine plus epinephrine. Both differences were statistically significant. Changes in hemodynamic parameters occurred most commonly in patients given lidocaine plus epinephrine (table). Epinephrine caused a significant increase in heart rate and a significant reduction in diastolic arterial pressure in both age groups. However, a significant reduction in systolic arterial pressure occurred only in middle-aged patients. None of the patients experienced hypotensive episodes, ECG changes, or cardiac dysrhythmias as a result of the use of epidural analgesia and epinephrine.

Hemodynamic Data (Mean ± SEM)

	Time in min				
	0	5	10	15	20
HR bpm					
M	62 ± 3	64 ± 3	64 ± 3	64 ± 3	64 ± 3
M-EP	70 ± 7	75 ± 7	76 ± 7^b	80 ± 7^a	75 ± 6^a
E	70 ± 6	69 ± 6	69 ± 6	69 ± 6	69 ± 6
E-EP	67 ± 2	70 ± 3^c	73 ± 3^c	73 ± 3^c	74 ± 4^c
SAP mmHg (kPa)					
M	$126 \pm 6 \ (16.8 \pm 0.8)$	$126 \pm 6 \ (16.8 \pm 0.8)$	$127 \pm 6 \ (16.9 \pm 0.8)$	$126 \pm 6 \ (16.8 \pm 0.8)$	$129 \pm 6 \ (17.2 \pm 0.8)$
M-EP	$130 \pm 8 \ (17.3 \pm 1.1)$	$124 \pm 9 \ (16.5 \pm 1.2)^b$	$125 \pm 8 \ (16.7 \pm 1.1)^a$	$121 \pm 8 \ (16.1 \pm 1.1)^c$	$120 \pm 8 \ (16.0 \pm 1.1)^d$
E	$131 \pm 6 \ (17.5 \pm 0.8)$	$132 \pm 6 \ (17.6 \pm 0.8)$	$132 \pm 6 \ (17.6 \pm 0.8)$	$129 \pm 6 \ (17.2 \pm 0.8)$	$129 \pm 7 \ (17.2 \pm 0.9)$
E-EP	$125 \pm 5 \ (16.7 \pm 0.7)$	$124 \pm 6 \ (16.5 \pm 0.8)$	$120 \pm 7 \ (16.0 \pm 0.9)$	$121 \pm 6 \ (16.1 \pm 0.8)$	$123 \pm 6 \ (16.4 \pm 0.8)$
MAP mmHg (kPa)					
M	$91 \pm 5 \ (12.1 \pm 0.7)$	$92 \pm 4 \ (12.3 \pm 0.5)$	$92 \pm 4 \ (12.3 \pm 0.5)$	$92 \pm 4 \ (12.3 \pm 0.5)$	$94 \pm 4 \ (12.5 \pm 0.5)$
M-EP	$93 \pm 5 \ (12.4 \pm 0.7)$	$89 \pm 6 \ (11.9 \pm 0.8)^b$	$89 \pm 6 \ (11.9 \pm 0.8)^a$	$86 \pm 6 \ (11.5 \pm 0.8)^c$	$84 \pm 5 \ (11.2 \pm 0.7)^d$
E	$90 \pm 4 \ (12.0 \pm 0.5)$	$91 \pm 4 \ (12.1 \pm 0.5)$	$92 \pm 4 \ (12.3 \pm 0.5)$	$91 \pm 3 \ (12.1 \pm 0.4)$	$91 \pm 4 \ (12.1 \pm 0.5)$
E-EP	$87 \pm 3 \ (11.6 \pm 0.4)$	$85 \pm 4 \ (11.3 \pm 0.5)$	$82 \pm 4 \ (10.9 \pm 0.5)$	$81 \pm 4 \ (10.8 \pm 0.5)^a$	$82 \pm 3 \ (10.9 \pm 0.4)^a$
DAP mmHg (kPa)					
M	$74 \pm 4 \ (9.9 \pm 0.5)$	$75 \pm 4 \ (10.0 \pm 0.5)$	$74 \pm 3 \ (9.9 \pm 0.4)$	$75 \pm 4 \ (10.0 \pm 0.5)$	$76 \pm 3 \ (10.1 \pm 0.4)$
M-EP	$75 \pm 4 \ (10.0 \pm 0.5)$	$71 \pm 5 \ (9.5 \pm 0.7)^a$	$71 \pm 5 \ (9.5 \pm 0.7)^a$	$69 \pm 5 \ (9.2 \pm 0.7)^b$	$66 \pm 4 \ (8.8 \pm 0.5)^{d}\dagger$
E	$70 \pm 3 \ (9.3 \pm 0.4)$	$71 \pm 3 \ (9.5 \pm 0.4)$	$72 \pm 3 \ (9.6 \pm 0.4)$	$72 \pm 3 \ (9.6 \pm 0.4)$	$72 \pm 3 \ (9.6 \pm 0.4)$
E-EP	$68 \pm 3 \ (9.1 \pm 0.4)$	$65 \pm 3 \ (8.7 \pm 0.4)$	$63 \pm 3 \ (8.4 \pm 0.4)$	$62 \pm 4 \ (8.3 \pm 0.5)^a$	$61 \pm 3 \ (8.1 \pm 0.4)^{a}\dagger$

Abbreviations: HR, heart rate; SAP, systolic arterial pressure; MAP, mean arterial pressure; DAP, diastolic arterial pressure; M, middle aged; M-EP, middle-aged with epinephrine; E, elderly; E-EP, elderly with epinephrine

[a] $p < .05$.
[b] $p < .02$.
[c] $p < .01$.
[d] $p < .001$ vs. values at 0 minutes by the 2-tailed paired *t*-test.
†$p < .05$ M-EP vs. M, E-EP vs. E, and E-EP vs. M by analysis of variance with the Student-Neuman-Keuls test.
(Courtesy of Tomoda MK, Ueda W, Hirakawa M: *Acta Anaesthesiol Scand* 33:647–651, 1989.)

The addition of epinephrine to the anesthetic lidocaine solution significantly improved the quality of surgical epidural analgesia. The hemodynamic reaction to epinephrine when injected into the epidural space together with lidocaine differed between middle-aged and elderly patients.

However, as none of the elderly patients experienced any harmful circulatory reactions to epinephrine administration, lidocaine-epinephrine solution at the concentration used in this study for epidural analgesia may be justified in the elderly.

▶ This study by Tomoda et al. has a very impressive but generally written (without data) abstract and, when you look at the data, they actually support the conclusions in the abstract. But the data in the absolutes are nowhere nearly as impressive as the conclusions in the abstract. For instance, the change in mean arterial pressure went from 130 to 120 in the middle-aged patients and from 125 to 120 in the elderly patients. That's not a very substantial change upon which to make a major conclusion. Similarly, the heart rate in those patients given epinephrine went from 70 to 80 in the middle aged as opposed to the elderly, in whom it went from 67 to 74. Again, not the kind of absolute numbers that cause you to sit up and take notice. The authors are careful to not make more of their data than exists, and we as readers need to be that careful also.—M.F. Roizen, M.D.

Cognitive and Functional Competence After Anaesthesia in Patients Aged Over 60: Controlled Trial of General and Regional Anaesthesia for Elective Hip or Knee Replacement

Jones MJT, Piggott SE, Vaughan RS, Bayer AJ, Newcombe RG, Twining TC, Pathy J, Rosen M (Univ of Wales, Cardiff; Univ Hosp of Wales, Cardiff)
Br Med J 300:1683–1687, 1990   8–11

It often is claimed that elderly patients are "never the same" after admission to the hospital, but the role, if any, of anesthesia in cognitive deterioration remains uncertain. The long-term effects of general and regional anesthesia were compared prospectively in 146 patients aged 60 years and older who had elective hip or knee replacement surgery. Seventy-two patients were assigned to receive general N_2O-halothane anesthesia supplemented by fentanyl and 74 received regional anesthesia with .5% bupivacaine. Several tests of cognitive function and functional competence were administered before and after surgery.

Both the recognition and response components of the choice reaction time test were improved 3 months after operation in patients given general anesthesia, compared with recipients of regional anesthesia. There were no other significant group differences. Eleven patients in the regional anesthesia group and 12 who received general anesthesia reported decreased memory and concentration after surgery, but testing failed to confirm such changes. Neither general nor regional anesthesia, when used with modern methods, appears to have significant long-term adverse effects on mental function in elderly patients.

▶ The findings of this study are reassuring (particularly as we grow older) that anesthetic technique, per se, does not appear to have long-term adverse effects on mental function in older patients. One wonders if the changes in mental status after operative procedures are related to other factors such as attention by nursing personnel, family members, and other associates, or to the environment in which postoperative recovery occurs? I believe these questions need to be addressed in future studies.—G.W. Ostheimer, M.D.

Age-Related Cognitive Recovery After General Anesthesia
Chung F, Seyone C, Dyck B, Chung A, Ong D, Taylor A, Stone R (Univ of Toronto)
Anesth Analg 71:217–224, 1990   8–12

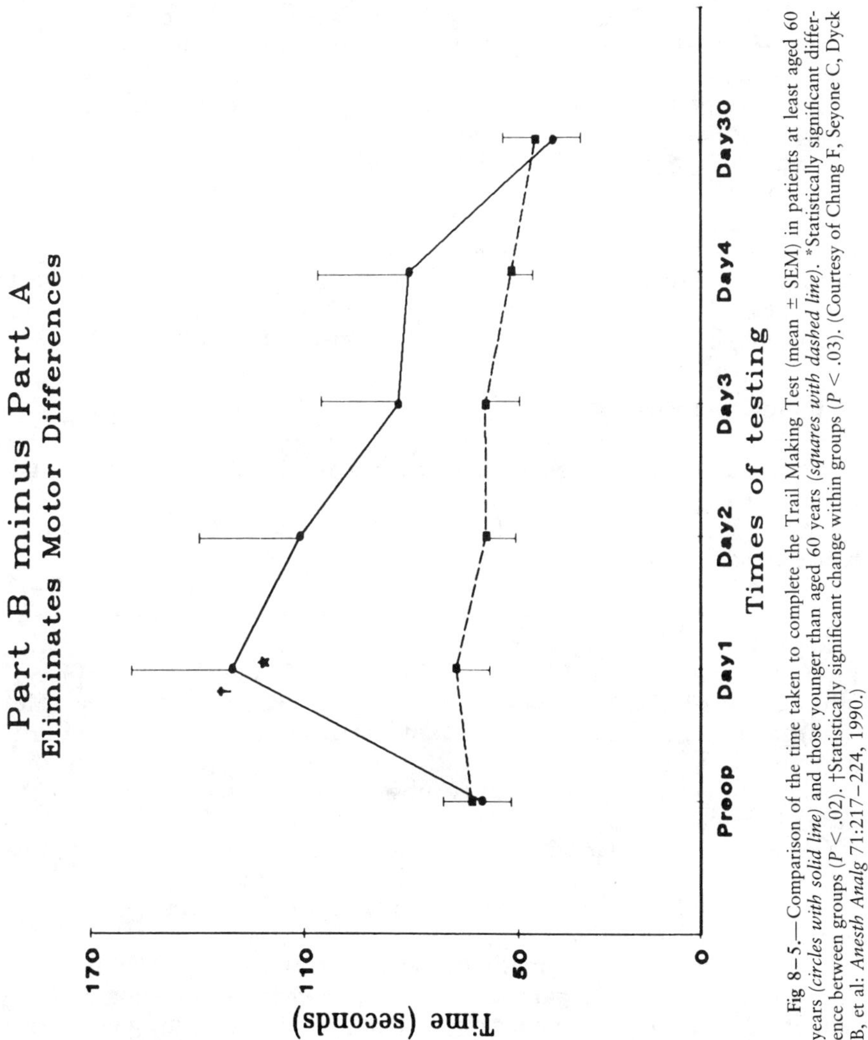

Fig 8–5.—Comparison of the time taken to complete the Trail Making Test (mean ± SEM) in patients at least aged 60 years (*circles with solid line*) and those younger than aged 60 years (*squares with dashed line*). *Statistically significant difference between groups ($P < .02$). †Statistically significant change within groups ($P < .03$). (Courtesy of Chung F, Seyone C, Dyck B, et al: *Anesth Analg* 71:217–224, 1990.)

An increasing number of older persons are having surgery. In an attempt to quantify the rate of mental recovery in elderly and young patients after general anesthesia for cholecystectomy, 15 patients older than age 60 years and 25 others whose mean age was 40 years were evaluated. The Mini Mental State Test, Symbol Digit Modalities Test, Digit Span Test, and Trail Making Test were used. Anesthesia was maintained with nitrous oxide/oxygen and volatile agents as needed.

Anesthetic doses were comparable in the 2 age groups. There were no significant group differences in results of the Mini Mental State Test or Digit Symbol Test postoperatively after correcting for baseline differences. The same was true for the Digit Span Test, but the Trail Making Test showed greater impairment in the older group on the first postoperative day (Fig 8–5). One patient, aged 60 years, was clinically confused in the early postoperative period in association with wound sepsis but recovered well.

Cognitive performance is impaired shortly after general anesthesia for cholecystectomy, even in younger patients. The elderly do not exhibit substantially more mental deterioration postoperatively than those who are younger.

▶ The results of this study are contrary to others that are available in the literature. Does the surgical procedure have an influence? Otherwise, I am at a loss how to explain why the elderly patients did not have a more delayed recovery of cognitive function as opposed to their younger counterparts.—R.D. Miller, M.D.

Diabetes Mellitus

Diabetic Nephropathy: Hemodynamic Basis and Implications for Disease Management
Noth RH, Krolewski AS, Kaysen GA, Meyer TW, Schambelan M (Univ of California, Davis; VA Med Ctr, Martinez, Calif)
Ann Intern Med 110:795–813, 1989   8–13

In 30% to 50% of patients with insulin-dependent diabetes mellitus, nephropathy eventually develops. In the United States, diabetic nephropathy accounts for 25% of patients undergoing chronic renal dialysis. Hemodynamic factors appear to have a major role in the initiation and progression of diabetic nephropathy. The incidence of hypertension in diabetic patients with nephropathy is substantially greater than that in the general population.

Glomerular vasodilation and hyperfiltration, mediated in part by prostaglandins, were thought to cause glomerular damage early in the course of diabetes. However, the result of studies with angiotensin converting enzyme inhibitors suggest that glomerular hypertension rather than glomerular hyperfiltration potentially causes glomerular injury. Therapy with antihypertensive drugs, particularly the angiotensin-converting enzyme inhibitors, has a major impact on delaying renal failure in hypertensive patients with established clinical diabetic nephropathy characterized by proteinuria of more than .3−.5 g/day. Clinical evidence indicates that antihypertensive drug therapy and dietary protein restriction can decrease the degree of albuminuria when still in its early microalbuminuria phase. Data on the long-term effects of antihypertensive drug therapy on disease progression when albuminuria is first treated in its early stage are not yet available.

The development of more sensitive immunologic assays for the detection of albumin in urine now allows a diagnosis of incipient nephropathy long before it would have been diagnosed using standard bromcresol green reagent strip testing. Even a small increase in urinary albumin excretion predicts the development of renal disease in patients with juvenile-onset diabetes. The ability to detect albuminuria much earlier in the course of diabetic nephropathy, plus the availability of therapies specifically directed against hemodynamic abnormalities throughout the course of diabetic renal disease, are having a positive impact on survival and the quality of life for patients with diabetic nephropathy.

▶ This review is fascinating. Two new major ideas are presented. First, you can prevent diabetic complications if you don't give protein. Well, we all know you shouldn't eat fat, so I guess the only thing we should consume is long-chain carbohydrates. Maybe baked potatoes are the ideal food.

The second new idea is that diabetes combined with hypertension is very bad for renal function, and the hypertension should be treated aggressively. But, as with many things, science lags behind clinical practice. For several years, clinicians have been using angiotensin-converting enzyme inhibitors such as captopril, and drugs that copy captopril, for their dramatic renal protective effects. What is the science behind this protection? No one knows for sure, and as you read through the article you'll find that a major controversy exists as to the mechanism of its protective effect. But it is clear that glomerular hypertension appears to be the cause of glomerular injury, and that captopril can reduce glomerular hypertension and the hyperfiltration that glomerular hypertension causes. This protective effect was found quite by accident when Berkman and Rifkin (1) reported the dramatic renal protective effect of critically narrowing 1 renal artery in a diabetic patient with renovascular hypertension.—M.F. Roizen, M.D.

Reference

1. Berkman J, Rifkin H: *Metabolism* 22:715, 1973.

Diabetes Mellitus and Ventilatory Capacity: A Five Year Follow-Up Study
Lange P, Groth S, Mortensen J, Appleyard M, Nyboe J, Schnohr P, Jensen G (Copenhagen)
Eur Respir J 3:288–292, 1990   8–14

Insulin-dependent diabetes has been associated with slight pulmonary dysfunction. A review was made of data from a prospective cardiovascular epidemiologic study of 11,135 Danish subjects to determine whether

Unadjusted Annual Decline of Forced Expiratory Volume in 1 Second (FEV_1) and Forced Vital Capacity (FVC) According to Sex and Diabetes

Decline of ventilatory function	Women			Men		
	Controls n=5,206	KDM n=67	NDM n=49	Controls n=3,845	KDM n=133	NDM n=77
ΔFEV_1 ml·yr^{-1}	26 (1)	23 (10)	54 (14)	35 (2)	42 (12)	57 (12)
ΔFVC ml·yr^{-1}	29 (2)	20 (13)	64 (15)	42 (3)	61 (13)	64 (13)

Mean values with SE in parentheses. ΔFEV_1: mean annual decline in forced expiratory volume in 1 second; ΔFVC: mean annual decline in forced vital capacity. **KDM**, known diabetes mellitus; **NDM**, new diabetes mellitus.
(Courtesy of Lange P, Groth S, Mortenson J, et al: *Eur Respir J* 3:288–292, 1990.)

the onset of diabetes coincides with impaired ventilatory capacity. The diabetic group included 126 subjects who had become diabetic or had a plasma glucose level above 11.1 mM/L at the second examination, and 200 others known at the outset to have diabetes or a high plasma level of glucose.

Subjects who became diabetic during observation had the steepest decrease in ventilatory function after controlling for age, gender, height, and tobacco use. Compared with nondiabetics, their forced vital capacity decreased by an average of 29 mL per year and their forced expiratory volume in 1 second by 25 mL. The decline in lung function in those who had diabetes throughout was not greater than in nondiabetics (table).

Patients with newly diagnosed diabetes experience an unusually large decline in ventilatory function, possibly because of cross-linking of pulmonary collagen. In more advanced diabetes, glycosylation of collagen tends to decelerate, and the effect on ventilatory function is smaller.

▶ Although the new onset of diabetes is shown by this study to decrease ventilatory function, the question of mechanism remains unsettled. Is it because protein synthesis in the diabetic is altered by the presence of nonenzymatic glycosylation? In any case, the study does show us that subjects with newly developed diabetes have a decline in ventilatory function that is greater than that in nondiabetic subjects. Why this is also greater than that of diabetics who have long-standing diabetes is not clear to me. Are these declines clinically significant? I can't tell: a 25-mL greater decline for the first 10 years wouldn't lead to a 250-mL decrease in the forced expiratory volume. That's a significantly greater decrease but a relatively minor effect compared to cigarette smoking for the same time period. It does again bring up the fact that diseases summate, and persons with diabetes probably shouldn't smoke and probably should have their hypertension treated aggressively.—M.F.Roizen, M.D.

Thyroid Disease

Thyroidectomy for Amiodarone-Induced Thyrotoxicosis
Farwell AP, Abend SL, Huang SKS, Patwardhan NA, Braverman LE (Univ of Massachusetts, Worcester)
JAMA 263:1526–1528, 1990   8–15

Amiodarone, an iodine-rich drug used to treat tachyarrhythmias, produces thyrotoxicosis in about 10% of patients who receive prolonged treatment with this medication and live in areas of moderate iodine deficiency. The drug has a prolonged half-life, and cardiac decompensation from underlying heart disease is frequent, making treatment difficult. Thyroidectomy was effective in 1 patient after several medical measures failed to control the hyperthyroid state.

Man, 54, had received 400 mg of amiodarone daily for nearly 3 years because of recurrent ventricular arrhythmia associated with idiopathic cardiomyopathy. One week before admission he had recurrence of mild palpitations, increased shortness of breath, decreased exercise tolerance, and a generalized lack of energy. Examination showed orthostasis and clinical thyrotoxicosis, confirmed by testing thyroid function. Thyrotoxicosis persisted despite replacement of amiodarone with quinidine and mexilitine, administration of methimazole, and the addition of dexamethasone and iopanoic acid. A near-total thyroidectomy was performed and the serum level of thyroxine fell rapidly. Degenerative and destructive follicular changes and diffuse fibrosis were noted in the specimen. Hypothyroidism was easily controlled with levothyroxine. Amiodarone later was reinstituted, and the patient remained euthyroid 11 months after operation taking .125 mg of levothyroxine daily.

It may take many weeks to control amiodarone-induced thyrotoxicosis medically. Radioactive iodine usually is not a viable option. Surgery is effective, providing permanent control in most cases. Near-total thyroidectomy appears to be reasonably safe in this setting.

▶ The use of amiodarone to treat dysrhythmias has been increasing, and perhaps there are some patients in whom the tachycardia and tachyarrhythmias that necessitate amiodarone are so severe that one would use amiodarone and thyroidectomy as a treatment option. However, I find it unusual, and I can't remember many other cases in the entire history of drug therapy in which a substantial surgical operation was done to allow a medical therapy to be used. But I think there are several places in cardiology where that is now being done, and perhaps even in orthopedics and cancer chemotherapy.—M.F. Roizen, M.D.

American Thyroid Association Guidelines for Use of Laboratory Tests in Thyroid Disorders
Surks MI, Chopra IJ, Mariash CN, Nicoloff JT, Solomon DH (Montefiore Med Ctr and Albert Einstein College of Medicine, Bronx; Univ of California, Los Angeles; Univ of Minnesota; Univ of Southern California)
JAMA 263:1529–1532, 1990   8–16

Tests for thyroid disease should be targeted to populations at risk including neonates, those with a strong family history of thyroid illness, elderly patients, postpartum women, and patients with autoimmune disorders. In testing for hypothyroidism, thyroxine (T_4)-binding globulin may be altered in the absence of thyroid disease in many different settings. Free T_4 estimates are preferred to determinations of total serum T_4. The free T_4 index is a function of total T_4 and the thyroid hormone-binding ratio. In most cases hypothyroidism reflects a disorder of the thyroid gland itself. Most patients have an increased serum concentration of thyrotropin. Laboratory tests can be helpful in monitoring levothyroxine therapy.

Hyperthyroidism can be confirmed by documenting elevated serum levels of thyroid hormone and a decreased serum level of thyrotropin. Occasionally, an elevated serum level of triiodothyronine (T_3) will aid in the diagnosis of hyperthyroidism. Nonthyroidal illnesses have a wide range of effects on thyroid hormone metabolism, circulating T_4 inhibitors, and serum thyroid hormone-binding proteins.

Some drugs such as phenytoin can lower serum levels of thyroid hormone. Some, including glucocorticoids and propranolol, can reduce the rate of reduction of T_3 by T_4 in peripheral tissues. Dopamine generally lowers the serum levels of sensitive thyrotropin, but most drugs do not affect this value.

▶ This article details the new use of thyroid function tests and the fact that the *free T_4 index* is now called the *free T_4 estimate,* which is usually obtained by multiplying the *total T_4 concentration* times the *thyroid hormone-binding ratio.*

The *thyroid hormone-binding ratio* was formerly called the *radioactive thyroid uptake*. So nothing has changed in the calculation—just the terms. The article also details factors that influence T_4-binding globulin and shows that, in sick patients—especially those in critical care units, the diagnosis of thyroid disease is difficult secondary to changes in thyroid-binding globulin and the fasting changes in thyroid-stimulating hormone. In mild to moderate illness, the free T_4 estimate is normal or elevated, with thyrotropin in the normal range. But in severe or chronic illness, the free T_4 estimate is down by 50% when determined by conventional assays but normal when determined by equilibrium dialysis. Thyrotropin may be normal or suppressed in severe chronic illness, especially if the patient has received steroids or dopamine. On the other hand, the thyrotropin level is transiently raised by acute illness.—M.F. Roizen, M.D.

9 Coagulation

The Role of Desmopressin in Reducing Blood Loss During Lumbar Fusions
Johnson RG, Murphy JM (Robert H Dedman Med Ctr, Dallas)
Surg Gynecol Obstet 171:223–226, 1990   9–1

Because desmopressin reduces blood loss in cardiac surgery and spinal fusion for scoliosis, this agent was evaluated in 97 patients having 115 lumbar fusion operations. In 52 operations on 42 patients, 20 µg of desmopressin were administered by slow infusion shortly after induction of anesthesia. Moderate hypotensive anesthesia was used in all cases.

The patient groups are compared in the table. Desmopressin had no apparent adverse effects. A lowering of blood pressure was countered by adjusting the depth of anesthesia and the infusion rate of intravenous fluid. Two control patients required homologous blood. Ten desmo-

Patient Data		
	Control group	*Desmopressin group*
No. of patients	55	42
No. of operations	63	52
Males to females	37:18	33:9
Age, yrs.		
Mean	38.4	38.2
Range	20 to 62	15 to 68
Weight, lbs.		
No. of males ≤200 . . .	20	25
>200	20	8
No. of females ≤150 . .	8	7
>150	15	2
Anterior to posterior		
approach	16:47	14:38
Internal fixation to no		
internal fixation	18:29	30:8
Levels fused per patient .	1.82	2.28
Intraoperative blood loss, ml.		
Mean	550	550
Range	100 to 3,000	100 to 1,350
Loss in Hemovac®		
drain, ml.	336	820
Autologous blood used,		
units per patient	0.70	0.29
Admitting hemoglobin and		
hematocrit level	13.8 and 39.8	13.8 and 39.9
Discharge hemoglobin and		
hematocrit	11.0 and 32.5	10.9 and 31.7

(Courtesy of Johnson RG, Murphy JM: *Surg Gynecol Obstet* 171:223–226, 1990.)

pressin-treated patients and 4 controls had a discharge hemoglobin level of less than 10 g/dL.

Desmopressin can lower intraoperative blood loss during lumbar fusion when expected bleeding exceeds 1 L. Its use should be considered on an individualized basis. Desmopressin may be helpful in a small patient having a lower preoperative hemoglobin level, and also when autologous blood is unavailable.

▶ When all of the publications regarding desmopressin are put together, the conclusion that it is an effective hemostatic agent is controversial.—R.D. Miller, M.D.

Low-Dose Preoperative Aspirin Therapy, Postoperative Blood Loss, and Transfusion Requirements

Taggart DP, Siddiqui A, Wheatley DJ (Royal Infirmary, Glasgow)
Ann Thorac Surg 50:425–428, 1990   9–2

Aspirin is used increasingly by patients awaiting coronary revascularization. The effects of regular daily aspirin in doses of 75, 150, and 300 mg were examined in 202 consecutive patients scheduled for elective coronary bypass graft surgery. All of the patients had chronic stable angina and were taking antianginal medication at the time of study. Half (101) had received aspirin daily for 6–9 months while awaiting surgery.

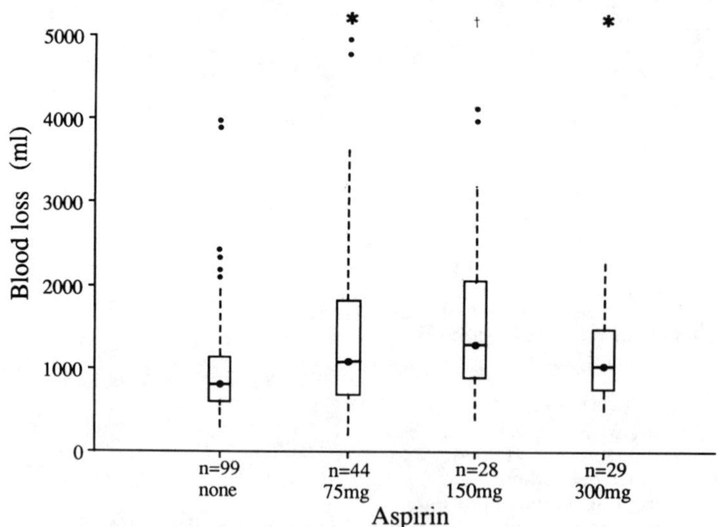

Fig 9–1.—Box-plot and whisker diagram shows total blood loss in the 4 groups of patients (*P < .05; † = P < .01 as compared with control group). Center box shows median and interquartile range with whiskers indicating range of data, except for outliers, which are marked individually *(solid dots).* (Courtesy of Taggart DP, Siddiqui A, Wheatley DJ: *Ann Thorac Surg* 50:425–428, 1990.)

Postoperative blood loss was higher in all aspirin-treated groups than in controls, but the increase was not dose related (Fig 9–1). Preoperative aspirin ingestion correlated only weakly with blood loss. Blood requirements increased by 2 units on average in patients given 75 mg or 150 mg of aspirin daily, and by 1 unit in those given 150 mg of aspirin daily. Seven aspirin-treated patients and 6 controls required reopening of the chest because of bleeding. Two control patients had surgical causes of bleeding. Aspirin use did not lengthen the hospital stay.

The regular use of low doses of aspirin does increase postoperative blood loss and transfusion requirements but does not prolong the hospital stay after coronary bypass surgery. Discontinuing aspirin for a week before surgery probably would not compromise graft patency.

► This study has multiple problems and is poorly controlled. Nevertheless, it does imply that aspirin therapy can increase blood loss and transfusion requirements.—R.D. Miller, M.D.

Ancrod (Arvin) as an Alternative to Heparin Anticoagulation for Cardiopulmonary Bypass

Zulys VJ, Teasdale SJ, Michel ER, Skala RA, Keating SE, Viger JR, Glynn MFX
(Toronto Gen Hosp)
Anesthesiology 71:870–877, 1989   9–3

Heparin has been the anticoagulant of choice for cardiopulmonary bypass (CPB). However, its use is associated with side effects and intolerance in some patients. An alternative anticoagulant is ancrod, derived from the venom of a pit viper. The safety and efficacy of ancrod anticoagulation were assessed in 20 patients undergoing elective CPB.

The concentration of fibrinogen reached a nadir in all patients during CPB but returned close to the preoperative value after patients were separated from CPB. The target plasma concentration of fibrinogen of .4 to .8 g/L was achieved within a mean of 13.3 hours of perfusion by using an average dose of ancrod of 1.65 units per g. Perfusion was without incident. The mean postoperative blood loss in the ancrod-treated group was 2,286 cc, compared to 1,737 cc in 20 matched heparin-treated controls. Blood product use consisted of a mean of 4.1 units of packed cells and 5.6 units of plasma in the ancrod-treated group. In the heparin-treated control group, a mean of 2.5 units of packed cells and 2.6 units of plasma were used. The difference in blood product use between these 2 groups was significant. There were no differences in the postoperative course or recovery period of these 2 groups.

The use of the defibrogenating agent ancrod is an effective method of anticoagulation for use during CPB. Although more experience with this agent is required before it can be recommended for routine use, when heparin is contraindicated, ancrod can be used successfully.

Ancrod Anticoagulation for Cardiopulmonary Bypass in Heparin-Induced Thrombocytopenia and Thrombosis

Teasdale SJ, Zulys VJ, Mycyk T, Baird RJ, Glynn MFX (Toronto Gen Hosp)
Ann Thorac Surg 48:712–713, 1989   9–4

Up to 15% of patients who receive heparin have thrombocytopenia. Although it usually resolves after discontinuation of heparin therapy, a small subset of patients have thrombosis and thromboembolism, even if heparin is withdrawn as soon as the syndrome is recognized. Ancrod is a defibrinogenating agent derived from Malayan pit viper venom. It can be used in cardiopulmonary bypass operations when heparin is contraindicated.

Man, 50, with a history of double aortocoronary bypass grafting, was admitted with acute myocardial infarction complicated by a ventricular septal defect (VSD) and circulatory failure. He underwent surgical closure of the VSD and single aortocoronary bypass grafting to the obtuse marginal artery. However, severe intraoperative thrombocytopenia developed complicated by microemboli that affected the lower extremities, leading to transmetatarsal amputation of the left forefoot. Three months later the patient was readmitted with deep vein thrombosis of the left lower extremity, which was successfully treated with warfarin sodium. Another 3 months later he was readmitted with increased angina and cardiac failure. Repeat cardiac catheterization revealed a persistent VSD. Repair of the VSD was attempted with an experimental low-molecular weight heparin, but thrombi were seen intraoperatively in the extracorporeal circulation, and the operation was aborted.

After referral to Toronto General Hospital, the patient underwent successful repair of the VSD with the use of ancrod infusion. Remnants of the previous VSD repair were removed, and the defect was patched with thick autogenous pericardium. The postoperative recovery was uneventful, and 2-dimensional echocardiography indicated no residual VSD. The patient was discharged from the hospital 10 days after operation.

The need for anticoagulation during cardiopulmonary bypass poses a special problem for patients with known sensitivity to heparin. Ancrod is a safe alternative to heparin anticoagulation in these cases.

▶ The authors emphasize the use of ancrod in patients who cannot be treated with heparin. A potentially more important use of this drug for the anesthesiologist is an alternative to protamine in highly sensitized patients (see Abstract 9–3). Nevertheless, allergic reactions to ancrod are also possible.—R.K. Stoelting, M.D.

Reversal of Protamine-Induced Catastrophic Pulmonary Vasoconstriction by Prostaglandin E₁

Whitman GJR, Martel D, Weiss M, Pochanapring A, See WM, Hopeman A, Harken AH, Dauber IM (Univ of Colorado; Univ of Washington)
Ann Thorac Surg 50:303–305, 1990   9–5

Protamine reversal of heparin can cause catastrophic pulmonary vasoconstriction in patients undergoing cardiopulmonary bypass. Complement activation and thromboxane release may play a role in this response. Reversal of the response was achieved by administration of prostaglandin E_1.

Man, 63, after aortic valve replacement, was given bovine heparin for anticoagulation. The patient was weaned from cardiopulmonary bypass with epinephrine and nitroglycerin. After protamine was administered peripherally for 10 minutes, the central venous pressure rose and global right ventricular dysfunction developed. Heparin was readministered and cardiopulmonary bypass reinstated. After bypass of a right coronary ostial dissection with a reverse saphenous vein graft, the patient could not be weaned from bypass. The left atrial pressure was 0 mm Hg. Epinephrine and nitroglycerin were unsuccessful systemically and when administered through the pulmonary artery. Hypoxic pulmonary vasoconstriction was not present. Prostaglandin E_1 injection into the pulmonary artery immediately elevated the left arterial pressure to 6 mm Hg. Prostaglandin infusion through the pulmonary artery was begun, with epinephrine given for systemic hypotension. Weaning from cardiopulmonary bypass was accomplished easily. Protamine was then administered for 1 hour. The patient's subsequent recovery was uneventful.

The patient's reaction appeared to be of type III, which may be mediated by nonimmunologic activation of complement from the heparin-protamine complex. Prostaglandin E_1 appears to be effective therapy for catastrophic pulmonary vasoconstriction that is unresponsive to standard vasodilators.

▶ Despite the almost daily use of protamine in my clinical practice, I have yet to observe drug-induced pulmonary vasoconstriction. When it does occur, however, I will remember this report for 2 reasons: the speculated value of prostaglandin E_1, and the subsequent uneventful injection of protamine at a slow rate (1 hour) to this patient.—R.K. Stoelting, M.D.

Desmopressin Acetate in Uncomplicated Coronary Artery Bypass Surgery: A Prospective Randomized Clinical Trial

Hedderich GS, Petsikas DJ, Cooper BA, Leznoff M, Guerraty AJ, Poirier NL, Symes JF, Morin JE (Royal Victoria Hosp, Montreal)
Can J Surg 33:33–36, 1990   9–6

Desmopressin acetate (DDAVP), a synthetic vasopressin analogue, may limit blood loss after surgery under cardiopulmonary bypass by releasing endogenous factor VIII:von Willebrand factor and promoting platelet aggregation. A prospective trial of DDAVP was undertaken in 62 consecutive patients having uncomplicated coronary bypass graft surgery. Half of the patients were assigned to receive DDAVP, .3 µg/kg, by infusion immediately after protamine administration.

Comparable numbers of DDAVP-treated patients and placebo recipients had received antiplatelet drugs in the week before surgery and the groups were hematologically comparable. Three DDAVP-treated patients and 1 in the placebo group were reexplored because of bleeding exceeding 200 mL/hr. There were no significant differences in total blood loss or amounts of red blood cells transfused. A small but significant fall in platelets occurred in the DDAVP-treated group. This prospective study fails to support the intraoperative use of DDAVP to limit perioperative bleeding in routine coronary bypass surgery.

▶ In the past there has been a plethora of articles showing that DDAVP given preoperatively to patients undergoing open cardiac procedures, especially congenital repairs, reduces bleeding. Most of these were historical studies, i.e., using historical controls. This randomized clinical trial shows that DDAVP is of no benefit in coronary artery bypass grafting and may be a risk. This study accentuates why controlled clinical trials are necessary; i.e., to either prove or disprove a point when all factors have been taken into account. In the discussion in the article, there is an excellent review of the complications of DDAVP; the possibility of premature vein graft thromboses and peripheral venous thromboemboli may well be increased in the DDAVP group.

Other factors that may be different in this study compared with the Salzman et al. study (1) are the different surgical technique used and the skill of the surgeons doing the operation. I don't know whether such factors influenced the benefit shown by Salzman and the lack of it here, or whether something else in the surgical technique or blood donation protocol is different between the Boston study and this Montreal study.—M.F. Roizen, M.D.

Reference

1. Salzman EW, et al: *N Engl J Med* 314:1402, 1986.

Anticoagulation for Noncardiac Procedures in Patients With Prosthetic Heart Valves: Does Low Risk Mean High Cost?
Eckman MH, Beshansky JR, Durand-Zaleski I, Levine HJ, Pauker SG (New England Med Ctr, Boston)
JAMA 263:1513–1521, 1990   9–7

Patients with prosthetic heart valves who require noncardiac surgery often have their hospital stay prolonged to receive intravenous heparin therapy to decrease the risk of thromboembolism. Because thromboembolic events are relatively infrequent and the period of increased risk is quite short, the cost can be great.

Cost-efficacy analysis was conducted by calculating the marginal cost per additional quality-adjusted year of life gained by avoiding thromboembolic events, and also the cost per death averted. A decision analytic model was used. The marginal cost of prolonging hospitalization to administer heparin appears to be prohibitively high compared with most current treatments, unless the most thrombogenic of valves is present. The marginal cost effectiveness of the first additional day of hospitalization ranges from $600,000 to $4.2 million per thromboembolic event averted.

Decisions on perioperative management should be individualized but, in general, heparin may be given intravenously postoperatively for 1 to 2 days after oral anticoagulation is restarted if the hospital stay is not prolonged as a result. A third day of heparin therapy is reasonable if a valve associated with a high risk of thromboembolism is present. Even if a hypercoagulable state is present, the cost of an added hospital day is prohibitive for all but the most thrombogenic valves.

▶ Conclusions I draw from this article are the following: There are no controlled studies on coagulation for noncardiac surgery in patients with prosthetic heart valves. The trade-offs are the risk of thromboembolism without anticoagulation versus the risk of bleeding with it. Clearly, mitral and ball valve prostheses result in a much greater risk of thromboembolism than aortic and disk valve prostheses. Thus, if you're going to change your practice, it's clear that anticoagulation in patients with aortic valves and disk valves probably should be changed first. Even if there is no risk or the risk is minimal, the authors estimate the cost of changing anticoagulation for noncardiac surgery in patients with a prosthetic heart valve to be between $111,000 and $1,000,000 per death prevented for anticoagulation on the first day, and twice as much for doing it on the second day postoperatively.

Are these figures correct? Why do they not reflect other morbidities prevented by anticoagulation, such as pulmonary embolism? Are any of the many assumptions made incorrect? Although, to come to a conclusion, some assumptions were necessary, I am not sure that all of them are correct. Because of the prestigious journal in which this article is published and the way the authors have done the study, however, these conclusions may become the standard of care unless we are careful to comment on the uncertainty of the assumptions made by the authors. You must understand that this is a cost-effectiveness analysis, not a benefit/risk analysis. Perhaps the benefit/risk analysis to find who should receive this therapy would be more meaningful. I hope that study is performed.—M.F. Roizen, M.D.

10 Postoperative Problems

Evaluation of a Forced-Air System for Warming Hypothermic Postoperative Patients
Lennon RL, Hosking MP, Conover MA, Perkins WJ (Mayo Clinic and Found, Rochester, Minn)
Anesth Analg 70:424–427, 1990   10–1

The efficacy of a forced-air patient heating system was compared with that of warmed cotton blankets in 30 adult surgical patients whose oral temperatures were 35° C or below at admission to the recovery room. Patients either were covered with blankets warmed to 37° C or were treated with the Bair Hugger system, which has a 400-W heating element and fan and a temperature controller limited to 43° C.

Neither method caused complications. Patients having forced-air warming were significantly warmer at all intervals than those kept in heated blankets. The latter patients spent significantly more time in the recovery room.

A forced-air warming system produces warming more rapidly than the use of heated cotton blankets and makes shivering less frequent. It also promotes earlier release from the recovery room. This system acts passively, i.e., without metabolically generated warming. It eliminates the major sources of heat loss in surgical patients—convection and radiation.

▶ I suppose the smart aleck response to this would be, "Why were the patients allowed to become hypothermic in the operating room at all?" But I think that's an inappropriate response, as we will probably be going to hypothermia intraoperatively more and more to protect vital organ function, especially the CNS. Warming patients in the operating room may be difficult, and systems such as this may be useful to warm them postoperatively when it is not possible to maintain temperature intraoperatively. My initial comment still holds, though; for the vast majority of patients, I believe intraoperative normothermia should be able to be maintained with simple maneuvers that are perhaps even less expensive than the ones proposed here. I was taught that it's good care to maintain things normal at all times rather than chase inadequate care from the beginning. Were my teachers wrong?—M.F. Roizen, M.D.

Episodic Arterial Oxygen Desaturation and Heart Rate Variations Following Major Abdominal Surgery

Rosenberg J, Dirkes WE, Kehlet H (Hvidovre Univ Hosp, Denmark; Univ of Cincinnati)

Br J Anaesth 63:651–654, 1989   10–2

Major operations, especially upper abdominal procedures, are followed by mild, constant arterial hypoxemia for up to 2 weeks. Preliminary studies have shown a new phenomenon of episodic sudden decreases in arterial oxygen saturation (SaO_2) to less than 80% during the first 16 hours after surgery. To determine whether severe sudden decreases in SaO_2 to less than 80% also occur in the late postoperative period, 20 patients (median age, 66 years) who underwent elective major abdominal operations were monitored continuously for heart rate and SaO_2 during the 2 nights before and the first 2 nights after operation. Arterial oxygen saturation was measured by pulse oximeter, using a finger probe.

The median increase in heart rate was 12 beats per $minute^{-1}$ on the first night after operation and 16 beats per $minute^{-1}$ on the second night, compared with preoperative values. The median decrease in SaO_2 was 2.3% on the first night after operation and 3.2% on the second night, compared with preoperative values (Fig 10–1). Before operation 4 patients had an episode of sudden decrease in SaO_2 to values less than 80%. After operation 3 patients had 1–8 episodes of decreased SaO_2 during the first night, and 8 patients had 1–372 episodes during the second night. Most episodes lasted less than 1 minute, but some lasted for 3–5 minutes.

One patient with 120 episodes spent 49% of the second postoperative night with an SaO_2 of less than 80%. The patient with 372 episodes spent 78% of the second night with an SaO_2 of less than 80%. This patient had severe cardiac arrhythmias on the third morning after operation. Oxygen administered by nasal catheter at 3 L/min^{-1} restored cardiac rhythm. In another patient who received oxygen therapy with 60%

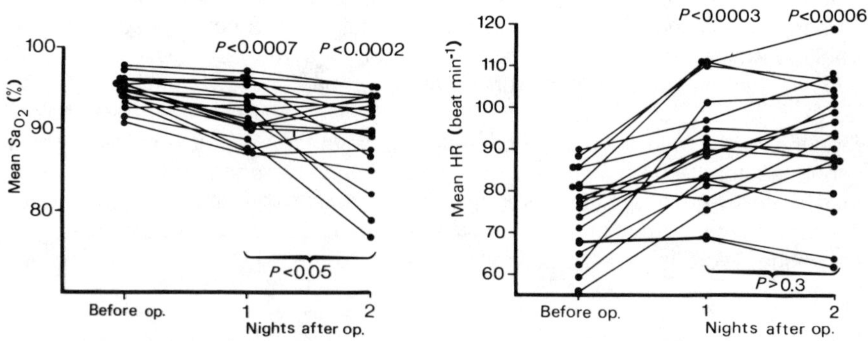

Fig 10–1.—Changes in mean SaO_2 and mean heart rate in 19 patients undergoing laparotomy. (Courtesy of Rosenberg J, Dirkes WE, Kehlet H: *Br J Anaesth* 63:651–654, 1989.)

oxygen, 15 L/min^{-1} by Hudson face mask on the second postoperative night, there was good correlation between SaO_2 and increase in heart rate during the entire night. A patient with 21 episodes during the second postoperative night died suddenly on the third postoperative day with signs of acute myocardial infarction. This patient had no history of ischemic heart disease. There was no correlation between opioid administration, heart rate, and SaO_2 disturbances. The clinical relevance of episodic arterial oxygen desaturation to values of less than 80% occurring in the late postoperative period is unknown, but these events may explain unexpected sudden death in patients with apparent uneventful postoperative recoveries.

Postoperative Myocardial Infarction and Episodic Hypoxaemia
Pateman JA, Hanning CD
Br J Anaesth 63:648–650, 1989   10–3

It was reported previously that perioperative invasive hemodynamic monitoring in patients who had a myocardial infarction (MI) within the preceding 3 months reduced the frequency of reinfarction from 36% to 5.7%. Because MI occurred most often on the third postoperative day, the period of invasive postoperative monitoring in the next study was extended to 96 hours and included patients who had an MI within the preceding 6 months. The reinfarction rate in that study was reduced from 3.8% after 24 hours of monitoring to 1.3% after 96 hours of monitoring. However, routine invasive monitoring for several days after operation is not justified. Rather, patients at increased risk for postoperative MI should be identified properly before operation. An analysis of the published literature yields several risk factors for postoperative MI that merit consideration.

Mechanisms other than intraoperative hemodynamic changes may be responsible for the peak of late postoperative MI, possibly perioperative withdrawal or alteration of drug therapy, and hypoxic episodes. Perioperative withdrawal or alteration of drug therapy occurs when cardiovascular-active drugs are suddenly withheld on the day of operation. Hypoxic episodes caused by sudden arterial oxygen desaturation occurring in the late postoperative period further contribute to the pathogenesis of MI in an already compromised myocardium.

Sleep patterns in the early postoperative period are severely disturbed. In patients in the intensive care unit, stages 3 and 4 and rapid eye movement sleep were almost completely suppressed during the first and second nights after operation. Any tendency to obstructive sleep apnea may be exacerbated in the early and late postoperative period, and may be associated with marked cardiovascular changes, including rapid increases in pulmonary and systemic arterial pressures and heart rate, arrhythmias, and left and right ventricular dysfunction.

Were all of these changes to occur during operation they would be treated vigorously on the grounds that they may cause myocardial ischemia and subsequent MI. However, events that are just as deleterious to the myocardium apparently occur after surgery when the patient and the surgeon are sleeping. Studies of the late postoperative period should therefore be extended, with special attention to the role of analgesics in the genesis of hypoxemia, to better identify those patients at increased postoperative risk for experiencing adverse cardiovascular events.

▶ I find the editorial (Abstract 10–3) and the article (Abstract 10–2) fascinating. Although on the surface the authors showed that patients experience episodic oxygen desaturation, they bring up many stimulating questions. Was the outcome of Rao et al.'s study (1), in which they put patients in the intensive care unit for 72 hours and placed pulmonary artery lines in an attempt to prevent perioperative myocardial infarction, related to wedge pressure measurements or to the fact that they gave those patients oxygen for 72 hours and thus prevented O_2 desaturation. Oxygen is cheap and effective and may reduce the incidence of perioperative myocardial infarction.

It's quite possible to use these studies to come to conclusions different from those of Rosenberg et al. or the editorial authors, Pateman and Hanning. This study also brings up the question of patient-controlled analgesia versus regional anesthesia. Because it appears that systemic narcotics are much more likely to be associated with episodic desaturation, perhaps related to the effect of muscle relaxation on pharyngeal muscles, this may imply that the patient should receive regional rather than intravenous narcotics. However, as 1 patient received 60% oxygen by face mask during the night, one wonders if this can be prevented simply by face mask oxygen. We aren't told whether the face mask was actually on the patient during the episodes of hypoxemia and myocardial ischemia. Later in the article, the authors stated that oxygen treatment with 3 L/min by nasal cannula was given and normal cardiac rhythym restored. Does this mean that the face mask was not on the patient at the other time? Again, like most good studies, this one stimulates more questions than it answers.—M.F. Roizen, M.D.

Reference

1. Rao TLK, et al: *Anesthesiology* 59:499, 1983.

The Experience of the Person Ventilating the Lungs Does Influence Post-operative Nausea and Vomiting
Hovorka J, Korttila K, Erkola O (Helsinki Univ)
Acta Anaesthesiol Scand 34:203–205, 1990
10–4

Mask ventilation may be a factor in postoperative nausea and vomiting by stretching the stomach or gut wall, but properly controlled studies are unavailable. The influence of the persons performing mask ventilation was assessed in a series of 198 patients requiring elective abdominal hysterectomy.

The patients, all ASA groups I and II and aged 35–55 years, were anesthetized with isoflurane in N_2O and oxygen. Either an experienced senior practitioner or an inexperienced junior member of the anesthetic team ventilated the patient before intubation. Patients were premedicated with pethidine and received fentanyl adjunctively.

Patients ventilated by an inexperienced person (group A) were comparable clinically with those managed by an experienced person (group B). Group B patients had less emesis within 2 hours after surgery and also in the first 6 hours (table). Group A patients required significantly more droperidol in the recovery room. An experienced anesthetist can lower

Percentage Incidence of Emesis in 2 Groups With Regard to Ventilation of Lungs in Women Undergoing Abdominal Hysterectomy Under Isoflurane Anaesthesia

Assessment	Group A (n = 124) Inexperienced person ventilating		Group B (n = 74) Experienced person ventilating	
Emesis (overall) 0–24 h after anaesthesia		79		66
Emesis 0–2 h after anaesthesia	54 †		35	
Nausea		27		27
Retching		19		7
Vomiting		8		1
Emesis 2–6 h after anaesthesia	40*		27	
Nausea		21		23
Retching		14		4
Vomiting		5		0
Emesis 6–12 h after anaesthesia	35		30	
Nausea		19		16
Retching		13		11
Vomiting		3		3
Emesis 12–18 h after anaesthesia	17		19	
Nausea		9		14
Retching		3		4
Vomiting		5		1
Emesis 18–24 h after anaesthesia	20		20	
Nausea		14		11
Retching		2		1
Vomiting		4		8

Emesis is defined as nausea, retching, or vomiting.
* = $P < .05$ and † = $P < .01$ vs Group B.
(Courtesy of Hovorka J, Korttila K, Erkola O: *Acta Anaesthesiol Scand* 34:203–205, 1990.)

the risk of nausea and vomiting in the early recovery period in patients given general anesthesia for abdominal hysterectomy.

▶ This study suggests that patients ventilated by inexperienced staff have a higher incidence of nausea, vomiting, and retching after surgery. Although that is so, the percentages of nausea were very high, 79% and 66%, in both groups; within the first 2 hours, 54% vomited and 35% retched in the group treated by inexperienced personnel, as did 40% and 27% of those treated by more experienced staff members. Probably these high percentages reflect the fact that the authors sought to maximize the percentage of patients vomiting by giving them 2 different types of narcotics preoperatively, by ventilating them with a mask once they were paralyzed, and by not emptying their stomachs at the end of surgery. Once again, Korttila and company have given us more information about a common condition, and a common problem, and have done it in a very nice fashion. The authors are to be congratulated for the excellence of this study.—M.F. Roizen, M.D.

Gastric Aspiration at the End of Anaesthesia Does Not Decrease Postoperative Nausea and Vomiting

Hovorka J, Korttila K, Erkola O (Helsinki Univ)
Anaesth Intensive Care 18:58–61, 1990   10–5

Despite advances in the techniques that are used, postoperative nausea and vomiting remain among the most common complications of general anesthesia. To determine whether gastric aspiration at the end of the operation would decrease the incidence of postoperative nausea and vomiting, studies were made in 201 women aged 35–55 years undergoing elective abdominal hysterectomy under general anesthesia with isoflurane in nitrous oxide and oxygen.

All of the women were randomly assigned to gastric aspiration at the end of anesthesia or to no gastric aspiration. Each patient was assessed for the incidence and severity of emesis for a 24-hour period postoperatively. The 2 groups of patients were well matched for age, weight, history of nausea and vomiting after previous anesthesia, duration of anesthesia, and drugs used during anesthesia (table).

The overall incidence of nausea and vomiting during the first 24 hours after operation was 79% in women whose stomach was aspirated after anesthesia, and 70% in those who did not have gastric aspiration. The difference was not statistically significant. Furthermore, the incidence of nausea and vomiting at all times during the 24-hour study period was similar in both groups. Vomiting was no longer severe after 12 hours and had nearly disappeared by 24 hours after anesthesia. Gastric aspiration at the end of general anesthesia for abdominal hysterectomy did not reduce the incidence of nausea and vomiting during the first 24 hours after surgery.

	Characteristics of Test Groups	
	Group A **Stomach** **aspirated**	**Group B** **Stomach not** **aspirated**
N	100	101
Age (yr)	43 (5)	43 (5)
Weight (kg)	64 (9)	65 (11)
Duration of anaesthesia (min)	94 (25)	96 (30)
Isoflurane concentration (%)		
Inspired	1.1 (0.2)	1.1 (0.2)
Expired	0.9 (0.2)	0.8 (0.2)
Alcuronium (mg)	16.4 (2.8)	16.9 (3.5)
Oxycodone for postoperative pain (total mg)	56 (14)	56 (16)
Droperidol for postoperative emesis		
total (mg)	1.2	1.2
range (mg)	0-7.5	0-6.25
number of patients	61	62

Note: Mean ± standard deviation.
(Courtesy of Hovorka J, Korttila K, Erkola O: *Anaesth Intensive Care* 18:58–61, 1990.)

▶ The results of this study are discouraging; I have had a very strong bias that this was an effective method of attenuating postoperative nausea and vomiting, especially in ambulatory surgery patients. Of course, if the anesthesiologists were very skillful in not pumping air into the stomach during induction of anesthesia, perhaps it is not an ineffective procedure.—R.D. Miller, M.D.

Anaesthesia, Movement and Emesis

Kamath B, Curran J, Hawkey C, Beattie A, Gorbutt N, Guiblin H, Kong A (City Hosp; Queens Med Ctr, Nottingham, England)
Br J Anaesth 64:728–730, 1990

10–6

Because motion sickness appears to dispose to postoperative nausea and vomiting, the effects of movement and of premedication were examined in 182 healthy women undergoing elective dilatation and curettage. Using a double-dummy technique, patients were randomly assigned to premedication with placebo; temazepam, 20 mg; or papaveretum, 20 mg, plus hyoscine, 400 μg. Anesthesia was induced with thiopental and maintained with nitrous oxide and halothane.

Patients given temazepam had significantly fewer episodes of postoperative nausea. Two thirds of the patients who identified a cause of nausea mentioned movement, and these patients appeared to be more susceptible than others to motion sickness on the basis of questionnaire responses. They also were more likely to have been treated previously for nausea or vomiting.

Temazepam reduced the risk of postoperative nausea in these generally healthy persons. It might be possible to identify susceptible patients preoperatively and to take measures to limit movement during recovery from anesthesia. The relationship between movement and nausea—vomiting requires further study.

▶ Considering the long list of drugs alleged to protect against nausea and vomiting, I find myself somewhat ambivalent about adding a drug to the list that is most often touted for its ability to offset insomnia.—R.K. Stoelting, M.D.

Nerve Injury Associated With Anesthesia
Kroll DA, Caplan RA, Posner K, Ward RJ, Cheney FW (Univ of California, Los Angeles; Virginia Mason Med Ctr, Seattle; Univ of Washington)
Anesthesiology 73:202–207, 1990
10–7

Nerve injuries continue to occur in anesthesiologic practice and result in medical malpractice claims for pain, suffering, and economic damage. A study of closed malpractice claims related to anesthetic care allowed the opportunity to explore the predisposing factors, severity, outcome, cost, and role of substandard care in such injuries.

The ASA Closed Claim Study included more than 1,500 claims for damages against anesthesiologists, 15% of which were for nerve injuries. About one third of the injuries were to the ulnar nerve; brachial plexus and lumbosacral nerve injuries were next in frequency. General anesthesia was used in 61% of the cases. Usually, the mechanism of injury was not apparent. Care was judged to be "standard" in nearly two thirds of cases. The severity of injury and payment for claims were lower in nerve damage cases compared with claims for other types of damage.

For disabling nerve injuries the median payment was $56,000, significantly lower than the $225,000 median payment for other types of disabling injuries. Payment was made in less than half of the nerve damage claims, compared with the 60% payment rate for other types of claims. Payment was just as likely to be made whether or not care was judged to be "standard."

The mechanisms of nerve injury described in the literature do not usually appear in claim files; mechanisms were identified in less than one third of the brachial plexus and lumbosacral root injuries, and even less frequently in ulnar nerve injuries. This finding suggests shortcomings in the medicolegal process or as yet unrecognized mechanisms of nerve injury.

▶ The appearance of peripheral neuropathy after operation is often attributed to the anesthetic technique or positioning. Consider the likely conversations between the anesthesiologist and surgeon when foot drop follows an operative procedure performed in the dorsal lithotomy position using regional anesthesia. Awareness and documentation of precautions taken to assure proper positioning, as well as describing the atraumatic institution of subarachnoid or epidural anesthesia, are highly useful in directing attention to the most likely explanation for peripheral nerve injuries.—R.K. Stoelting, M.D.

11 Ventilation

Indications for Pulmonary Function Testing
Zibrak JD, O'Donnell CR, Marton K (New England Deaconess Hosp, Boston; Harvard Med School)
Ann Intern Med 112:763–771, 1990   11–1

To assess the role of preoperative pulmonary function testing in predicting postoperative outcome, a MEDLINE search of English-language articles from 1966 to 1987 was undertaken using the following medical subject headings: respiratory function tests, lung, lung diseases, and preoperative care. Studies were subdivided by operative site and those in which pre- and posttest probabilities of morbidity, mortality, sensitivity, and specificity could be determined were included.

Presently available data indicate that preoperative pulmonary function testing provides measurable benefit in predicting the postoperative outcome in patients undergoing lung resection. In addition, persistently increased PCO_2 values, defined as more than 45 mm Hg, may predict increased mortality in patients undergoing coronary artery bypass surgery and those undergoing lung resection. Except for patients undergoing lung resection, an increased PCO_2 is not an absolute contraindication, as some patients with increased PCO_2 can have coronary artery bypass surgery and other major procedures successfully.

Split perfusion lung scanning and pulmonary exercise testing appear to be useful preoperative tests in selected patients undergoing lung surgery, but further studies are warranted before these procedures can be recommended routinely. There is no strong evidence that preoperative pulmonary function tests are of measurable benefit in identifying patients at risk for postoperative complications after upper abdominal or cardiac surgery, and other surgical procedures.

Most of these studies were limited by methodologic difficulties, including poor study design and insufficient data. Further studies are warranted before a consensus can be reached on the role of preoperative pulmonary function testing in evaluating patients before all surgical procedures, except for lung resection. A careful general history and physical examination with emphasis on respiratory complaints may identify those in whom pulmonary function testing may assist in making a specific pulmonary diagnosis and assessing the degree of impairment before surgery.

▶ I have thought and taught for many years that preoperative pulmonary function tests (except for planned pulmonary resection) are largely a waste of time unless the anesthesiologist firmly believes that the results will affect management of the anesthetic (i.e., whether bronchodilators are indicated, selecting the pattern of intraoperative ventilator support, and so on). This article substantiates the fact that very few good data are available to support "routine" spirometry, even in patients with chronic obstructive pulmonary disease.—R.R. Kirby, M.D.

Lidocaine-Induced Bronchoconstriction in Asthmatic Patients: Relation to Histamine Airway Responsiveness and Effect of Preservative
McAlpine LG, Thomson NC (Western Infirmary, Glasgow)
Chest 96:1012–1015, 1989   11–2

Inhalation of nebulized lidocaine, which is used to produce anesthesia of the respiratory tract before bronchoscopy, may cause bronchoconstriction in some asthmatic patients. To determine whether the degree of histamine airway responsiveness can predict the development and extent of lidocaine-induced bronchoconstriction and to examine the role of the methylparaben preservative in causing this response, 20 patients with asthma underwent a histamine inhalation test and a lidocaine inhalation challenge (6 mL of lidocaine 4%) on separate days.

The mean concentration of histamine that produced a 20% fall in the forced expiratory volume in 1 second (FEV_1) was .58 mg/mL. In the group overall, a mean fall in FEV_1 of 7.53% occurred after lidocaine

---

Patient Characteristics and Results of Airway Responses to Histamine and Lidocaine

Subject No.	Age/Sex	Atopy	Current Treatment	FEV_1, % pred	$PC_{20}H$, mg/ml	Max Change in FEV_1 Post-lidocaine
1	41/F	+	B,S,T	72	0.19	− 16.3
2	44/F	+	B,S	84	0.16	20.0
3	51/M	+	B,S,T	54	0.29	− 13.2
4	37/F	+	B,S,T	94	0.34	− 16.1
5	59/F	+	B,S	100	0.36	− 7.8
6	58/F	−	B,S	83	0.33	− 30.1
7	71/M	−	B,S,N	62	0.92	28.2
8	43/M	+	B,S	107	3.44	− 10.5
9	30/F	+	B	123	1.00	− 4.4
10	24/M	+	B,S	77	4.17	− 21.6
11	27/M	+	B,S	90	0.24	− 13.3
12	47/M	+	B,S	94	0.71	9.5
13	30/F	−	B,S	73	0.65	− 9.7
14	27/M	+	B,S	88	0.5	− 42.1
15	44/M	−	B,S	113	0.48	− 7.6
16	59/F	+	B,S	67	1.10	− 6.4
17	63/F	+	B,S	59	0.25	9.4
18	28/F	+	B,S	61	0.27	− 14.9
19	26/F	+	B	99	2.00	− 9.0
20	23/M	+	B,S	103	0.98	− 9.1

Abbreviations: BB, inhaled β-agonist: *S*, inhaled steroid; *T*, oral theophylline; *N*, inhaled nedocromil sodium; $PC_{20}H$, concentration of histamine provoking 20% fall in FEV_1.
(Courtesy of McAlpine LG, Thomson NC: *Chest* 96:1012–1015, 1989.)

challenge, but 5 patients (25%) had a bronchoconstrictor response to lidocaine (fall in FEV_1 of greater than 15%) (table). There was no correlation between the maximum percentage change in FEV_1 after inhalation of lidocaine and histamine responsiveness, even after considering the 5 patients with a reduction in FEV_1 of more than 15%.

Three subjects with a bronchoconstrictor response to lidocaine were rechallenged with the commercial 4% lidocaine preparation and with a 4% preservative-free lidocaine solution. Bronchoconstriction occurred similarly with both solutions.

Inhaled topical lidocaine induces bronchoconstriction in a significant number of asthmatic patients. This bronchoconstrictor response to lidocaine cannot be predicted from histamine responsiveness and is not related to the preservative in the lidocaine preparation.

▶ Is this effect really related to lidocaine, or is it simply a foreign body response? Even distilled water can induce bronchospasm when aspirated by susceptible individuals. Historically, in the 1960s and early 1970s lidocaine was advocated to "break" refractory bronchospasm, although such treatment has never become a mainstay of asthma therapy. I don't think this paper establishes that lidocaine is contraindicated in asthmatics. The authors' final point, however, is that caution should be exercised when topical lidocaine is used to anesthetize the airways.—R.R. Kirby, M.D.

Naloxone Administration and Laryngospasm Followed by Pulmonary Edema

Olsen KS (Central Hosp of Kristianstad, Kristianstad, Sweden)
Intensive Care Med 16:340–341, 1990   11–3

Pulmonary edema has been described after postoperative naloxone administration, and it also can be a complication of laryngospasm.

Woman, 59, with a history of hoarseness, underwent laryngeal biopsy under general anesthesia with fentanyl, and received naloxone, .4 mg, when spontaneous breathing failed to return after succinylcholine infusion was halted. Laryngospasm was evident when respiration resumed and recurred after succinylcholine administration; obstruction was nearly complete. Diazepam, fentanyl, and succinylcholine were then given and intubation was carried out for mechanical ventilation. Frothy pink fluid poured from the endotracheal tube during attempts to let the patient breathe spontaneously. Positive end expiratory pressure was added, and the pulmonary edema was treated with aminophylline, furosemide, morphine, and glyceryl trinitrate. Bilateral interstitial edema was noted on chest radiography. The patient was extubated the next day.

It is not clear how laryngospasm produces pulmonary edema, but capillary damage from a large negative transpulmonary pressure is a possible factor. Both naloxone and laryngospasm may have contributed to pulmonary edema in the present patient. Naloxone should be used cautiously, especially in patients with preexisting heart disease who have recently had severe laryngospasm.

▶ I strongly disagree that it is not known how laryngospasm produces pulmonary edema. So-called negative-pressure pulmonary edema has been recognized and described for many years. One does not have to implicate naloxone as a causative factor here; the airway obstruction alone is sufficient explanation.—R.R. Kirby, M.D.

12 Intravenous Fluid Therapy

Blood Transfusion—General

Elective Surgery Without Transfusion: Influence of Preoperative Hemoglobin Level and Blood Loss on Mortality
Spence RK, Carson JA, Poses R, McCoy S, Pello M, Alexander J, Popovich J, Norcross E, Camishion RC (Univ of Medicine and Dentistry of New Jersey, Camden; East Tennessee State Univ, Johnson City)
Am J Surg 159:320–324, 1990   12–1

In the past preoperative blood transfusion was routine. However, concerns about increasingly scarce supplies, rising costs, and the possibility of transmitting fatal diseases have made it necessary to reevaluate this practice. The influence of preoperative levels of hemoglobin and operative blood loss on survival after surgery was studied by analyzing the results of 113 major elective surgeries performed on 107 consecutive Jehovah's Witness patients. Forty-one procedures were performed on male patients and 72 on female patients. The age range was 8–88 years (mean, 47 years).

Preoperative levels of hemoglobin ranged from 6 g/dL to 16.7 g/dL (mean, 11.4 g/dL). Ninety-three patients had preoperative levels higher than 10 g/dL and 20 had levels between 6 and 10 g/dL. All patients had

Mortality, Preoperative Level of Hemoglobin, and Blood Loss	
	No./Total (%)
Preoperative hemoglobin*	
>10 g/dL	3/93 (3.2)
6–10 g/dL	1/20 (5)
Blood loss†	
>500 mL	4/54 (7.4)
<500 mL	0/59 (0)
Preoperative hemoglobin and blood loss‡	
>10 g/dL + >500 mL	3/44 (6.8)
>10 g/dL + <500 mL	0/49 (0)
6–10 g/dL + >500 mL	1/10 (10)
6–10 g/dL + <500 mL	(0/10) (0)

*P > .25.
†P < .025.
‡P < .025.
(Courtesy of Spence RK, Carson JA, Poses R, et al: *Am J Surg* 159:320–324, 1990.)

had blood loss or anemia, or both, for at least 2 weeks. Surgery was performed on the basis of need, regardless of the level of hemoglobin. Estimated blood loss ranged from 0 to 5,600 mL, with a median loss of 500 mL and a mean loss of 750 mL. Fifty-two percent of patients had blood losses of less than 500 mL and 78% had blood losses of less than 1,000 mL. Volume resuscitation during surgery was principally crystalloid.

Four of 113 patients died, for a mortality rate of 3.5%. Mortality is stratified in the table for preoperative level of hemoglobin and estimated blood loss. Mortality was unaffected by preoperative levels of hemoglobin but was significantly increased by blood loss of more than 500 mL. The 4 who died had preoperative hemoglobin levels ranging from 6.1 g/dL to 15.2 g/dL and in 3 the levels were above 10 g/dL. However, all 4 had operative blood losses ranging from 800 mL to 5,600 mL.

Mortality in elective surgery seems to be dependent more on estimated blood loss than on preoperative levels of hemoglobin. Apparently, elective surgery can be performed safely in patients with preoperative levels of hemoglobin as low as 6 g/dL if estimated blood loss does not exceed 500 mL.

▶ Although the conclusions of this study state the obvious, I wanted to include it because it appeared in the surgical literature and no doubt could influence many surgeons.—R.D. Miller, M.D.

Transfusion of Fresh Whole Blood Stored (4° C) for Short Period Fails to Improve Platelet Aggregation on Extracellular Matrix and Clinical Hemostasis After Cardiopulmonary Bypass

Golan M, Modan M, Lavee J, Martinowitz U, Savion N, Goor DA, Mohr R (Chaim Sheba Med Ctr, Tel Hashomer; Tel Aviv Univ, Israel)
J Thorac Cardiovasc Surg 99:354–360, 1990   12–2

The hemostatic effect of 1 unit of fresh whole blood is equivalent to 8–10 platelet units. Because preparing fresh whole blood for transfusion within 8 hours of donation is a complicated logistic problem for most blood bank units, the effects of short periods of cold storage (4° C) on the hemostatic effects of fresh whole blood were investigated. At random, 36 patients undergoing coronary artery bypass grafting received transfusions of unrefrigerated fresh whole blood (group A), fresh whole blood after 5 hours' storage at 4° C (group B), or fresh whole blood after 24 hours' storage at 4° C. Platelet function was studied on a extracellular matrix with a scanning electron microscope and graded 1–4, with normal being grade 4.

The 24-hour blood loss from chest drains was significantly less in group A than in groups B and C. Consequently, group A received significantly fewer blood units than groups B and C. There was a nonsignificant trend for a lower percentage of grade 4 platelet aggregation in group

B (17%) compared with group A (42%), whereas none (0%) in group C achieved grade 4. Posttransfusion platelet count and mean platelet volume were not significantly different in any of the groups. These data show that storage of fresh whole blood at 4° C, even for a short period of 5 hours, markedly diminishes its hemostatic effect, probably by decreasing platelet aggregability.

▶ My experience in Viet Nam was that warm, fresh whole blood has a tremendous hemostatic effect. This study confirms that its hemostatic effect is reduced by storage in a cold temperature.—R.D. Miller, M.D.

Blood Transfusion—Autologous

Immediate Preoperative Phlebotomy With Autologous Blood Donation for Aortic Replacement

Paty PSK, Shah DM, Chang BB, Kaufman JL, Feustel PJ, Leather RP (Albany Med College, NY)
Surg Gynecol Obstet 171:326–330, 1990   12–3

The use of autologous blood can decrease the need for homologous blood transfusion in patients undergoing extensive elective surgery. The blood is usually obtained by intraoperative isovolemic hemodilution or phlebotomy 1–2 weeks before operation. Immediate preoperative phlebotomy was studied in an attempt to minimize the intraoperative time delay or preoperative period between phlebotomy and surgery.

Preoperative isovolemic hemodilution was performed in 69 patients several days before elective aortic replacement for infrarenal aneurysmal disease. A mean of .57 L of whole blood was obtained. Volume was replaced with lactated Ringer's solution. Hematocrit levels dropped from a mean value of 42.9% to 33.7%. The mean intraoperative blood loss was 1.2 L. Hemodynamic parameters were stable in the perioperative and intraoperative periods.

The effect of the technical modification of exclusion aneurysmorrha-

Transfusion Requirements According to Aortic
Replacement Technique

	Exclusion	*Open*	*Level of significance*
No. of patients	50	19	
Blood loss, ml.	920±90	2,030±250	p<0.001
Autologous blood transfused, ml.	550±25	580±60	NS
Homologous blood transfused, ml.	175±35	570±119	p<0.05

Values expressed as mean ± S.E.M.; Student's *t* test.
(Courtesy of Paty PSK, Shah DM, Chang BB, et al: *Surg Gynecol Obstet* 171:326–330, 1990.)

phy in 50 patients and open aneurysmorrhaphy in 19 on reduction of intraoperative homologous blood transfusion was assessed. Seventy-two percent of those in whom aneurysms were excluded received no homologous blood intraoperatively. Blood loss was less in the excluded group than in the open aneurysmorrhaphy group, as was the need for homologous blood transfusion. The mortality was 2.9%. There was no increase in morbidity (table).

Preoperative isovolemic hemodilution is an acceptable way to obtain autologous blood for intraoperative use, thereby decreasing dependence on homologous blood transfusion. Exclusion aneurysmorrhaphy may also decrease such dependence in elective aortic replacement for aneurysm.

▶ This is a different approach to obtaining autologous blood. To utilize isovolemic hemodilution 1–2 days preoperatively is an attractive approach that could be used for many kinds of surgery. The only disadvantage is that it requires hospitalization. Will it be possible to have patients admitted 1 or 2 days preoperatively to use this approach?—R.D. Miller, M.D.

Increased Preoperative Collection of Autologous Blood With Recombinant Human Erythropoietin Therapy
Goodnough LT, Rudnick S, Price TH, Ballas SK, Collins ML, Crowley JP, Kosmin M, Kruskall MS, Lenes BA, Menitove JE, Silberstein LE, Smith KJ, Wallas CH, Abels R, Von Tress M (Case Western Reserve Univ; RW Johnson Pharmaceutical Research Inst, Raritan, NJ; Puget Sound Blood Ctr, Seattle; Jefferson Med College; Univ of North Carolina; et al)
N Engl J Med 321:1163–1168, 1989   12–4

To determine whether recombinant human erythropoietin increases the amount of autologous blood collectable before surgery, 47 adults scheduled for elective orthopedic operations received either erythropoietin, 600 units per kg, intravenously or a placebo twice weekly for 3 weeks. Up to 6 units of blood were collected during this time. The patients also received iron sulfate. Those with a hematocrit of less than 34% were excluded from donation.

A mean of 5.4 units was collected for the erythropoietin patients and 4.1 units for placebo patients. The mean red blood cell volume donated was 41% greater in the erythropoietin group. All but 1 of 23 erythropoietin recipients were able to donate 4 or more units, compared with 7 of 24 placebo recipients. Adverse effects were comparable in the 2 groups.

Recombinant erythropoietin promotes the ability of elective surgical patients to donate autologous blood, and significant adverse effects are not a problem. Women and children, who have smaller blood volumes, and anemic patients are the most likely to benefit from this measure.

► The outcome of this study speaks for itself. Clearly, any approach that increases collection of autologous blood should be encouraged.—R.D. Miller, M.D.

Blood Transfusion—Immune

Effect of Blood Transfusions on Immune Function: Part VI. Effect on Immunologic Response to Tumor

Waymack JP, Fernandes G, Yurt RW, Venkatraman JT, Burleson DG, Guzman RF, Mason AD Jr, Pruitt BA Jr (US Army Inst of Surgical Research, San Antonio; Univ of Texas, San Antonio; Cornell Univ, New York)
Surgery 108:172–178, 1990   12–5

In animal studies, transfusions reportedly increase the risk of tumor metastasis clinically and enhance primary tumor growth. It is possible, however, that patients with more advanced tumors receive more transfusions. The effects of transfusion were studied on host responses to both primary tumor growth and metastasis growth in rats bearing 3 types of tumor (two 1,2-dimethylhydrazine-induced poorly differentiated colon cancers and a rapid-growing solid tumor induced by the same agent).

With both the slow- and rapid-growing colon cancers, there were no significant differences in tumor size or tumor infiltration by leukocytes in rats given Ringer's lactate and those given blood at the time of tumor challenge. There was no difference in the T lymphocyte subpopulations in these groups. Survival was somewhat shorter in transfused animals (Fig 12–1), and natural killer cell lysis of tumor cells was less. If transfusion impairs natural killer cell function by countering interleukin-2 production, administration of interleukin-2 with blood might block or correct the immunosuppressive effect of transfusion.

► This study provides further confirmation of the adverse effects of blood transfusion on immune function and tumor growth.—R.D. Miller, M.D.

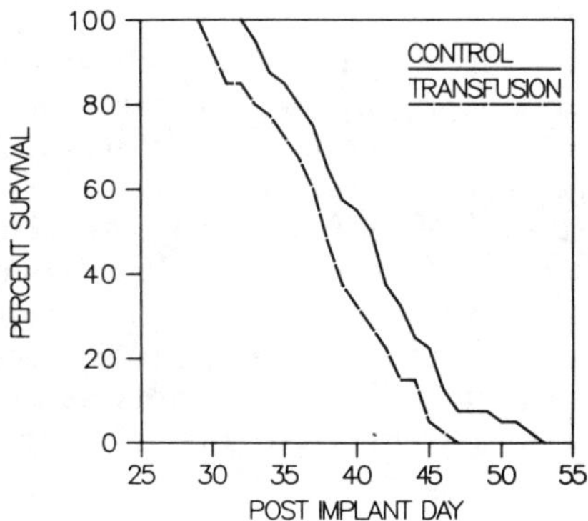

Fig 12–1.—Survival curves for rats administered blood transfusions or lactated Ringer's solution at the time of challenge with 1×10^6 tumor cells administered intravenously. (Courtesy of Waymack JP, Fernandes G, Yurt RW, et al: *Surgery* 108:172–178, 1990.)

Recurrence Rates After Radical Hysterectomy in Transfused and
Untransfused Patients and Influence of Histology

Histology	Transfused/ recurred (%)	Untransfused/ recurred (%)	P
Squamous cell	43/7 (16.3%)	38/1 (2.6%)	.06
Adeno.	12/1 (8.33%)	14/1 (7.14%)	NS
Adenosquamous	4/0	2/0	NS
Clear cell	4/1 (25%)	1/0	NS
Anaplastic	5/1 (20%)	3/0	NS
Total	68/10 (14.7%)	58/2 (3.4%)	.035

Abbreviations: Adeno, adenocarcinoma; *NS*, not significant.
(Courtesy of Eisenkop SM, Spirtos NM, Montag TW, et al: *Obstet Gynecol* 76:110–113, 1990.)

The Clinical Significance of Blood Transfusion at the Time of Radical Hysterectomy

Eisenkop SM, Spirtos NM, Montag TW, Moossazadeh J, Warren P, Hendrickson M (Stanford Univ; Women's Cancer Ctr, San Jose and Burlingame, Calif; Ctr for Gynecologic Oncology, Encino, Calif; St Joseph's Hosp, Denver)
Obstet Gynecol 76:110–113, 1990   12–6

Although blood transfusion contributes to the safety of major surgery, it can have immunosuppressive effects. The clinical significance of perioperative transfusion at the time of radical hysterectomy with retroperitoneal lymphadenectomy for stage IB cervical cancer was evaluated in a review of data on 126 patients. These patients had clear surgical margins, negative retroperitoneal lymph nodes, no lymph-vascular space involvement in the hysterectomy specimen, no perioperative radiation therapy, no history of immunosuppression with medication, and at least 18 months of follow-up.

The distributions of age, weight, operative time, nodal yields, mean lesion diameters, median depths of invasion, and histologic subtypes were not statistically different between the transfused and nontransfused groups. The average estimated blood loss in the transfused group was 1,104 mL, compared to 764 mL in the nontransfused group. There were 10 recurrences among the 68 transfused patients, compared with 2 recurrences among the 58 patients who did not receive transfusions. There was also a nonsignificant trend toward recurrence in patients with squamous cell lesions (table). Transfusion appears to have an adverse effect on the outcome of radical hysterectomy for stage IB cervical cancer.

The Effect of Packed Cells and Whole Blood Transfusions on Survival After Curative Resection for Colorectal Carcinoma

Wobbes T, Joosen KHG, Kuypers HHC, Beerthuizen GIJM, Theeuwes AGM
(Univ Hosp Nijmegen, The Netherlands; Catholic Univ, Nijmegen)
Dis Colon Rectum 32:743–748, 1989   12–7

Perioperative blood transfusion may contribute to a higher recurrence rate and lower survival in cancer patients, possibly through a potentially immunosuppressive effect. A distinct relationship has been shown between the kind and amount of blood components transfused and the incidence of recurrence and death in patients with colorectal carcinoma. In a retrospective study the effect of perioperative blood transfusion on survival after curative resection for colorectal carcinoma was evaluated in 137 men and 133 women (mean age, 62 years). Eighty-six patients (32%) did not receive perioperative blood transfusion, 110 (41%) received packed cells, and 74 (27%) received at least 2 units of whole blood.

The 5-year disease-free survival was 58% in the transfused group and 78% in the nontransfused group. The overall 5-year survival rates were 57% and 72%, respectively. The differences between groups were highly significant. Among the transfused patients, there were no statistically significant differences in disease-free survival and overall survival among those who received whole blood or a combination of whole blood and packed cells (51%) and those who received only packed cells (63%). However, the 5-year disease-free survival rate was significantly worse among patients who received more than 6 units of blood, as compared to those who received smaller volumes. Cox regression analysis showed that the amount of blood was a factor significantly related to the disease-free period. Perioperative blood transfusions have a significant detrimental effect on survival after curative resection for colorectal carcinoma, and this effect is not enhanced by transfusion of whole blood.

▶ It is increasingly clear that blood transfusions have an immunosuppressive effect that decreases the survival rate with patients with cancer. It has also been suggested that packed red blood cells depress the immune system less than whole blood. However, this retrospective study was unable to confirm a difference using packed red blood cells as opposed to whole blood with regard to effect on survival in cancer patients. This is in contrast to the Wobbes et al. study (see Abstract 12–9).—R.D. Miller, M.D.

Association Between Transfusion With Plasma and the Recurrence of Colorectal Carcinoma

Marsh J, Donnan PT, Hamer-Hodges DW (Univ of Edinburgh; Western Gen Infirmary, Edinburgh)
Br J Surg 77:623–626, 1990   12–8

Numerous studies have shown that perioperative blood transfusions given during surgery for malignancy adversely affect tumor recurrence. Additional studies have shown that whole blood is more harmful in this respect than packed cells. A retrospective study was carried out to determine whether the use of different blood transfusion components alters the risk of tumor recurrence.

Between 1980 and 1984, 132 patients with Dukes' stage B or C colorectal cancer underwent potentially curative operations. Extracted from the records were patient characteristics, including the main prognostic variables known to affect tumor recurrence; the amount of whole blood, packed cells and plasma given during the 30-day perioperative period; the time relative to the start of operation when these products were given; and the duration of recurrence-free postoperative survival. Sixty-two patients received transfusions of some blood component, 57 received a fluid containing red blood cells, and 23 received a blood component containing significant plasma.

The relative risk of tumor recurrence for patients receiving plasma was 2.44; for patients receiving whole blood, 2.47; and for all patients receiving either whole blood or plasma, 2.39. Thus the risk of tumor recurrence for patients receiving a transfusion of either plasma or whole blood was more than twice that for patients who did not receive protein-containing blood components. The transfusion of packed red blood cells did not increase the risk of tumor recurrence. There was no significant difference in risk of tumor recurrence for patients receiving transfusions before, during, or after operation.

Age was significantly associated with time to recurrence indicating that older patients had a shorter time to recurrence, with a relative risk of 1.05 for each year of age. No other variable was significantly associated with an increased risk of tumor recurrence.

▶ In contrast to the Wobbes et al. study, this study indicates that removing the plasma (i.e., packed red blood cells) would be safer than the use of whole blood in regard to recurrence of cancer.—R.D. Miller, M.D.

Risk of Postoperative Septic Complications After Abdominal Surgical Treatment in Relation to Perioperative Blood Transfusion

Wobbes Th, Bemelmans BLH, Kuypers JHC, Beerthuizen GIJM, Theeuwes AGM (Univ Hosp Nijmegen; Catholic Univ of Nijmegen, The Netherlands)
Surg Gynecol Obstet 171:59–62, 1990   12–9

Risk factors for postoperative sepsis were examined in a series of 548 patients undergoing elective intra-abdominal operations between 1980 and 1987. At least 1 complication occurred in 36% of these patients. The postoperative mortality was .9%.

Positive blood cultures were present in 3.8% of patients in this series. Wound infection was diagnosed in 6.9% of the patients, urinary tract infection in 14.4%, and respiratory tract infection in 14.1%. Also, 6% of the patients had intra-abdominal sepsis. Univariate analysis indicated that blood transfusion was a significant factor in postoperative sepsis (table). Both the duration of surgery and the total amount of blood given

Univariate Analysis of Factors Significantly Related to Postoperative
Septic Complications

Septic complications	*N*	*Per cent*
Blood transfusion		
Yes	260	40.5*
No	288	29.1
1 to 3 units	198	35.9
>3 units	62	55.7
Serum protein missing	296	36.8
<60 gm./L	104	42.3*
>60 gm./L	148	24.3
Gastric malignant disease	57	54.4*
Other	78	43.6
Colonic malignant disease	157	31.8
Inflammatory intestinal disease	190	29.5
Other	66	27.3
Total gastrectomy	35	65.7*
Partial gastrectomy	100	42.0
Colonic resections	382	30.6
Other	31	22.6
Anastomotic dehiscence		
Yes	16	87.5
No	532	31.9
Diabetes		
Yes	24	54.2[†]
No	524	33.6
Staff surgeon	307	38.4[†]
Resident	241	29.5
Perioperative antibiotics		
Yes	263	29.7[†]
No	285	39.0

*$P < .01$, chi-square test.
†$.01 < P < .05$, chi-square test.
(Courtesy of Wobbes Th, Bemelmans BLH, Kuypers JHC, et al: *Surg Gynecol Obstet* 171:59–62, 1990.)

were significantly associated with septic complications. Administration of more than 3 units of blood was a significant independent risk factor. Perioperative blood administration can increase the risk of sepsis developing after intra-abdominal surgery.

▶ The retrospective reviews that have appeared in recent years implicate blood transfusion as causing immunosuppression and thus increasing the risk of septic complications. In none of these analyses did the data show that sicker patients or those having more extensive operations were the ones who needed blood transfusions. This article attempts to deal with that by looking at one transfusion or a transfusion as a yes/no, and then comparing 1–3 units with no units. They found no significant difference in survival whether patients received 1 unit or no units, but there was an increased risk with big operations, which obviously are associated with more bleeding and a greater risk of surgical dissection. Although the findings somewhat support the belief that survival is determined by extent of disease and not by transfusion, if one looks at the actual data of the study some increased risk is nevertheless associated with transfusion. If they had done this study in 200 more patients and the trends continued, they would have found that transfusion of 1–3 units in fact increases the risk relative to no transfusion.

Does this mean that transfusions are immunosuppressive to the extent that they inhibit survival? We don't know. Studies such as this retrospective study are helpful, but we need a definitive investigation before saying that blood transfusion per se results in immunocompromise, increasing the risk of sepsis or lack of survival.—M.F. Roizen, M.D.

Nutritional

Nutritional Support in Surgical Practice: Part II
Meguid MM, Campos AC, Hammond WG (State Univ of New York, Syracuse)
Am J Surg 159:427–443, 1990   12–10

Well-nourished patients who require interruption of oral nutrition either because of the effects of surgical treatment or because of the effects of disease, or both, can tolerate starvation for brief periods. However, to allow starvation to be added to the stresses of disease and treatment in seriously ill, malnourished patients is not sensible from a therapeutic standpoint. Therefore, correction of malnutrition, either before initiating therapy or concomitant with treatment, is likely to benefit these particular patients.

Patients with nonspecific inflammatory bowel disease or gastrointestinal tract fistulas who are potential candidates for surgical intervention should be considered high-risk patients in whom the prompt initiation of preoperative enteral or parenteral nutrition may reduce postoperative morbidity and mortality. Although substantial nutritional support in these patients has little or no direct effect on the pathogenesis of the disorder, the discontinuance of oral intake may well have a beneficial effect on the basic disease process.

Parenteral nutrition probably has no beneficial effect on the pathogenetic process in patients admitted with acute pancreatitis. Although parenteral nutrition is not likely to be of significant benefit in patients with mild or moderate pancreatitis, the prompt and vigorous use of parenteral nutrition in those with severe pancreatitis, particularly in chronic alcoholics in whom nutritional status is already compromised, may well be crucial for survival.

In patients with organ system failure, including acute renal failure, liver failure, or pulmonary failure, appropriate nutritional support may help the patient to cope with the abnormal intermediary metabolism resulting from such failure until satisfactory organ system function returns. With the readily available modern techniques and personnel for nutritional support, protein-calorie malnutrition can be eliminated from the list of factors with which the seriously ill patient must cope.

▶ Because we are anesthetizing increasingly ill patients, anesthesiologists must be familiar with the various approaches to nutritional support in surgical patients. This is not a study per se; rather, it is an excellent review regarding the whole issue of nutritional support in the surgical patient and is highly recommended for reading.—R.D. Miller, M.D.

Continuous Enteral Feeding: A Major Cause of Pneumonia Among Ventilated Intensive Care Unit Patients

Jacobs S, Chang RWS, Lee B, Bartlett FW (Riyadh Armed Forces Hosp, Riyadh, Saudi Arabia)

J Parenter Enteral Nutr 14:353–356, 1990   12–11

Fatal nosocomial pulmonary infection is frequent in patients in the intensive care unit who required mechanical ventilation. Because continuous enteral feeding is commonly practiced in this setting, the relationship between lung infection and enteral feeding was studied in a series of 24 ventilated patients who received Ensure continuously for longer than 3 days.

Pneumonia occurred in 54% of these patients, with 12 of 13 who had a persistently high morning gastric pH being affected. In 11 cases (Fig 12–2), the causative organism was isolated from the stomach, oropharynx, or trachea before pneumonia supervened. The effect of enteral feeding appeared to be distinct from that of administration of ranitidine. The patients who had a morning gastric pH above 3.5 had a mortality 1.6 times that expected from the Apache II score.

These findings suggest that continuous enteral feeding can lead to a persistently high gastric pH and colonization by a single organism that

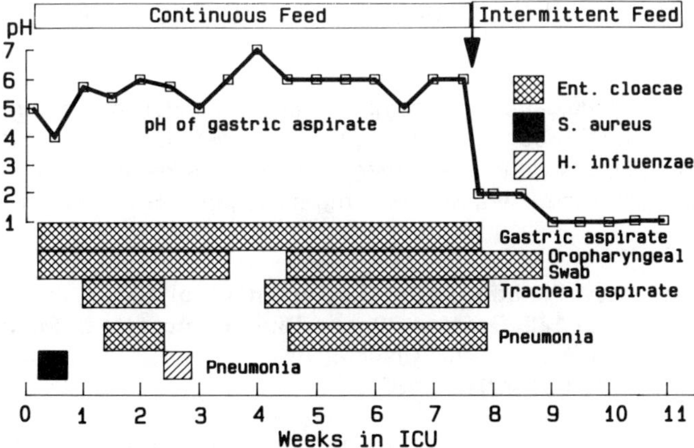

Fig 12–2.—Relationship between gastric pH and incidence of pneumonia in patient with Guillain-Barré syndrome. (Courtesy of Jacobs S, Chang RWS, Lee B, et al: *J Parenter Enteral Nutr* 14:353–356, 1990.)

can produce pneumonia. Intermittent feeding may reduce the risk of pneumonia yet still protect against gastric ulceration.

► I'd like to see more confirmation of this work before concluding that continuous enteral feeding is deleterious. The figures cited, however, are impressive.— R.R. Kirby, M.D.

Colloids

Hemodynamic and Oxygen Transport Response to Modified Fluid Gelatin in Critically Ill Patients
Edwards JD, Nightingale P, Wilkins RG, Faragher EB (Univ Hosp of South Manchester, Manchester, England)
Crit Care Med 17:996–998, 1989   12–12

In Europe, collagen derivatives, (e.g., modified fluid gelatin, or MFG), are used extensively as plasma substitutes. In a prospective study the hemodynamic and oxygen transport effects of the rapid infusion of 500 mL of MFG were studied in 10 critically ill adults with acute cardiorespiratory failure and hypovolemia.

Rapid infusion of MFG resulted in significant increases in mean arterial pressure, pulmonary artery wedge pressure, stroke volume index, cardiac index, and oxygen delivery. There were no significant changes in heart rate, shunt fraction, or systemic vascular resistance. Significant reductions occurred in the hemoglobin concentration and arterial oxygen content, whereas oxygen consumption appeared to increase but did not reach statistical significance.

An ideal synthetic plasma substitute should resemble the properties of human serum albumin. Experiences in Europe suggest that MFG fulfills these requirements and compares favorably with other available artificial colloids. The overall circulatory effects of MFG are beneficial in critically ill patients.

► This study investigates yet another plasma expander, but it suffers in that there is no control group or other plasma expanders evaluated. This omission makes comparisons difficult. Furthermore, what is needed is a plasma expander that can also carry and deliver more oxygen.— R.D. Miller, M.D.

Cardiorespiratory Function After Replacement of Blood Loss With Hydroxyethyl Starch 120, Dextran-70, and Ringer's Acetate in Pigs
Linko K, Mäkeläinen A (Helsinki Univ)
Crit Care Med 17:1031–1035, 1989   12–13

A medium-molecular weight hydroxyethyl starch (HES) (MW 120,000) (HES 120) has recently been introduced. Its effects on hemodynamics and oxygen transport were compared with those of dextran-70 (DEX) and Ringer's acetate (RA) in a standardized hemorrhagic-trauma model that resembled a situation of extensive surgery and massive blood loss.

The small intestines of 20 anesthetized healthy pigs were exteriorized in saline-moistened gauze to simulate an intra-abdominal operation. During a 2-hour period 4% of the animal's body weight was bled in 6 increments using an arterial cannula and replaced immediately with a 6% solution of HES 120, a 4.6% solution of DEX-70, or RA. The amount of fluid infused was equal to the amount of blood withdrawn in the colloid groups but increased by fourfold in the RA group. The control animals were not bled and received no fluid replacement.

There were no significant cardiorespiratory changes in the control animals. Hydroxyethyl starch and DEX caused reductions in hemoglobin of 41% and 44%, respectively, whereas RA caused only a 25% reduction. One animal died of hypovolemic shock 3 hours after infusion of RA. Cardiac output increased significantly in the HES and DEX groups after hemodilution. In both groups cardiac output was maintained at above initial values throughout the 5-hour observation period. In contrast, cardiac output did not increase in the RA group during hemodilution, and it decreased consistently during the follow-up period. Stroke volume and mean arterial pressures were increased in the colloid groups but decreased in the RA group. Oxygen consumption and delivery were highest in the HES group and lowest in the RA group. Arteriovenous oxygen difference increased slowly in the RA group throughout the study.

Both HES and DEX are superior to RA in blood replacement regimens. The new HES-120 has slightly better cardiorespiratory effects than a 4.6% solution of DEX-70 when used for replacement of blood loss.

▶ I have no experience with HES-120. However, the advantages claimed for it sound remarkably similar to those claimed for dextran 40, compared to dextran 70 some 20 or so years ago. Only time will tell whether this new addition will be useful.—R.R. Kirby, M.D.

Albumin Supplementation in the Critically Ill: A Prospective, Randomized Trial
Foley EF, Borlase BC, Dzik WH, Bistrian BR, Benotti PN (Harvard Univ Med School; New England Deaconess Hosp, Boston)
Arch Surg 125:739–742, 1990   12–14

Hypoalbuminemia is an accurate prognostic indicator of poor outcomes in a variety of clinical settings. Albumin replacement to correct it in critically ill patients is controversial. In a prospective, randomized trial, 25% albumin was administered to 18 hypoalbuminemic, critically ill patients to achieve and maintain serum levels of 25 g/L or more. Twenty-two others served as controls and were given no concentrated albumin.

No clinical benefit from albumin therapy could be found with regard to the mortality or major complication rate. Mortality in the treatment

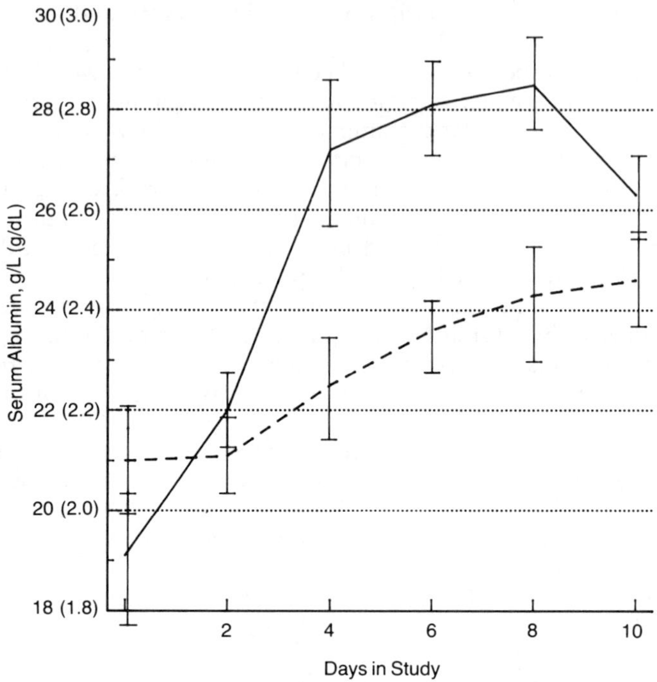

Fig 12–3.—Mean (± SEM) serum albumin concentrations in the treatment *(solid line)* and nontreatment *(broken line)* groups over the first 10 days of study. (Courtesy of Foley EF, Borlase BC, Dzik WH, et al: *Arch Surg* 125:739–742, 1990.)

group was 39% and in the control group, 27%. Major complication rates were 89% in the treatment group and 77% in the control group. There were also no between-group differences in length of hospitalization, stay in the intensive care unit, ventilator dependence, or tolerance of enteral feeding, despite significant increases of albumin in the treatment group (Fig 12–3).

Albumin therapy in hypoalbuminemic critically ill patients has no beneficial impact on a variety of outcome variables, despite its value in raising serum albumin concentrations. Albumin treatment is a costly intervention that does not appear to be justified in this patient population.

▶ Colloid enthusiasts will be disappointed and crystalloid enthusiasts elated at the results of this study. However, it's unlikely that either side will change its point of view. Unfortunately, this very expensive and unproven form of support will continue. Only the manufacturers will benefit.—R.R. Kirby, M.D.

Effectiveness of Hypertonic Saline-Dextran 70 for Initial Fluid Resuscitation of Major Burns

Onarheim H, Missavage AE, Kramer GC, Gunther RA (Univ of California, Davis)
J Trauma 30:597–603, 1990   12–15

An effective small-volume regimen of fluid treatment would be helpful for the prehospital treatment of patients in shock. The efficacy of an initial bolus infusion of hypertonic saline-dextran (HSD) solution, 4 mL/kg, on cardiovascular function was evaluated in anesthetized sheep given a 40% scald burn injury. Resuscitation with either 7% saline in 6% dextran 70 or the same volume of normal saline began 1 hour after injury. Ringer's lactate was then infused to maintain the cardiac output at 90% of baseline.

Infusion of HSD rapidly restored the cardiac output and mean arterial pressure to levels greater than those achieved with the same volume of normal saline. Hemodynamic improvement, however, was short lived. The need for further fluid was delayed by only 38 minutes on average, and total fluid needs for the first 6 hours were not significantly reduced by the initial HSD infusion. Skin edema was no less prominent in the HSD group than in animals given normal saline.

Resuscitation with a small volume of HSD improved cardiovascular function after burn injury in this study but only transiently. This probably is explained by a sustained increase in vascular permeability and continued plasma leakage after thermal injury.

▶ Would a larger volume of HSD have produced more than a transient response, particularly if administered over a longer period of time? Let's face it—A 4 mL/kg infusion of any substance in the management of major burn or trauma (280 mL in a 70-kg patient) is unlikely to be of much benefit if a deficit of several liters exists.—R.R. Kirby, M.D.

Synthetic Oxygen-Carrying Substances

The Efficacy of Polymerized Pyridoxylated Hemoglobin Solution as an O_2 Carrier

Gould SA, Sehgal LR, Rosen AL, Sehgal HL, Moss GS (Michael Reese Hosp, Chicago; Univ of Chicago)
Ann Surg 211:394–398, 1990   12–16

An experimental study in baboons showed that stromafree hemoglobin solution (SFH) with a hemoglobin (Hb) concentration of 7 g/dL can support life in primates in the absence of red blood cells. Although the animals survived the total exchange transfusion with SFH, oxygen consumption, mean arterial pressure (MAP), and cardiac output at zero hematocrit were significantly decreased and heart rate (HR) was significantly increased from baseline values. Because it is possible that these hemodynamic changes resulted from the low Hb level in the SFH solution, a study was conducted using an SFH solution with a higher Hb concentration.

Because SFH solutions with high Hb concentrations have unacceptable colloid osmotic pressure (COP), a polymerized pyridoxylated hemoglobin solution (Poly SFH-P) equal to 14 g/dL of Hb with normal COP was prepared and tested for its ability to support hemodynamics and oxygen transport in the absence of red blood cells.

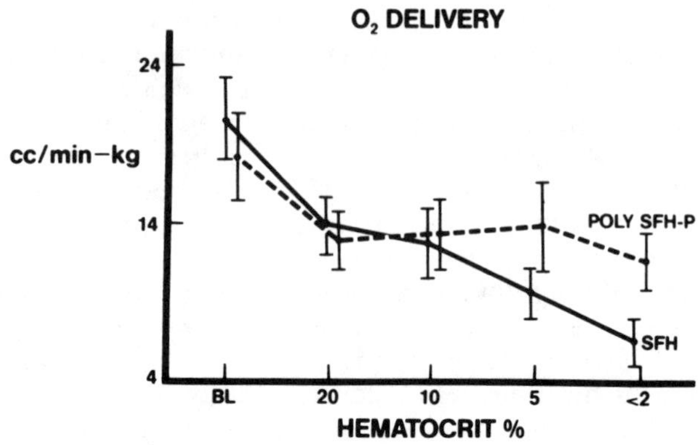

Fig 12–4.—Total O_2 delivery vs. hematocrit. Data presented as mean ± SEM. (Courtesy of Gould SA, Sehgal LR, Rosen AL, et al: *Ann Surg* 211:394–398, 1990.)

Under ketamine anesthesia, 6 adult baboons underwent total exchange transfusions with Poly SFH-P. Whole blood was removed in 50-mL aliquots and replaced with approximately equal volumes of the infusate. The exchange was stopped at hematocrits of 20%, 10%, 5%, and less than 2% to obtain hemodynamic measurements.

All animals receiving Poly SFH-P survived the total-exchange transfusion. At the end of the exchange at zero hematocrit, the mean MAP, HR, cardiac output, and oxygen consumption remained at baseline values (Fig 12–4). The final plasma Hb was 9.7 g/dL, compared with a final plasma Hb of only 4 g/dL reported in the earlier study. Thus Poly SFH-P appears to be an effective oxygen carrier having greater potential as a useful red blood cell substitute than the unmodified SFH solution used in the previous study.

▶ This and other groups have been working for years to develop an oxygen-carrying solution that can be stored for long periods and does not transmit disease. Most such solutions cause toxicity, usually to the kidney. Probably the most encouraging solution has been developed by a company called Somatogen, which has applied molecular engineering techniques to develop a hemoglobin molecule that will not transmit disease, can be stored for long periods of time, and will not require type and cross-matching.—R.D. Miller, M.D.

Rat Maze Performance After Resuscitation With Cross-linked Hemoglobin Solution

Pryzbelski RJ, Kant GJ, Bounds MJ, Slayter MV, Winslow RM (Walter Reed Army Inst of Research, Washington, DC; Washington Hosp Ctr, Washington, DC; Letterman Army Inst of Research, San Francisco)
J Lab Clin Med 115:579–588, 1990   12–17

Earlier studies have indicated that unmodified stroma-free hemoglobin solution produces neurotoxicity and behavioral impairment in rats. Subsequently, infusion of a clinically relevant dose of a modified (diaspirin α-α cross-linked) 14% hemoglobin (HbXL) solution caused no memory degradation or learning impairment in nonhemorrhaged rats and the brains were free of pathologic changes.

The HbXL solution was examined for evidence of neurobehavioral toxicity after infusion into hemorrhaged rats that were bled to 50% of their total body volume under anesthesia after they were trained to swim a water alley maze. The rats were then resuscitated with 14% HbXL solution (45 mL/kg), Ringer's lactate (RL) (60 mL/kg), or autologous shed blood (BLD). They were then retested in the water maze and examined histologically for evidence of neurotoxicity.

None of the HbXL- or BLD-infused rats died during resuscitation, but 20% of those resuscitated with RL died. Overall, there were no significant differences in the water maze performance among the treatment groups. Animals resuscitated with HbXL or BLD were free of pathologic changes in the brain at necropsy 10 days after treatment, but ischemic brain lesions were observed in 3 of the 12 surviving rats resuscitated with RL solution. Renal cortical tubular regeneration suggestive of previous damage was present in all treatment groups. There was a significant correlation between the total pathology in the 5 organs examined and maze errors. These findings suggest that resuscitation with 14% HbXL solution does not cause neurotoxicity in this lethal hemorrhage model.

▶ This is another study trying to find an oxygen-carrying solution that can be stored for a long period of time. Because of several problems, this solution probably will not be used on a widespread basis clinically. I hope that my opinion is incorrect, as we desperately need an oxygen-carrying solution that does not transmit disease.—R.D. Miller, M.D.

13 Critical Care

General

Clinical Assessment of Hemodynamic Values in Two Surgical Intensive Care Units: Effects on Therapy
Celoria G, Steingrub JS, Vickers-Lahti M, Teres D, Stein KL, Fink M, Friedmann P (Baystate Med Ctr, Springfield, Mass; Univ of Massachusetts School of Public Health, Amherst; Univ of Massachusetts Med Ctr, Worcester)
Arch Surg 125:1036–1039, 1990   13–1

Data on 115 survivors seen at 2 centers were studied prospectively to determine the impact of pulmonary artery catheterization in the surgical intensive care unit. Surgical residents predicted hemodynamic status and planned treatment before catheterization; the charts were later reviewed by a panel of intensive care specialists and a general surgeon.

Rates of correct classification of pulmonary wedge pressure, cardiac output, and systemic vascular resistance ranged from 47% to 55%. The catheterization findings led to a major change in treatment planning in half of the patients. Changes were more often necessary for patients having vascular surgery and less often for trauma patients.

Pulmonary artery catheterization frequently provides information important in planning treatment in patients under surgical intensive care. Nevertheless, it is necessary to assess the potential benefit of the study and the morbidity and mortality risks in each patient.

▶ In the complex and unpredictable situations presented by critically ill patients, it will always be difficult to prove that a single monitor made a difference in survival. Perhaps the best approach is to accept the fact that pulmonary artery catheters inherently expand the clinician's diagnostic and therapeutic capabilities with minimal associated risk. If this is true, we can direct future efforts to comparison of noninvasive monitors with pulmonary artery catheters and the accuracy of the derived information.—R.K. Stoelting, M.D.

APACHE II Score Does Not Predict Multiple Organ Failure or Mortality in Postoperative Surgical Patients
Cerra FB, Negro F, Abrams J (Univ of Minnesota)
Arch Surg 125:519–522, 1990   13–2

Use of the acute physiology and chronic health evaluation (APACHE) II system in the surgical intensive care unit has been proposed on the assumption that physiologic abnormalities seen within 24 hours of admission to the unit accurately reflect the later course and outcome. During a

1-year period the ability of this system to predict the development of multiple organ failure syndrome was studied in 92 patients.

Sixty-nine patients had multiple organ failure syndrome and 68 of them died. The APACHE II scores failed to predict to a clinically useful extent either multiple organ failure or death. Scores significantly underestimated the potential for development of organ failure syndrome. Factors that did help in predicting multiple organ failure syndrome and mortality included the ratio of Pa_{O_2} to inspired oxygen fraction, the serum level of lactate, and the levels of creatinine and bilirubin.

In multiple organ failure syndrome the extent of organ injury is manifest several days after admission to the intensive care unit. A useful predictive severity index would have to take into account the particular disease process, previous treatment used to stabilize the patient, and the time required for injury to become physiologically apparent.

▶ The results of this study should come as no surprise to those who have reviewed predictive indices scoring systems since their inception. The basic problem with all of those proposed thus far is that they cannot take into account incidents that have not yet occurred when the initial score is determined. Thus tension pneumothorax on the tenth day of intensive care unit admission, when the patient had not been intubated or mechanically ventilated at admission, cannot be predicted nor its impact on outcome assessed. This intrinsic defect in all systems renders them at best suspect and at worst useless.—R.R. Kirby, M.D.

Effective Measures for Reducing Blood Loss From Diagnostic Laboratory Tests in Intensive Care Unit Patients

Foulke GE, Harlow DJ (Univ of California, Davis, Sacramento)
Crit Care Med 17:1143–1145, 1989   13–3

In a prospective study blood loss as a result of diagnostic testing (DBL) was studied in 151 patients admitted to the medical intensive care unit (ICU) during 2 consecutive 10-week periods. A general policy was implemented of using small-volume, pediatric-size phlebotomy tubes and reduced volumes for arterial blood gas specimens for routine laboratory tests. During the second period, the DBL was displayed on each ICU flow sheet.

Total DBL and DBL per day were significantly lower than they would have been had standard volume tubes been used. This represented an average savings of 33%. The frequency with which blood had to be redrawn as a result of this policy was 1%. During the first period 8 patients with no evidence of major blood loss had a reduction in hematocrit value of at least 2% and required transfusion. The average number of units of blood transfused was 3.25, with the patient DBL representing an average of 17% of transfusion requirements. In contrast, during the second period only 1 of 70 patients required such transfusion. In addition, the number of routine tests ordered per day was significantly lower in the second period.

Diagnostic blood loss is a major problem in patients in the ICU. The use of small specimen volumes in this setting, as well as a reduction in the number of tests ordered, will reduce DBL. The latter can be monitored by recording DBL in the ICU database.

▶ Although the reduction of hematocrit attributed to blood sampling was significant, it's not immediately clear why a decrease of 2% or more should necessitate transfusion. What is important, however, is the reminder that blood can be lost in excessive amounts for often meaningless tests.—R.R. Kirby, M.D.

Propofol for Long-Term Sedation in the Intensive Care Unit: A Comparison With Papaveretum and Midazolam
Harris CE, Grounds RM, Murray AM, Lumley J, Royston D, Morgan M (Royal Postgrad Med School, Hammersmith Hosp, London)
Anaesthesia 45:366–372, 1990   13–4

The agent used to provide sedation in patients who require artificial ventilation in the intensive care unit (ICU) should ideally be short acting and noncumulative to allow rapid recovery for neurologic assessment and early weaning. The suitability of propofol to provide sedation in patients who require mechanical ventilation in the ICU was compared with the standard method of sedation in the unit, i.e., an infusion of papaveretum supplemented with bolus injections of midazolam. In 15 patients, propofol was given as a continuous infusion at a rate of 1–3 mg/kg/hr, preceded by a bolus of 1 mg/kg if indicated clinically; analgesia was provided by bolus doses of papaveretum. Twelve patients received papaveretum plus midazolam.

The levels of sedation were generally satisfactory in both groups, although 6 patients given propofol required neuromuscular blocking agents to achieve synchronization with the ventilator, compared with none given papaveretum plus midazolam. Several patients in both groups required inotropic support because of the severity of their illness, but there were no significant differences in respiratory and hemodynamic variables between groups. There was no evidence of adrenocortical suppression in the propofol-treated group. These data show that propofol can be a very useful sedative agent in the ICU, but sedative regimens should be tailored to individual patient requirements.

▶ We've been pleased with propofol as an adjunct to achieving ventilator support in our surgical ICU. It's been particularly useful when rapid assessment necessitates a rapidly awakened and responsive patient. My personal experience has involved continuous infusion for up to 10 days without any noted adverse effects. Obviously, reasonable hemodynamic stability is a prerequisite for successful use. Bear in mind, however, that when used this way, it's *very* expensive.—R.R. Kirby, M.D.

Predictors of Death Following ICU Discharge

Latour J, Lopez-Camps V, Rodriguez-Serra M, Giner JS, Nolasco A, Alvarez-Dardet C (Hosp Gen de Elche; Residencia Sanitaria de Sagunto; Hosp Luis Alcanyis de Játiva, Spain; Universidad de Alicante, Spain)
Intensive Care Med 16:125–127, 1990　　　　　　　　　　　13–5

Although the main objective of intensive care units (ICUs) is to increase survival, early after-discharge mortality occurs in a proportion of patients. An attempt was made to identify groups at high risk of dying shortly (within 2 months after admission) after discharge from the ICU.

The study group was composed of 700 patients older than 14 years who were consecutively discharged alive from the ICUs of 3 general hospitals in the Valencia region of Spain. Most had sustained acute myocardial infarction (45%) or had other cardiovascular diagnoses (24%). Patients were assessed according to 8 variables that could influence prognosis: age, simplified acute physiologic score (SAPS), therapeutic intervention scoring system in the first day of stay, organ or system failure, length of stay in the ICU, socioeconomic status, educational level, and marital status.

The observed early after-discharge mortality rate was 7.3%. Patients in the noncardiovascular group had a higher rate of mortality (15.4%) than those with myocardial infarction (4.2%) or other cardiovascular disease (3.3%). There was a strong association between mortality and all of the variables assessed except for marital status and socioeconomic level. Organ and system failure, SAPS higher than 10, and advanced age were the most sensitive criteria. The SAP score and advanced age (>65 years) had the strongest associations with mortality in multiple logistic regression analysis.

The variables have a low positive predictive value and thus are not suitable for individual predictions. However, these simple clinical and demographic prognostic criteria allow identification of groups of ICU survivors at high risk of early after-discharge mortality.

▶ Frequently, ICU physicians gauge the adequacy of their efforts based on successful ICU discharge of their patients. Often we don't follow up on what happens to them once they reach the ward. As this study shows, a significant percentage do not survive hospitalization (and many others may die not long after hospital discharge). Perhaps an analysis of total mortality, say up to a year after the ICU stay, is more realistic to gauge success or failure of a very limited and extremely costly resource.—R.R. Kirby, M.D.

Shock

Effects of Naloxone on Splanchnic Perfusion in Hemorrhagic Shock

Tuggle DW, Horton JW (Univ of Oklahoma; Univ of Texas, Dallas)
J Trauma 29:1341–1345, 1989　　　　　　　　　　　13–6

A substance that could maintain vital organ perfusion would be ideal when there is no immediate access to volume resuscitation for persons in hemorrhagic shock. The effects of using the opiate receptor antagonist naloxone alone were compared with the effects of using incomplete volume resuscitation in dogs bled to a mean arterial pressure of 35 mm Hg for 2 hours. Shed blood was returned to 8 animals, 8 others received a bolus of naloxone, 2 mg/kg, followed by 2 mg/kg/hr in normal saline; and 7 controls received normal saline.

Dogs given either shed blood or naloxone all survived to the end of the experiment (180 minutes). Dogs in the control group had a mean survival time of 18.6 minutes. Severe hemorrhagic shock impaired splanchnic perfusion to a significant degree. Both return of shed blood and naloxone increased the mean arterial pressure, cardiac output, and stroke volume. Colonic blood flow was 40% higher in dogs given shed blood than in those given naloxone. Hepatic arterial flow rose 70% above baseline in both groups. Blood flow to the diaphragm was significantly better in the naloxone-treated animals.

Naloxone improves cardiovascular function and survival in dogs in profound shock, but adequate volume replacement remains the major goal in treating hemorrhagic shock. The means by which the opiate receptor blockade improves regional blood flow and survival remains to be determined.

▶ Is naloxone staging a comeback in the treatment of hemorrhagic shock? This abstract seems to imply that it is. I remain unconvinced (but willing to listen), chiefly because the precise role that the release of endogenous opiate peptides plays in the pathogenesis of shock has not been elucidated. A 180-minute survival period in treated dogs cannot be construed to mean that human survival will be enhanced. The authors are correct, however, in stating that volume replacement is the mainstay of shock therapy.—R.R. Kirby, M.D.

A Comparison of the Cerebral and Cardiovascular Effects of Complete Resuscitation With Isotonic and Hypertonic Saline, Hetastarch, and Whole Blood Following Hemorrhage
Ducey JP, Mozingo DW, Lamiell JM, Okerburg C, Gueller GE (Brooke Army Med Ctr, Fort Sam Houston, Tex)
J Trauma 29:1510–1518, 1989   13–7

Hemorrhagic shock was induced in swine to lower the mean arterial pressure to less than 30 mm Hg. The animals then received 6% or .9% saline, 6% hetastarch, or whole blood until normal oxygen delivery was documented. Cranial pressures were measured in the presence of an epidural mass that was created by inflating a balloon in the epidural space.

Lower intracranial pressures resulted from resuscitation with hypertonic saline, and cerebral perfusion pressure remained normal throughout. Animals given physiologic saline had lower cerebral perfusion pressures. Intracranial elastance fell significantly in hypertonic saline-treated animals, particularly in the presence of an epidural mass. There were no significant histopathologic differences between the various treatment groups.

Hypertonic saline had no apparent benefit over the other materials studied when normalization of oxygen delivery served as the end point of resuscitation. It may, however, have a role in treating hemorrhagic shock if closed head injury has occurred. In this setting it may help by lowering intracranial pressure and minimizing the effects of an intracranial mass.

▶ When all is said and done, it may be that the ultimate benefit of hypertonic solutions will relate to areas such as decreased intracranial pressure and decreased edema formation elsewhere in the body. I'm still inclined to believe that intravascular volume resuscitation is an important effect, but studies such as this one do cast doubt on that presumption.—R.R. Kirby, M.D.

Molecular Biology of Circulatory Shock: II. Expression of Four Groups of Hepatic Genes Is Enhanced After Resuscitation From Cardiogenic Shock
Buchman TG, Cabin DE, Vickers S, Deutschman CS, Delgado E, Sussman MM, Bulkley GB (Johns Hopkins Med Insts)
Surgery 108:559–566, 1990   13–8

Some patients who are successfully resuscitated from circulatory shock nevertheless experience multiple organ failure (MOF). The changes associated with shock and MOF include altered gene expression that can affect such functions as albumin and procoagulant synthesis.

An attempt was made to characterize MOF-associated changes at the cellular level by obtaining sequential liver biopsy specimens from swine with cardiogenic shock associated with MOF. Pre-shock and postresuscitation biopsy specimens served to create a complementary DNA library and allow screening for genes whose expression is enhanced by at least fivefold after resuscitation from shock. Twelve enhanced genes were identified by RNA hybridization and 9 by sequencing.

Both acute-phase genes and heat-shock genes are enhanced after resuscitation of swine from cardiogenic shock. Expression of acute-phase genes is liver specific and necessary for systemic homeostasis. The expression of heat-shock genes, common to all cells, is important for intracellular homeostasis. The synthesis of acute-phase proteins is independent, and possibly exclusive, of heat-shock gene expression.

▶ Molecular biology is even getting into cardiogenic shock. This study is an example of the increasing trend toward melding molecular biology and clinical medicine.—R.D. Miller, M.D.

Hypertonic Saline Solution-Hetastarch for Fluid Resuscitation in Experimental Septic Shock

Armistead CW Jr, Vincent J-L, Preiser J-C, De Backer D, Minh TL (Erasme Univ Hosp, Brussels)
Anesth Analg 69:714–720, 1989   13–9

Hypertonic saline solution is used effectively to resuscitate patients with severe hypovolemia, but its role in treating septic shock is less clear. Combining hypertonic saline solution with colloid has been proposed to enhance the vascular effects of these fluids.

The hemodynamic and metabolic effects of 6% hydroxyethyl starch (HES) in .9% saline solution or in 7.5% hypertonic saline solution were compared in a canine model of endotoxic shock. Hydroxyethyl starch, 10 mL/kg, was given 30 minutes after administration of *Escherichia coli* endotoxin. Thereafter, physiologic saline was given in a volume needed to keep the pulmonary artery balloon-occluded pressure at baseline level.

The total sodium load was greater in animals that were given hypertonic saline with HES. Hematocrit values and levels of protein were consistently lower in these animals. Cardiac filling pressures, cardiac output, and oxygen delivery-consumption were greater than when animals received HES in physiologic saline. Vascular resistance was similar in the 2 groups. The rate of survival did not differ significantly. Hypertonic colloid solutions offer a way of rapidly restoring hemodynamic stability in septic shock, but the hemodynamic improvement is largely transient despite persistent effects on blood volume.

▶ What this study shows is that septic shock obviously is much more complex than simple hemorrhagic shock. The high incidence of multiorgan system failure in the former entity is pretty convincing evidence that much more than a simple perfusion defect is operative. Thus restoration of perfusion (by improved volume expansion) alone will not improve outcome. One should not conclude, however, that such therapy, in combination with other approaches, is not beneficial.—R.R. Kirby, M.D.

Prospective, Controlled, Randomized Trial of Naloxone Infusion in Early Hyperdynamic Septic Shock

Safani M, Blair J, Ross D, Waki R, Li C, Libby G (Med Ctr of Long Beach, Calif)
Crit Care Med 17:1004–1009, 1989   13–10

To determine whether naloxone infusion is effective in patients with severe hyperdynamic septic shock, a prospective study was conducted in which 22 patients were randomly assigned to receive naloxone or placebo.

Patients were treated approximately 12 hours after the onset of shock. The mean arterial pressure was 63 mm Hg. All patients had clinical evidence of an infectious process and were given dopamine, 20 µg/kg/min.

Five (46%) of the 11 patients in the naloxone-treated group and 1 (9%) of the 11 patients given placebo responded clinically. The mean arterial pressure of the responders increased from 62 mm Hg to 89 mm Hg within 20 minutes of naloxone treatment; this response was sustained throughout the patients' clinical course. The mean arterial pressure did not change significantly in patients who did not respond to naloxone or in patients given placebo. Although the survival rate among responders was 100%, the overall survival in all groups was essentially the same. Naloxone produced no adverse effects, except for mild agitation in some patients.

Naloxone infusion is clinically effective in some patients with severe early hyperdynamic septic shock. Almost half of the patients in this series had improved hemodynamic profiles. However, naloxone treatment does not appear to increase the overall survival rate.

▶ Seemingly, the same old story: brief, often dramatic, hemodynamic improvement, but no effect in terms of improved survival. One cannot help but see in naloxone a repeat of the steroid experience from the 1960s through the 1980s, at least where shock and sepsis are concerned. If naloxone were truly effective, wouldn't well-designed studies have demonstrated this efficacy after more than a decade of research? However, compare this study with that of Tuggle et al. (1).—R.R. Kirby, M.D.

Reference

1. Tuggle DW, et al: *J Trauma* 29:1341, 1989.

Treatment of Uncontrolled Hemorrhagic Shock With Hypertonic Saline Solution

Gross D, Landau EH, Klin B, Krausz MM (Hadassah Univ Hosp, Jerusalem)
Surg Gynecol Obstet 170:106–112, 1990   13–11

Although hypertonic saline solution (HTS) has been recommended as an initial treatment for hemorrhagic shock, it may not be safe for patients with "uncontrolled" shock. Uncontrolled hemorrhagic shock (UCHS), as induced in an animal model by incision of branches of the ileocolic artery, leads to continuous free intra-abdominal hemorrhage. The effect of HTS on UCHS was observed in 2 groups of rats.

In the first group, the abdomen was closed immediately after induction of hemorrhage and before HTS administration. These rats were then divided into 6 subgroups; 1 group was not treated with HTS and 5 were treated at times ranging from 5 to 120 minutes after closure of the abdomen. In the second group, which was divided into identical subgroups, the abdomen was kept open to observe the bleeding response after HTS therapy.

In the first group, UCHS was followed by a decrease in mean arterial

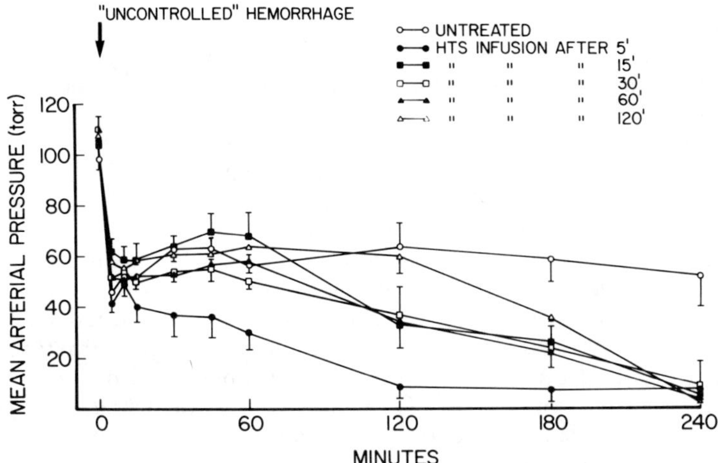

Fig 13–1.—Mean arterial pressure in uncontrolled hemorrhagic shock treated by HTS at different time periods after abdominal injury in rats with abdominal closure. (Courtesy of Gross D, Landau EH, Klin B, et al: *Surg Gynecol Obstet* 170:106–112, 1990.)

pressure from 99 torr to 46 torr within 5 minutes, with a gradual increase to 63 torr after 30 minutes. The survival rate was 80%. Treatment with HTS led to further decreases in mean arterial pressure and increased mortality (Fig 13–1). In group 2, the response of mean arterial pressure was similar to that in group 1 given HTS infusion after 5, 60, and 120 minutes. The amount of shed blood was greater at these periods than after 15 minutes and 30 minutes.

The increase in arterial blood pressure and peripheral vasodilation brought about by HTS treatment may increase blood loss. Although HTS restores arterial blood pressure and prevents mortality in controlled hemorrhagic shock, its use in treating victims in hemorrhagic shock after abdominal trauma should be reconsidered. The adverse response to HTS occurs as late as 2 hours after the hemorrhagic insult.

▶ This paper follows up a similar study by the same authors published in 1988 in the *Journal of Trauma* (1) and reviewed in the 1990 YEAR BOOK OF ANESTHESIA (2). My comments then are still applicable. Based on these results, anesthesiologists should use a demonstrably less effective means of fluid resuscitation, i.e., one that does not increase blood pressure as effectively, to reduce uncontrolled blood loss. Nevertheless, these investigators have done a good job and have provided us with much food for thought.—R.R. Kirby, M.D.

References

1. Gross D, et al: *J Trauma* 28:751, 1988.
2. 1990 YEAR BOOK OF ANESTHESIA, pp 257–258.

Trauma

Early Physiologic Predictors of Injury Severity and Death in Blunt Multiple Trauma
Siegel JH, Rivkind AI, Dalal S, Goodarzi S (Maryland Inst for Emergency Medical Services Systems, Baltimore; Univ of Maryland)
Arch Surg 125:498–508, 1990   13–12

Predictors of mortality risk were derived from data on 185 patients who sustained blunt traumatic hepatic injury among other injuries. The model derived from studying these patients was then tested in 323 patients with multiple trauma whose index injury was pelvic fracture. None of this group had blunt liver injury. The variables used included the admission Glasgow Coma Score (GCS), base excess or deficit, arterial level of lactate, Injury Severity Score, and initial 24-hour volume of blood required by replacement.

In all 2-variable combinations the GCS was significantly predictive, reflecting the influence of brain injury on mortality. As single variables both base excess and the initial 24-hour volume of blood required were highly significant. The combination of admission GCS and base excess was the most accurate predictor of death or survival, and it was a significantly early predictor of outcome in the group of patients with pelvic fractures.

Two readily obtained measures, the GCS and base excess, provide a quantitative assessment of the risk of death in a patient with multiple injuries. The base excess reflects the severity of perfusion-related hypovolemic ischemic shock, and the GCS is the best immediately available measure of neurologic function.

▶ This provocative article suggests that determination of the GCS score and base excess is valuable. Pertinent comments concerning this study were provided by Donald B. Trunkey, M.D., an internationally renowned trauma expert. He noted, for example, that the death rate from blunt liver trauma in this series was 31%, rather than the usually reported 10% to 20% in other large series. The higher death rate may have influenced some of the findings. In addition, he noted that hypoxia and hypovolemia contribute significantly as "secondary injuries" to the GCS. Clearly, hypoxia and ischemia will be reflected in a base excess abnormality and make it unlikely that variables such as blood pressure and heart rate (both related to perfusion) can be dismissed out-of-hand. Nevertheless, this study deserves careful further evaluation because it seems to overcome some of the deficiencies recognized in APACHE II and other predictive scoring systems.—R.R. Kirby, M.D.

The Effect of Preexisting Conditions on Mortality in Trauma Patients
Morris JA Jr, MacKenzie EJ, Edelstein SL (Vanderbilt Univ; Health Services Research and Development Ctr, Baltimore)
JAMA 263:1942–1946, 1990   13–13

The presence of preexisting disease, independent of age, may define a subgroup of trauma patients at increased risk of dying. A case-control study was done to test this hypothesis.

Cases were all 3,074 trauma deaths occurring in 1983 in any of the 331 acute care hospitals in California. Three or 4 control patients (9,869 total) who were trauma survivors were matched to each case on the basis of injury severity, age, and individual hospital. Hospital discharge data were reviewed. Conditional logistic regression analysis was used to estimate the relative odds of dying among patients with and without 1 or more of 11 chronic conditions potentially deterimental to outcome.

Conditions that significantly increased the risk of dying were cirrhosis, congenital coagulopathy, ischemic heart disease, chronic obstructive pulmonary disease, and diabetes. The relative odds for these conditions were 4.5, 3.2, 1.8, 1.8, and 1.2, respectively.

These findings support the recommendation of the American College of Surgeons that the presence of underlying disease should be considered in decisions to triage and transfer patients to trauma centers. These findings also stress the significance of underlying disease in the case-mix adjustment of case-fatality rates and identification of unexpected deaths for quality assurance reviews.

▶ Frequently, however, those involved with initial triage management and disposition don't have any information regarding preexisting disease. By the time such facts come to light, the patient is already in the system.—R.R. Kirby, M.D.

Thoracotomy During Trauma Resuscitations—An Appraisal by Board-Certified General Surgeons
Hoyt DB, Shackford SR, Davis JW, Mackersie RC, Hollingsworth-Fridlund P
(Univ of California, San Diego)
J Trauma 29:1318–1321, 1989   13–14

The impact of resuscitative thoracotomy done by board-certified surgeons was evaluated during a 4.5-year period in 113 patients. Thoracotomy was performed on patients in cardiac arrest within 20 minutes of hospital arrival, and 64 (57%) had thoracotomy done immediately on admission.

None of the patients survived a blunt mechanism injury, even with thoracotomy. The probability of survival among those with penetrating injuries was .48. Most patients who died of penetrating injuries had severe and advanced physiologic derangements at the time of hospitalization.

The use of resuscitative thoracotomy for patients who sustain penetrating wounds is supported. It allows direct access to the injury for repair or permits temporary occlusion of the thoracic aorta.

▶ These investigators are well established and careful in what they study and report. I've also noted increased enthusiasm for resuscitation thoracotomy, although the results in the cases I've observed have not been as good as those reported here.— R.R. Kirby, M.D.

Critical Care

Noninvasive Mechanical Ventilation for Acute Respiratory Failure
Elliott MW, Steven MH, Phillips GD, Branthwaite MA (Brompton Hosp, London)
Br Med J 300:358–360, 1990   13–15

Intermittent positive-pressure ventilation (IPPV), delivered noninvasively via a nasal mask, can relieve chronic respiratory failure. This approach was used in 6 patients with acute life-threatening exacerbations of respiratory disease. All 6 were confused or obtunded and severely hypoxic and hypercapnic. Three had deteriorated acutely because of infection. A Respironics nasal mask and either a Lifecare PLV 100 or Brompton Pneupac ventilator were used. The median tidal volume was 1.25 L.

All patients improved initially, with a rise in the median arterial oxygen tension from 4.4 kPa to 8.7 kPa. A normal level of consciousness returned within 12–24 hours in 5 patients and a rapid diuresis ensued. One patient died after declining intubation and conventional ventilation. Four patients were discharged home and were well 5–22 months later. One continued to use nasal IPPV during sleep at home. One patient remained hospitalized awaiting heart-lung transplantation and used the ventilator for 12–16 hours a day.

Nasal IPPV is feasible in patients with acute-on-chronic respiratory failure when intubation is inappropriate or difficult weaning is anticipated. This method may also be used when long-term ventilatory support may be necessary. If intubation proves to be necessary, nasal IPPV may aid the return of spontaneous breathing.

▶ Although it is of interest, this study suffers from the lack of other treatment groups with which to compare the outcome, i.e., patients treated more conservatively with oxygen, "stir-up" regimens, and the like, and those who are intubated and mechanically ventilated. The number of patients studied—6—is too small to allow final judgments. Additional study is warranted.— R.R. Kirby, M.D.

Oxygen Delivery in Patients With Adult Respiratory Distress Syndrome Who Undergo Surgery: Correlation With Multiple-System Organ Failure
Cryer HG, Richardson JD, Longmire-Cook S, Brown CM (Univ of Louisville; Humana Hosp Univ, Louisville)
Arch Surg 124:1378–1385, 1989   13–16

Mortality from adult respiratory distress syndrome (ARDS) has not declined appreciably in the past 2 decades. To identify factors that contribute to sepsis, multisystem organ failure, and death, data were studied on 52 consecutive patients with ARDS who had surgery during the reversible phases of the syndrome. Mortality was 62% in this series.

Multivariate analysis indicated that oxygen delivery and the alveolar-arterial oxygen gradient 3 days after ARDS was diagnosed were the most important correctable correlates of mortality. Both factors influenced the development of multisystem organ failure and survival. The variables were not significant on day 1 or 7. Even when patients dying of disease unrelated to ARDS were included, day 3 oxygen tension and the alveolar-arterial oxygen gradient accounted for 42% of total variability between survivors and nonsurvivors.

Optimization of oxygen delivery and the alveolar-arterial oxygen gradient after the onset of ARDS may promote resolution of the disorder and prevent further organ dysfunction. Survival should improve as a result. The alveolar-arterial oxygen gradient is minimized through an optimal level of positive end-expiratory pressure. Arterial oxygen saturation is maximized and cardiac output is increased by optimizing preload, providing inotropic support, and occasionally by reducing afterload.

▶ These results are surprising in view of numerous papers in the past decade purporting to show that arterial oxygenation and the various indices used to describe it (PaO_2/FiO_2/PA-a O_2, shunt, and so on) are of little value in discriminating survivors from nonsurvivors and predicting outcome. That oxygenation and oxygen delivery are important cannot be denied. Whether they are the major determinants of outcome in ARDS and multiorgan system failure awaits further validation.—R.R. Kirby, M.D.

Prostacyclin for the Treatment of Pulmonary Hypertension in the Adult Respiratory Distress Syndrome: Effects on Pulmonary Capillary Pressure and Ventilation-Perfusion Distributions
Radermacher P, Santak B, Wüst HJ, Tarnow J, Falke KJ (Heinrich-Heine-Univ, Düsseldorf; Freie Univ, Berlin)
Anesthesiology 72:238–244, 1990   13–17

An important component of the management of adult respiratory distress syndrome (ARDS) is reducing pulmonary vascular pressures. Because endothelial injury with diffuse pulmonary vasoconstriction and microthrombosis are probable causes of pulmonary hypertension in ARDS, prostacyclin (PGI_2), a naturally occurring vasodilator produced by endothelial cells with antiplatelet aggregation and cytoprotective abilities, may prove beneficial in treatment. To test the hypothesis that PGI_2 might decrease the pulmonary capillary pressure (PCP) and improve systemic oxygen delivery in ARDS, 9 patients in whom pulmonary artery hypertension developed during ARDS were treated with an infusion of PGI_2, 12.5–35 ng/kg/min.

Pulmonary artery pressure was reduced significantly from 35.6 mm Hg to 28.8 mm Hg after PGI_2 infusion. This was associated with a significant reduction in PCP, obtained by analysis of the pressure decay curve after pulmonary artery occlusion, from 22.9 mm Hg to 19.7 mm Hg. The mean contribution of pulmonary venous resistance to total pulmonary vascular resistance did not change during PGI_2 infusion. The cardiac index increased during PGI_2 infusion because of an increase in heart rate and stroke volume. There was a significant increase in the venous admixture because of marked deterioration of ventilation-perfusion matching. However, PGI_2 infusion did not significantly alter the PaO_2 because of an increased mixed venous oxygen content, indicated by an augmented mixed venous PO_2. This caused a significant increase (35%) in the systemic oxygen delivery rate.

Short-term infusion of PGI_2 attenuates pulmonary artery hypertension and lowers PCP in patients with ARDS, without deleterious effects on arterial oxygenation. It may be a useful drug to reduce pulmonary vascular pressures in patients with ARDS.

▶ This report is encouraging, but prostacyclin has been tried in ARDS models for a decade. If it has obvious beneficial effects, why has it not become a mainstay of therapy? I would like to see this study repeated in a large number of patients—9 is not enough of a sample size from which to draw any far-reaching conclusions.—R.R. Kirby, M.D.

Improved Survival in ARDS Patients Associated With a Reduction in Pulmonary Capillary Wedge Pressure

Humphrey H, Hall J, Sznajder I, Silverstein M, Wood L (Univ of Chicago Hosps and Clinics)
Chest 97:1176–1180, 1990

13–18

Adult respiratory distress syndrome (ARDS) continues to cause a high rate of mortality, even with aggressive supportive therapy. The acute lung injury that initiates ARDS leads to alveolar flooding and mechanical and gas exchange abnormalities in the lung. In animal studies, decreasing hydrostatic pressures in the pulmonary circulation, as judged by the measured pulmonary capillary wedge pressure (Ppw), reduces lung edema and improves gas exchange. To determine whether lowering the Ppw is associated with increased survival or a decreased stay in the intensive care unit (ICU), data on 20 men and 20 women (mean age, 46 years) were studied retrospectively. At study entry, the mean Ppw for all patients was 12 mm Hg.

Patients were divided into 2 groups; in the 16 patients in group 1 a Ppw reduction of at least 25% was achieved; the 24 patients in group 2 did not experience this reduction (Table 1).

Survival was significantly different in the 2 groups, even after stratification by age or severity of illness. Twelve patients in group 1 survived, but only 7 patients in group 2 survived. Stay in the ICU was shorter for patients in group 1, but not significantly so (Table 2).

During the first 5 days after lung injury, ARDS can be considered a reversible condition. Patients who still require mechanical ventilatory support after 1–2 weeks often manifest extensive pulmonary fibrosis and

TABLE 1.—Characteristics of Patients With ARDS (N = 40)*

		Group 1 (N = 16)		Group 2 (N = 24)	
		Mean	Range	Mean	Range
Age, yr		35	(16-78)	53	(21-81)
Prob die, % (by APACHE II)		15	(13-17)	14	(1315)
Mean Ppw					
Entry		13.0	(9.0-17.0)	11.4	(9.4-13.4)
24 hours		6.5	(2.0-11.0)	13.0	(8.0-18.0)
48 hours		7.7	(6.2-9.2)	13.0	(6.9-19.1)
Heart rate	at 0	126	(88-165)	111	(70-163)
Heart rate	at 24	124	(94-158)	109	(60-144)
Heart rate	at 48	111	(84-130)	107	(64-140)
MAP (mm Hg)	at 0	86	(64-127)	85	(57-138)
	at 24	83	(51-122)	80	(52-119)
	at 48	91	(77-114)	80	(42-110)
PEEP	at 0	9	(0-15)	6	(0-15)
	at 24	9	(0-15)	8	(0-20)
	at 48	10	(0-15)	10	(0-20)
FIO_2	at 0	0.86	(0.5-1.0)	0.72	(0.4-1.0)
	at 24	0.65	(0.3-1.0)	0.62	(0.4-1.0)
	at 48	0.60	(0.4-1.0)	0.55	(0.4-1.0)
Creatinine	at 0	1.9	(0.9-2.9)	1.8	(1.0-2.6)
	at 24	1.7	(0.8-2.7)	2.0	(0.9-2.9)
	at 48	1.9	(0.8-2.9)	1.8	(0.9-2.4)

*Data point for Ppw, heart rate, mean arterial pressure *(MAP)*, *(PEEP)*, fractions of inspired oxygen *(FIO_2)*, and creatinine are taken at 0 (entry), 24 hours, and 48 hours into therapy.

(Courtesy of Humphrey H, Hall J, Sznajder I, et al: *Chest* 97:1176–1180, 1990.)

distortion of lung architecture. Thus reducing lung edema in the early stages may shorten the duration and intensity of supportive therapy and improve outcome. Intervention directed at the reduction of Ppw should increase survival in these patients.

▶ The problem here is that ARDS patients frequently need increased Ppw to support perfusion of other organ systems. Lowering the Ppw as a primary goal

TABLE 2.—Survival and Length of Stay in ICU

	Group 1 (N = 16)	Group 2 (N = 24)
Survived	12 (75%)	7 (29%)*
ICU length of stay (days)	8.9 ± 8	14.8 ± 11.4 days

*$P < .02$ χ^2, Mantel-Haenzel.
(Courtesy of Humphrey H, Hall J, Sznajder I, et al: *Chest* 97:1176–1180, 1990.)

of therapy in ARDS seems risky unless such therapy is very selectively applied. I'd also like to see this work done prospectively. There are too many unknowns that can be omitted inadvertently in a retrospective study.— R.R. Kirby, M.D.

Physiology of Aging Related to Outcome in the Adult Respiratory Distress Syndrome
Gee MH, Gottlieb JE, Albertine KH, Kubis JM, Peters SP, Fish JE (Jefferson Med College)
J Appl Physiol 69:822–829, 1990   13–19

Most studies of adult respiratory distress syndrome (ARDS) indicate that patients who die within 30 days are older than those who survive. To identify potential age-related changes in organ system function that could help explain this association, 39 patients with ARDS were studied; 17 patients were younger than 60 years and 16 were 60 years or older. Six patients whose body temperatures were 97.5° F or less at the outset were analyzed separately.

Mortality was 12% in the younger group and 69% in older patients who were not hypothermic. All 6 initially hypothermic patients died. Older patients tended to have a higher ratio of arterial oxygen pressure to inspired oxygen fraction and a lower positive end-expiratory pressure than younger patients. They also had a lower cardiac output, but systolic blood pressure did not differ with age. Both older patients and those who were hypothermic had relatively high serum urea nitrogen and creatinine levels.

Age-related impairment of normal regulatory mechanisms may well contribute to a blunted response to treatment and thereby to a poor outcome of ARDS. It may be necessary to stratify patients by age in future studies of ARDS.

▶ The impact of age on outcome of therapy for ARDS has been argued for years. This study supports the seemingly intuitive prediction that elderly patients will do worse. However, the numbers of patients evaluated are too small to allow any definite conclusions.— R.R. Kirby, M.D.

Respiratory Care

Ventilatory Muscle Support in Respiratory Failure With Nasal Positive Pressure Ventilation
Carrey Z, Gottfried SB, Levy RD (Royal Victoria Hosp, Montreal; Montreal Chest Hosp; McGill Univ)
Chest 97:150–158, 1990   13–20

Intermittent positive pressure ventilation through a tightly fitted nasal mask (NPPV) is a noninvasive alternative method of providing chronic intermittent ventilatory support. Its effects on inspiratory muscle activity were evaluated in 3 normal subjects and 4 women and 5 men with acute or chronic respiratory failure caused by restrictive (4 patients) or obstructive (5 patients) respiratory disorders.

Application of NPPV significantly reduced the phasic diaphragm electromyogram amplitude to 6.7% of values obtained during spontaneous breathing in normal subjects, to 6.4% in the restrictive group, and to 8.3% in the obstructive group. Simultaneous reductions in accessory respiratory muscle activity also were observed. The presence of positive intrathoracic pressure swings on inspiration in all subjects also supports the finding that NPPV suppressed inspiratory muscle activity. Oxygen saturation and end-tidal and arterial PCO_2 remained stable or improved with NPPV, compared with values obtained during spontaneous breathing.

Nasal positive pressure ventilation can provide adequate ventilatory support in a noninvasive fashion while reducing the energy expenditure of inspiratory muscles in patients with restrictive or obstructive respiratory disorders. It appears that long-term assisted ventilation with NPPV improves ventilatory performance by resting chronically fatigued inspiratory muscles.

▶ Continuous positive airway pressure (CPAP) has been applied successfully by both mask and nasal prongs. Nasal positive pressure ventilation, however, has had only limited clinical trials. This report indicates some efficiency, although improvements in gas exchange were not overly impressive. Whether the technique will find widespread application is difficult to assess. Problems such as aspiration of gastric contents, gastric distention, effective alarm systems, and so on require additional investigation. However, the same was true when face mask CPAP was introduced in the 1970s. Any noninvasive ventilatory support technique that is effective deserves a close look.—R.R. Kirby, M.D.

A New Device That Allows Synchronous Intermittent Inspiratory Chest Tube Occlusion With Any Mechanical Ventilator
Blanch PB, Koens JC Jr, Layon AJ (Univ of Florida, Gainesville)
Chest 97:1426–1430, 1990   13–21

Massively leaking bronchopleural fistulas (BPFs) can be difficult to control. Combined with acute respiratory failure, BPFs result in an 81% mortality. Intermittent inspiratory chest tube occlusion (IICTO) is an effective way to control even the largest BPF. However, IICTO is difficult to use for a variety of reasons. In 2 patients, BPF associated with acute respiratory failure was managed with a simple new device that allows IICTO application with any mechanical ventilator.

The device consists of a pressure-amplifying valve connected between a supply of gas and exhalation valve that functions as the dynamic component of the IICTO system. This pressure-amplifying valve is considered normally to be closed, meaning that a trigger or signal pressure is required to open the device to actuate the exhalation valve. The triggering pressure required is 3 cm H_2O. Loss of this pressure closes the pressure

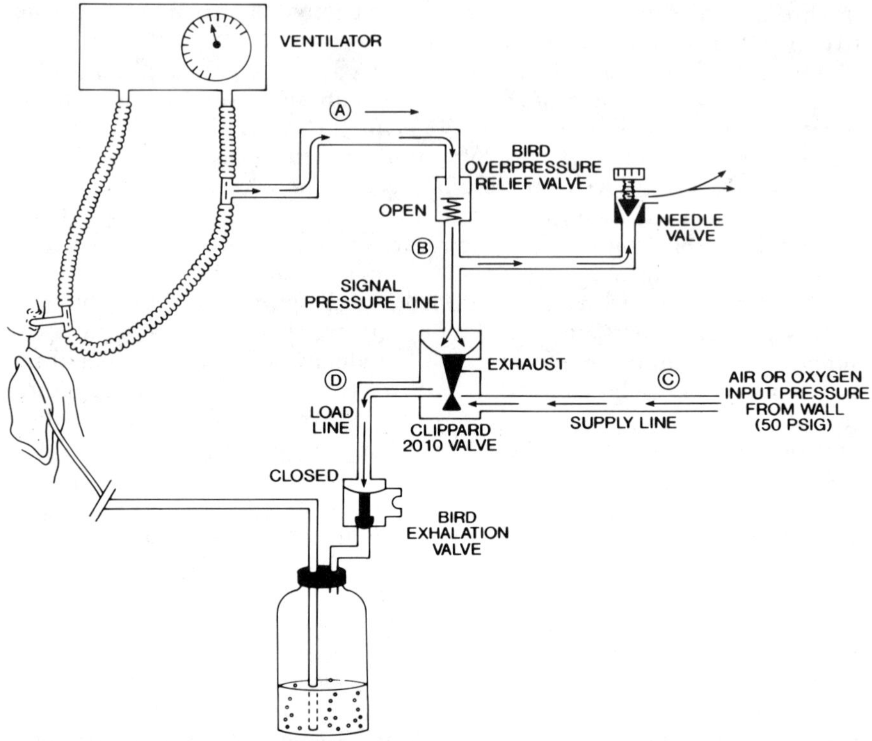

Fig 13–2.—Inhalation phase of the system used to control BPF air leaks during mechanical ventilation. Increased pressure generated during mechanical inhalation allows gas *(A)* to be directed through an overpressure relief valve (Bird) to a pressure-amplifying valve (Clippard 2010) *(B)* where a diaphragm is pressurized that causes the pressure amplifier to open and thus permits 50 psig of oxygen or air *(C)* to flow through and pressurize and close an exhalation valve *(D)*. The exhalation valve occludes the outlet of the underwater seal and thus provides intermittent inspiratory chest tube occlusion. (Courtesy of Blanch PB, Koens JC Jr, Layon AJ: *Chest* 97:1426–1430, 1990.)

amplifier and depressurizes the exhalation valve through an exhaust port in the former valve (Figs 13–2 and 13–3). Triggering is provided by attaching a line with an overpressure relief valve into the inspiratory limb of the ventilator breathing circuit proximal to the humidifier. The overpressure relief valve is adjusted to relieve pressure at about 5 cm H_2O above the level of continuous positive airway pressure.

Initiation of mechanical inhalation increases airway pressure, opens the overpressure governor, triggers the pressure amplifier, and closes the exhalation valve to occlude the chest tube. A needle valve dissipates the triggering pressure during the expiratory phase.

This device is clearly effective and may have played a role in the eventual recovery of 1 of the patients with BPF. It is extremely versatile and can provide IICTO with most ventilators. If further study shows this technique to be without serious risk, it may have a place in the treatment of patients with BPF associated with acute respiratory failure.

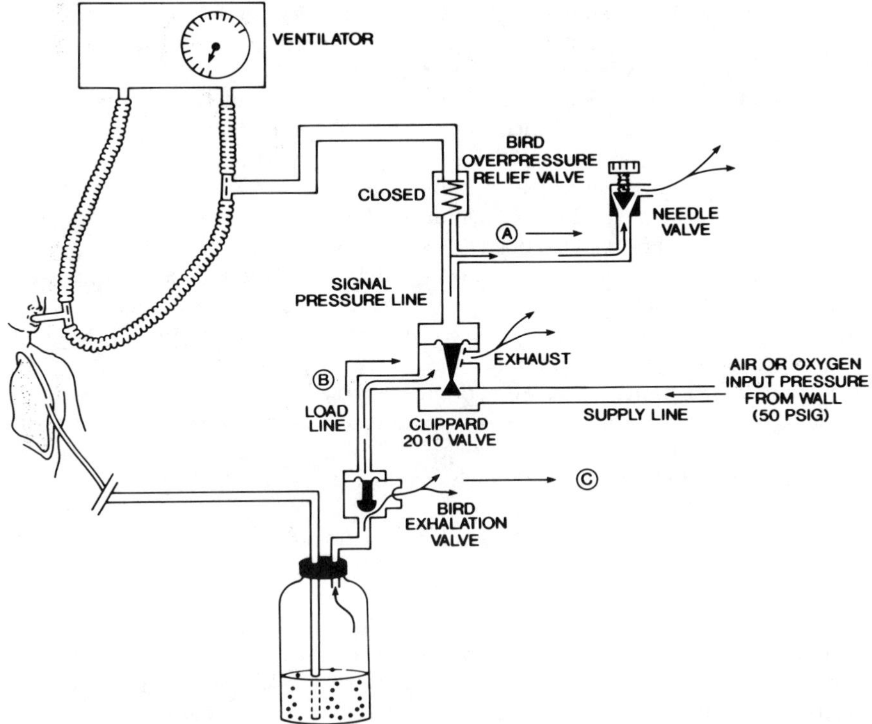

Fig 13–3.—During the exhalation phase, airway pressure decreases and causes the overpressure relief valve to close. The pressure loading the diaphragm *(A)* in the amplifier valve dissipates via a needle valve that closes the amplifier valve. Thus the exhalation valve opens and allows the chest tube and the underwater seal apparatus to function in the normal manner. (Courtesy of Blanch PB, Koens JC Jr, Layon AJ: *Chest* 97:1426–1430, 1990.)

▶ I've had a great deal of experience with this device and a number of its predecessors since 1974. In selected patients they can be life-saving. This particular model is particularly helpful because it can be used with any ventilator currently manufactured. Good patient selection is the key to success, together with very careful monitoring.—R.R. Kirby, M.D.

Difficulty in Weaning From Respiratory Support in a Patient With the Intermediate Syndrome of Organophosphate Poisoning

Routier RJ, Lipman J, Brown K (JG Strijdom Hosp; Univ of the Witwatersrand, Johannesburg)
Crit Care Med 17:1075–1076, 1989   13–22

A patient was treated for the intermediate syndrome of organophosphate poisoning (OPP) and levels of acetylcholinesterase were documented.

Man, 33, was found stuporous and with respiratory arrest that required intubation and mechanical ventilation. He had bilateral ptosis, meiosis, bronchospasm with copious secretions, and diarrhea. He was tachycardic and hypertensive and had muscle fasciculations. Based on excessive cholinergic activity, OPP was suspected and later confirmed by decreased levels of serum acetylcholinesterase (S-AChe) (229 mU/mL of serum) and erythrocyte acetylcholinesterase (E-AChe) (1,089 mU/μmol of hemoglobin). Atropine was given and symptoms resolved within the next 72 hours. On day 5 the patient had a second episode of severe muscle weakness that affected the muscles of respiration, proximal limb muscles, neck flexors, and muscles innervated by the palatal, facial, and external ocular motor cranial nerves. Respiratory muscle weakness was severe, as evidenced by a negative inspiratory force (NIF) or -18 cm of H_2O. The levels of S-AChe (188 mU/mL of serum) and E-AChe (1,153 mU/μmol of hemoglobin) remained low. The patient required continued ventilatory support until 10 days after admission when he was successfully extubated. At this time the NIF had increased to -70 cm of H_2O, and activity of S-AChe (855 mU/mL of serum) and E-AChe (1,968 mU/μmol of hemoglobin) remained low.

The intermediate syndrome of OPP occurs within $24-96$ hours after acute poisoning and lasts for $5-18$ days. It is characterized by acute onset of second muscle weakness that typically involves classic muscle groups. Ventilatory support is necessary during this period, and weaning can be achieved safely by monitoring respiratory muscle performance, such as NIF, irrespective of E-AChe activity. A pathologic change may occur at the motor-end plate, producing failure of neuromuscular transmission.

▶ That such an intermediate syndrome should occur is not surprising in view of the "irreversible binding" of organic phosphates to acetylcholinesterase. However, this problem generally is not well recognized, hence the reason for inclusion of this abstract.—R.R. Kirby, M.D.

Reevaluation of Hemodynamic Consequences of Positive Pressure Ventilation: Emphasis on Cyclic Right Ventricular Afterloading by Mechanical Lung Inflation
Jardin F, Delorme G, Hardy A, Auvert B, Beauchet A, Bourdarias J-P (Hôp Ambroise Paré, Boulogne, France)
Anesthesiology 72:966–970, 1990   13–23

During controlled ventilation, the reduced right ventricular (RV) stroke volume during inflation is usually attributed to the decrease in venous return resulting from increased intrathoracic pressure. However, during lung inflation the transpulmonary pressure is suddenly increased, and may thereby increase the resistance to flow in all vessels exposed to alveolar pressure. This would exert an opposite effect, namely, increased RV output impedance. To evaluate the cyclic changes in RV function induced by controlled ventilation, right heart catheterization and 2-dimensional

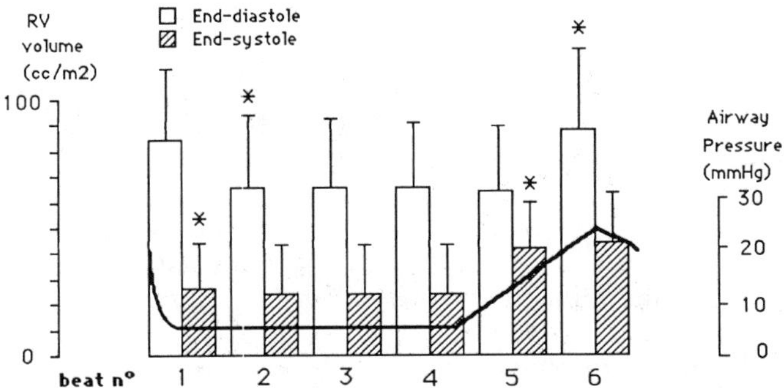

Fig 13–4.—Changes in RV volumes throughout the respiratory cycle, identified by the mean airway pressure change. Beats 1–4 occurred during expiration and beats 5 and 6 occurred during inspiration. Corresponding ejection fractions are as follows: .71,* .64,* .63, .37,* and .50*. *P < .05 vs. preceding beat. (Courtesy of Jardin F, Delorme G, Hardy A, et al: *Anesthesiology* 72:966–970, 1990.)

echocardiography were performed in 20 patients requiring respiratory support for acute respiratory failure. Simultaneous measurements of RV pressure, RV stroke output, and RV dimensions permitted a beat-to-beat evaluation of RV function throughout the mechanical respiratory cycle.

Compared with expiration, mechanical lung inflation produced a cyclic increase in RV systolic pressure and end-systolic volume, an increase in RV end-diastolic volume with no change in RV diastolic pressure, and markedly reduced RV ejection fraction (Fig 13–4). These data suggest that mechanical lung ventilation substantially affects RV function, primarily by increasing RV afterload during inflation.

▶ The data also may suggest that the patient was being excessively ventilated. Tidal volumes were 8–12 mL/kg and the shunt fraction was 35 ± 14%. These values suggest that certain lung areas probably were overventilated, with maximal pressure transmission to the involved pulmonary vasculature. This comment is not intended to decrease emphasis on the importance of right ventricular function and afterload; it is intended simply to point out that the way patients are ventilated plays an important role in how they respond clinically.— R.R. Kirby, M.D.

A Clinical Comparison of Indices of Pulmonary Gas Exchange With Changes in the Inspired Oxygen Concentration

Herrick IA, Champion LK, Froese AB (Queen's Univ, Kingston, Ont)
Can J Anaesth 37:69–76, 1990   13–24

Because precise estimation of the physiologic shunt fraction is difficult, several indices have been suggested as convenient substitutes in assessing pulmonary gas exchange. Various indices were compared relative to the behavior of the physiologic shunt as the inspired oxygen fraction (FiO$_2$) is altered clinically. Twelve adults receiving postoperative ventilatory support participated in the study. The mean age was 65 years. All patients but 1 were assessed within 2–6 hours after surgery.

The 10 hemodynamically stable patients had a mean physiologic shunt fraction of .166; 6 of them had a value exceeding .2 at some time. None of the indices (arterial-alveolar oxygen tension ratio, arterial oxygen tension-inspired oxygen concentration ratio, respiratory index, alveolar-arterial oxygen tension difference) consistently paralleled the behavior of the physiologic shunt as the FiO_2 changed. The mean difference in calculated shunt fraction using mixed rather than central venous blood gas tensions was .01.

No reliable index of physiologic shunt fraction is available in hemodynamically stable patients. Under less optimal clinical conditions, the indices probably are even less reliable. It remains necessary to calculate the physiologic shunt fraction when accurate evaluation of pulmonary gas exchange is critical.

▶ The question is whether a reliable index is necessary for good patient care. At present, calculation of the physiologic shunt fraction means that a pulmonary artery catheter must be inserted to obtain mixed venous blood. Although such monitoring is probably useful in selected patients, it is applied indiscriminately far too often. Curiously, I find that if the "numbers" agree with the clinical impression, they are incorporated into the decision-making process. If they don't, they are usually ignored, making one question why the catheter was inserted in the first place.—R.R. Kirby, M.D.

Continuous Positive Airway Pressure by Face Mask in *Pneumocystis carinii* Pneumonia
Gregg RW, Friedman BC, Williams JF, McGrath BJ, Zimmerman JE (George Washington Univ)
Crit Care Med 18:21–24, 1990   13–25

Eighteen men with AIDS who were in hypoxic respiratory failure because of *Pneumocystis carinii* pneumonia received continuous positive airway pressure (CPAP) by mask as a temporizing measure. The apparatus (Fig 13–5) sometimes was modified to provide a high inspired oxygen fraction at flow rates up to 90 L/min. Treatment began with 5 cm of water of CPAP and 100% oxygen at a flow rate of 60 L/min. Flow was adjusted until pressure variations throughout the respiratory cycle were less than 2 cm of water.

Of the 18 patients, 8 were hypoxemic when treatment began. The average time of mask CPAP was 4.5 days. All of the patients tolerated treatment, but conjunctivitis or skin necrosis on the nasal bridge developed in some patients because of mask leakage. Of the 18 patients, 7 died in the intensive care unit and 3 others died before hospital discharge. The only factor predictive of death was failure of CPAP; all 5 patients who required mechanical ventilation died in the hospital.

Continuous positive airway pressure by mask can support lung func-

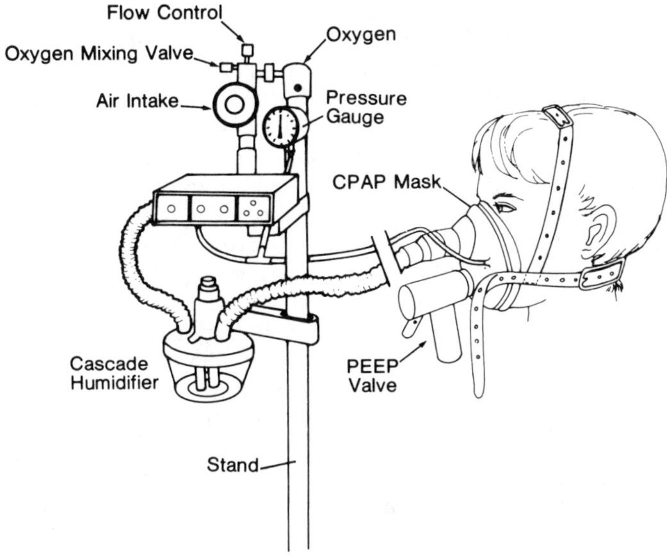

Fig 13–5.—Humidified oxygenated air is delivered to the patient at high flow, monitored by the pressure gauge, an oxygen monitor (not shown), and an alarm system to detect disconnections. The air intake may be connected to a 10-cm length of ventilator tubing to reduce noise. (Courtesy of Gregg RW, Friedman BC, Williams JF, et al: *Crit Care Med* 18:21–24, 1990.)

tion in patients with *P. carinii* pneumonia who are in hypoxic respiratory failure, and can allow conversation. The treatment can preclude the need for mechanical ventilation in those who choose to receive unlimited treatment.

▶ Face mask CPAP is useful in many forms of acute respiratory insufficiency. In view of the very negative connotation of tracheal intubation in patients with AIDS, an effective, largely noninvasive approach is welcome.—R.R. Kirby, M.D.

Positive Pleural Pressure Decreases Coronary Perfusion

Fessler HE, Brower RG, Wise R, Permutt S (Johns Hopkins Med Insts)
Am J Physiol 258:H814–H820, 1990   13–26

Maneuvers that increase pleural pressure raise pressure surrounding the heart (P_{SH}). This may reduce left ventricular oxygen demand by decreasing left ventricular afterload. However, coronary flow may also be directly impeded by positive P_{SH}. The effects of positive P_{SH} on coronary perfusion were assessed.

Pressure surrounding the heart was raised in 10-mm Hg increments from 0 to 60 mm Hg in an isolated canine heart-lung preparation with constant venous return, arterial pressure, and lung volume. Increased P_{SH} produced a rapid significant drop in left atrial transmural pressure (P_{LATM}) of up to a mean of 1.28 mm Hg. The drop was interpreted as a reflection of reduced left ventricular afterload with constant venous return and lung volume. However, at P_{SH} levels of more than 30 mm Hg, initial drops in P_{LATM} were followed by sustained increases, which suggests deterioration in cardiac function despite the lower level of afterload. Increased P_{SH} was also associated with reductions in circumflex coronary artery flow. When the circumflex coronary artery was dilated maximally with adenosine, P_{SH} effects were amplified, suggesting that positive P_{SH} mechanically impeded coronary flow. The aortic-coronary sinus lactate concentration difference dropped from .71 to .1 mM when P_{SH} was increased to 60 mm Hg for 90 seconds, suggesting myocardial ischemia.

Pressure surrounding the heart elevated at a constant cardiac output and arterial pressure produced evidence of myocardial ischemia. Thus, even in the absence of clinically apparent hemodynamic changes, increased pleural pressure may have unanticipated adverse effects on the balance of supply and demand for coronary perfusion.

▶ In any clinical setting the ultimate effect of an increase of P_{SH} depends on the balance of good effects (decrease of left ventricular afterload) and bad ones (decrease of coronary perfusion). It would be rare to have sustained P_{SH} of 30–60 mm Hg in the absence of cardiac tamponade, but intermittent increases to this level can certainly occur with positive-pressure mechanical ventilation.— R.R. Kirby, M.D.

Maximal Inspiratory Pressure Is Not a Reliable Test of Inspiratory Muscle Strength in Mechanically Ventilated Patients

Multz AS, Aldrich TK, Prezant DJ, Karpel JP, Hendler JM (Albert Einstein College of Medicine, Bronx)
Am Rev Respir Dis 142:529–532, 1990   13–27

Maximal inspiratory pressure (MIP) is a clinical test generally used to help predict whether weaning from ventilatory support will be successful. Although MIP has been validated as a reliable measure of inspiratory strength in normal subjects, it is not certain that it is reliable in patients receiving mechanical ventilation.

The reproducibility and reliability of MIP were evaluated in 14 patients receiving mechanical ventilation, all of whom were stable and capable of spontaneous inspiratory efforts. Maximal inspiratory pressure was assessed using the technique described by Marini and associates. Measurements were made in triplicate, by 1 to 5 experienced pulmonary physicians, on 1–7 successive days for each patient. A total of 396 measurements were performed.

The triplicate measurements had a coefficient of variation of 12 ± 1%. There was a wide range in the MIP results for a given patient on a given day among the various investigators (Fig 13–6). The difference between high and low estimates in a single patient on a single day averaged 40 ± 4% of the high estimate. Analysis of variance showed significant effects on MIP of patient, day of study, and investigator, but not of time of day.

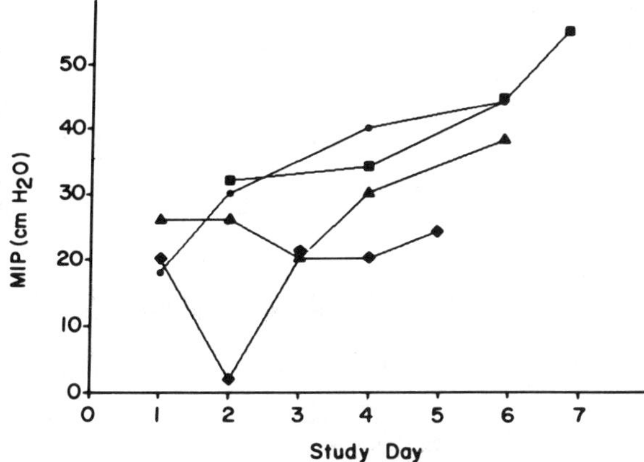

Fig 13–6.—Best MIP reported by each of 5 investigators for a patient over 7 consecutive days. The reported MIP values varied widely between different investigators and different days. The same investigator did not always report the best (or worst) MIP. (Courtesy of Multz AS, Aldrich TK, Prezant DJ, et al: *Am Rev Respir Dis* 142:529–532, 1990.)

Despite satisfactory reproducibility of MIP measurements on a single patient by a single investigator, the reliability of this measurement among patients receiving mechanical ventilation is poor. In many cases, differing MIP reports by different investigators of the same patient would have resulted in different estimates of weaning prognosis. Because "true" MIP is equal to or greater than measured MIP, the findings imply that MIP is often underestimated in these patients.

▶ I've been concerned for some time that the MIP not only is not a valid predictor of weaning ability but is also potentially dangerous. Prolonged inspiratory effort against an occluded airway, the method by which the test is performed, may predispose to so-called negative-pressure pulmonary edema. This potential complication may be increasingly problematic in patients who have already sustained some form of pulmonary damage that necessitated ventilatory support in the first place.— R.R. Kirby, M.D.

Efficiency of Airway Heat and Moisture Exchangers in Anesthetized Humans

Bickler PE, Sessler DI (Univ of California, San Francisco)
Anesth Analg 71:415–418, 1990   13–28

The efficiency of 5 commercially available airway heat and moisture exchangers was assessed in tracheally intubated patients receiving isoflurane-nitrous oxide-oxygen anesthesia during controlled ventilation. The Humid-Vent Filter, Humid-Vent 1, Pall Conserve, Siemens 150, and ThermoVent 600 were compared.

Each filter was placed between the Y-piece of the circle system and the endotracheal tube for 40 minutes. The parameters compared included absolute respiratory water loss, time to peak efficiency, and water-conserving ability during changing airway temperature.

All of the filters reached nearly maximum efficiency in reducing water loss within 10 minutes of application. The Humid-Vent Filter and Siemens 150 were the most efficient. Airway temperature rose rapidly by up to 8° C during all trials. Higher temperatures were reached with those filters that conserved water most efficiently. The respiratory heat conserved by the filters represented 5.5% to 7.2% of estimated total metabolic heat production during anesthesia. In practice, filter performance may vary because incompletely dried inspired gases tend to decrease actual heat loss, and because differing fresh gas flows may alter the temperature or humidity of inspired gas, and therefore the amount of heat lost.

▶ Bear in mind, however, that such devices produce an inordinate increase in both the inspiratory and expiratory work of breathing, thus significantly reducing their usefulness in spontaneously breathing patients and those treated with moderate to high levels of PEEP/CPAP.—R.R. Kirby, M.D.

Comparison of Conventional Mechanical Ventilation and High-Frequency Ventilation: A Prospective, Randomized Trial in Patients With Respiratory Failure
Hurst JM, Branson RD, Davis K Jr, Barrette RR, Adams KS (Univ of Cincinnati; Children's Hosp Med Ctr, Cincinnati)
Ann Surg 211:486–491, 1990   13–29

There are many reports attesting to the advantage of using high-frequency ventilation (HFV) in treating acute respiratory failure. The use of conventional mechanical ventilation was compared with the use of percussive HFV in a prospective series of 100 patients admitted to surgical intensive care. All were at risk for acute respiratory failure. The therapeutic end point consisted of a pH over 7.35, a $PaCO_2$ of 35–45 torr, and a $PaCO_2/FiO_2$ ratio exceeding 225.

Thirty-two patients on HFV and 28 on conventional respiration had acute respiratory failure. Patients on HFV reached the therapeutic end point at lower levels of continuous positive airway pressure and mean airway pressure, but there were no differences between the 2 groups in mortality, time in surgical intensive care, cardiovascular interventions, or incidence of barotrauma. Four patients failed to reach the therapeutic end point, and 3 died despite transfer to the other mode of ventilatory support. High-frequency ventilation offers no clear advantage over conventional mechanical ventilation in patients with adult respiratory distress syndrome, and its use should be limited to patients who are resistant to conventional ventilatory measures.

▶ High-frequency ventilation is now in its 23rd year of formal study and still has no clearly defined use in adult respiratory care. This is a well-written article with a careful analysis of data. It will not convince the proponents of such therapy that their faith is misplaced; I'm sure they will continue to search for a disease to be treated, and I will continue to await their results.—R.R. Kirby, M.D.

Heat and Moisture Exchangers and Vaporizing Humidifiers in the Intensive Care Unit
Martin C, Perrin G, Gevaudan M-J, Saux P, Gouin F (Hôp Sainte Marguerite, Marseille, France; Hôp Salvator, Marseille)
Chest 97:144–149, 1990   13–30

Mechanical ventilation with an endotracheal tube or tracheostomy in place bypasses the normal heat and moisture exchanging process. In a prospective study the use of a Pall Ultipor breathing circuit filter (PUBCF), a heat and moisture exchanger, was compared with the use of heated hot water systems (HHWSs) in 73 patients in the intensive care unit who required controlled mechanical ventilation. (The study ended when a patient with a PUBCF died of total obstruction of the tracheostomy tube.)

Six patients in the PUBCF group had tracheostomy tube occlusions, but none of those in the HHWS group had this complication. Thick, tenacious bronchial secretions also occurred only in the PUBCF group, and hypothermia was more frequent in this group. Contamination of breathing circuits was much more frequent in the HHWS group (54% vs. 11%).

The PUBCF did not adequately humidify inspired gases in this study. It did protect to some extent against contamination of breathing circuits, but about 10% of patients remained at risk for this complication. Use of the PUBCF may increase the occurrence of tracheal tube occlusion. This complication occurred only in patients whose minute ventilation was 10 L/min or higher.

► To the already well-documented problem of increased circuit resistance caused by heat and moisture exchangers, we must add the danger of airway obstruction. The old adage, "When something seems to be too good to be true, it probably isn't," seems to apply here. These devices are already commonplace in the operating room and are increasingly found in the intensive care unit. If they are used, it should only be with great care and probably for short periods of intrahospital transport. They simply are not as good as standard heated humidifiers, even though they are simple and inexpensive.—R.R. Kirby, M.D.

Cardiopulmonary Resuscitation

Buffer Agents Do Not Reverse Intramyocardial Acidosis During Cardiac Resuscitation
Kette F, Weil MH, von Planta M, Gazmuri RJ, Rackow EC (Univ of Health Sciences/The Chicago Med School, North Chicago)
Circulation 81:1660–1666, 1990   13–31

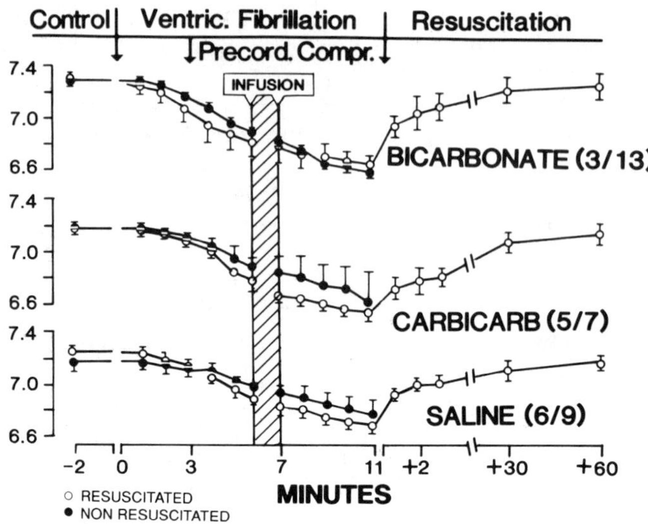

Fig 13−7.—Plot of effects of hypertonic sodium bicarbonate, Carbicarb, or sodium chloride on myocardial pH. No changes occurred in myocardial pH, and no differences in myocardial pH occurred between resuscitated and nonresuscitated animals. (Courtesy of Kette F, Weil MH, von Planta M, et al: *Circulation* 81:1660−1666, 1990.)

Buffer agents have been used aggressively during closed-chest cardiac resuscitation to neutralize decreases in myocardial pH and improve myocardial resuscitability. Results of a previous study using a porcine model of cardiac arrest suggested that sodium bicarbonate might augment the carbon dioxide load, exacerbating intracellular acidosis. To further investigate the effects of buffer agents, 2 of these agents were infused into the right atrium of pigs during cardiac resuscitation.

The animals were given sodium bicarbonate (a carbon dioxide-generating buffer), Carbicarb (a carbon dioxide-consuming buffer), or hypertonic sodium chloride (control solution). Continuous measurement of intramyocardial pH showed a progressive decrease from an average value of 7.26 before ventricular fibrillation to 6.87 before infusion of buffers.

After administration of the 2 buffer agents, systemic circulation and great cardiac vein pH significantly increased. Intramyocardial pH, however, continued to decline to an average of 6.62 after 11 minutes of ventricular fibrillation, a decline not affected by either buffer solution or the saline control (Fig 13−7). Resuscitability was closely related to coronary perfusion pressure at the time of direct-current countershock but not to pH, a finding reported in previous studies.

Under controlled experimental conditions of cardiac arrest, the administration of buffer agents had little benefit. Because these agents do not alter myocardial pH during the time frame of cardiopulmonary resuscitation, their use as a means of counteracting myocardial acidosis is of questionable value.

▶ Another nail in the coffin of sodium bicarbonate therapy during cardiopulmonary resuscitation. The peculiar observation I've made, however, is that many, if not most, clinicians continue to administer large amounts of this drug despite the adverse publicity from a multitude of studies since 1986. Even if one doesn't feel that bicarbonate causes additional problems such as worsening intramyocardial acidosis, *no* data show that its administration improves outcome. Enough is enough!—R.R. Kirby, M.D.

Effects of Bicarbonate Therapy on Tissue Oxygenation During Resuscitation of Hemorrhagic Shock

Mäkisalo HJ, Soini HO, Nordin AJ, Höckerstedt KAV (Helsinki Univ Central Hosp)
Crit Care Med 17:1170–1174, 1989   13–32

Transfusion of colloids assists hemodynamic recovery in hypovolemic shock. Hydroxyethyl starch (hetastarch) is effective in the treatment of hypovolemic shock of pigs, although acidosis resolves slowly. The effects of a 7.5% dose of bicarbonate on tissue oxygenation during treatment of hypovolemic shock with hetastarch were investigated in 12 piglets.

The 6 animals receiving colloid alone and the 6 receiving colloid plus bicarbonate recovered hemodynamically. However, tissue oxygen measurements recovered more slowly in the bicarbonate-treated group. The changes in cardiac output and mean arterial pressure are compared with oxygen pressure in Figure 13–8. Pulmonary artery wedge pressure and the arterial bicarbonate concentration were higher in the group given bicarbonate during early resuscitation than in the control group. Arterial plasma lactate levels were higher in the bicarbonate group at the end of the 40-minute follow-up period.

Bicarbonate adjunct therapy for hypovolemic shock has no beneficial effect on hemodynamics. The addition of bicarbonate may be harmful to tissue oxygenation when resuscitation involves hetastarch.

▶ This study adds to the growing body of literature suggesting that bicarbonate therapy in resuscitation is actually counterproductive. Published data increasingly suggest that such therapy treats a "number" (decreased pH) and may give the physician a sense of "doing something," but it is of little benefit and may actually be harmful to the patient.—R.R. Kirby, M.D.

Effects of Alkaline Buffer Administration on Survival and Myocardial Energy Metabolism in Pigs Subjected to Ventricular Fibrillation and Closed Chest CPR

Wiklund L, Ronquist G, Stjernström H, Waldenström A (Univ Hosp, Uppsala, Sweden)
Acta Anaesthesiol Scand 34:430–439, 1990   13–33

Bicarbonate administration can maintain the function of many enzyme systems, but rapid administration has produced metabolic alkalosis and impaired survival in patients requiring cardiopulmonary resuscitation (CPR). Bicarbonate was assessed in anesthetized piglets with ventricular

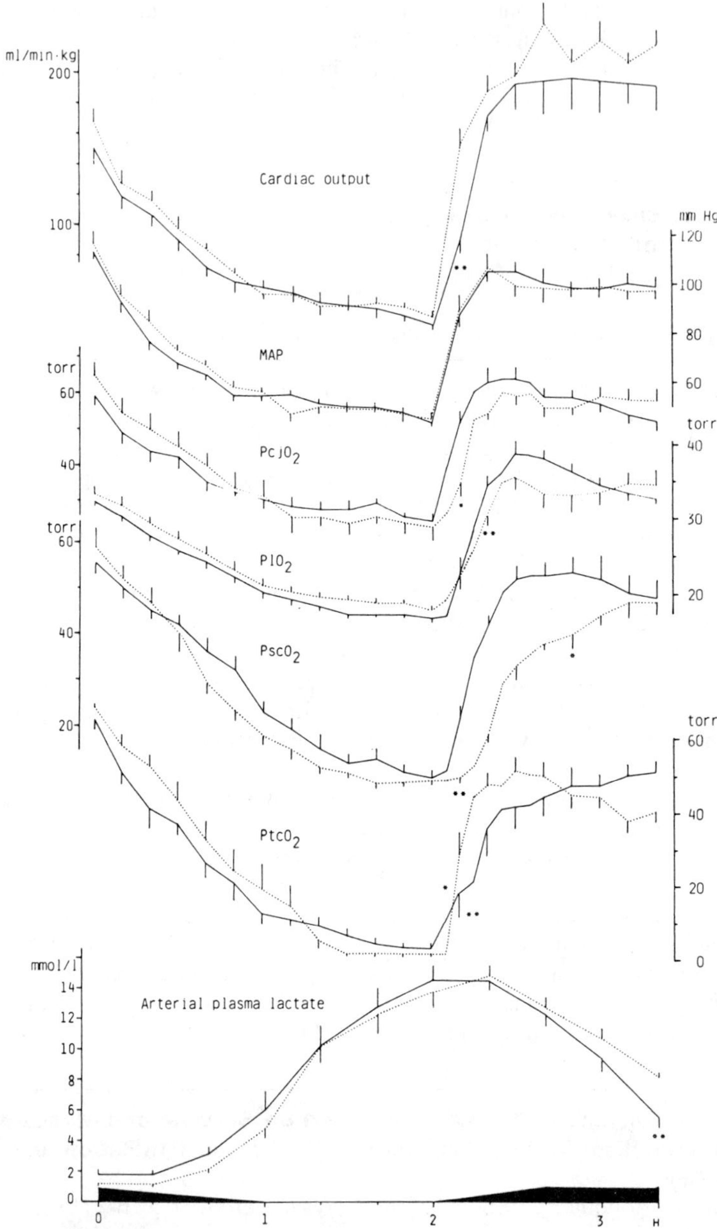

Fig 13–8.—Cardiac output, mean arterial pressure *(MAP)*, conjuctival oxygen pressure (Pcjo$_2$) liver tissue oxygen pressure (Plo$_2$) subcutaneous oxygen pressure (Psco$_2$) transcutaneous oxygen pressure (Ptco$_2$), and arterial plasma lactate values during the experiment. The 4 periods of the experiment are: bleeding (0–1 hour), shock (1–2 hours), volume restoration (2–2.67 hours), and follow-up (2.67–3.34 hours). Volume correction with hetastarch (control group (n = 6), *solid lines*), or hetastarch and sodium bicarbonate (NaHCO$_3$) (bicarbonate group (n = 6), *dotted lines*).Values are mean ± SEM. *Asterisk* indicates $P < .05$; *double asterisk*, $P < .01$; *triple asterisk*, $P < .001$. (Courtesy of Mäkisalo HJ, Soini HO, Nordin AJ, et al: *Crit Care Med* 17:1170–1174, 1989.)

fibrillation induced by a transthoracic DC shock. A 10-minute period of CPR followed induction of ventricular fibrillation. After 1 minute of CPR, animals received 50 nmol of either sodium bicarbonate or tris buffer mixture within 5 minutes. Other animals received normal saline. All groups received epinephrine.

Cardiopulmonary resuscitation was more often successful in animals given saline or tris buffer mixture. Survival correlated with a low myocardial creatine phosphate content and low base excess in blood. The myocardial adenosine triphosphate content did not correlate directly with survival. Bicarbonate administration produced higher base excess and carbon dioxide pressure values. The tris buffer mixture had a greater intracellular alkalinizing effect.

A tris buffer mixture appears to provide effective intracellular buffering while avoiding an excessive increase in carbon dioxide tension or base excess. Rapid infusion of bicarbonate can create excessive alkalosis and a high carbon dioxide pressure.

▶ Again, bicarbonate administration is shown to be deleterious. We shouldn't assume from this work that tris buffer is beneficial, however, because saline injection produced the same results. The message from this and other studies seems to be that bicarbonate therapy for cardiac arrest is bad. Other attempts at alkalinization don't make the problem worse, but they also don't make things better. Can we assume that buffer therapy during CPR is going the way of the dodo? How many patients have died as a result of what seems to be misdirected therapy?—R.R. Kirby, M.D.

Cardiac Effects of Carbon Dioxide-Consuming and Carbon Dioxide-Generating Buffers During Cardiopulmonary Resuscitation
Gazmuri RJ, von Planta M, Weil MH, Rackow EC (Univ of Health Sciences/ Chicago Med School, North Chicago)
J Am Coll Cardiol 15:482–490, 1990   13–34

The administration of sodium bicarbonate has long been recommended for correction of metabolic acidosis in patients undergoing cardiopulmonary resuscitation (CPR). But bicarbonate dissociates into carbon dioxide (CO_2) and water, thus potentially increasing CO_2. Because of the increased CO_2 load, administration of sodium bicarbonate is likely to decrease myocardial cell pH despite an increase in coronary pH. The hypothesis that buffer agents consuming, rather than generating, CO_2 would be more successful in reversing myocardial acidosis was tested.

The effects of hypertonic solutions of either the CO_2-"generating" sodium bicarbonate buffer, a mixture of sodium carbonate and sodium bicarbonate (Carbicarb) acting as a CO_2-"consuming" buffer, or saline placebo were compared during CPR in 25 miniature pigs. The animal model was designed to stimulate a typical "sudden death" event, with resuscitation initiated after 5 minutes and defibrillation within 13 minutes. Sodium bicarbonate and Carbicarb were administered to 8 pigs each and sodium chloride placebo to 9 pigs.

Neither the carbon dioxide pressure nor the lactate content of coronary vein blood was favorably altered by either buffer therapy. Each of the hypertonic solutions brought about a transient decrease in coronary perfusion pressure during precordial compression, a critical determinant of resuscitability. Four animals treated with bicarbonate, 5 treated with Carbicarb, and 6 receiving placebo were successfully resuscitated and had a comparable 24-hour survival rate.

Under experimental conditions, neither CO_2-generating nor CO_2-consuming buffers altered coronary vein carbon dioxide pressure or improved the outcome of CPR. Thus the routine use of these buffers is not supported.

▶ Carbicarb has seemed to be an attractive alternative to bicarbonate therapy and, in theory, might be expected to improve CPR outcome. Unfortunately, this study does not provide an optimistic viewpoint. A lot more work must be done in this area before any type of alkalinizing solution can be recommended.—R.R. Kirby, M.D.

Age-Related Effects of Compression Rate and Duration in Cardiopulmonary Resuscitation

Dean JM, Koehler RC, Schleien CL, Berkowitz I, Michael JR, Atchison D, Rogers MC, Traystman RJ (Johns Hopkins Med Insts)
J Appl Physiol 68:554–560, 1990   13–35

Few researchers have systematically studied the optimal compression rate and duration during cardiopulmonary resuscitation (CPR). The effects of various compression rate and duration combinations on chest geometry and cerebral perfusion pressure during CPR were studied in immature swine.

Pentobarbital-anesthetized piglets, 2 weeks and 8 weeks old, were given CPR after ventricular fibrillation. Duty cycle was increased from 10% to 80% by 10% increments at compression rates of 40, 60, 80, 100, 120, and 150/min. Pulsatile displacement, mean aortic and sagittal sinus pressures, and anterior chest wall deformity were evaluated.

A rising duty cycle increased cerebral perfusion pressure until chest relaxation time was compromised. In both age groups, inadequate chest recoil, development of static chest deformation, and limitation of pulsatile chest wall movement were seen when relaxation times were very short. These chest geometry changes correlated with deterioration of cerebral perfusion pressure in the 8-week-old piglets only. In the younger animals, perfusion pressures reached a plateau but did not deteriorate.

Duty cycle significantly affects cerebral perfusion pressure during conventional CPR in 2- and 8-week-old piglets. These findings stress the importance of duty cycle in generating cerebral perfusion pressure and suggest that younger animals can tolerate high compression rates, except at very long duty cycles.

▶ The problem of compression rate and duration has been argued for a good part of the past decade. A difference in the response of infants and young animals, compared to adults and older animals, does seem to exist. However, how effectively these observations can be translated into clinically useful algorithms has not yet been resolved.—R.R. Kirby, M.D.

Do Brainstem Auditory Evoked Potentials Detect the Actual Cessation of Cerebral Functions in Brain Dead Patients?

Barelli A, Della Corte F, Calimici R, Sandroni C, Proietti R, Magalini SI (Catholic Univ of the Sacred Heart, Rome)
Crit Care Med 18:322–323, 1990   13–36

Recording the brain stem auditory evoked potential (BAEP) is useful in detecting brain stem dysfunction and in predicting the neurologic outcome after severe head injury. To determine whether BAEPs can persist over the long term in postanoxic brain-dead patients, potentials were recorded in 18 such patients who lacked all evidence of cerebral or brain stem function. Most of the patients had head injuries.

There were no recognizable waveforms on either side in 4 patients. Wave I was present bilaterally in 6 patients; in 3 patients wave II also was recorded on at least 1 side. There was evidence of all peaks (of waveforms I–V) present bilaterally in 2 patients. It was possible for the BAEP waveforms to persist despite fulfillment of a complete set of brain death criteria (Fig 13–9).

Clinical findings such as apnea and brain stem areflexia only partially reflect the anatomofunctional state of the brain stem, and they are not sufficient for declaring brain death after a hypoxic cerebral insult. All patients with postanoxic encephalopathy should undergo BAEP recording before brain death is declared.

▶ The conclusion reached in this study is tenable only if one does not accept apnea and brain stem areflexia (with other tests including cerebral perfusion

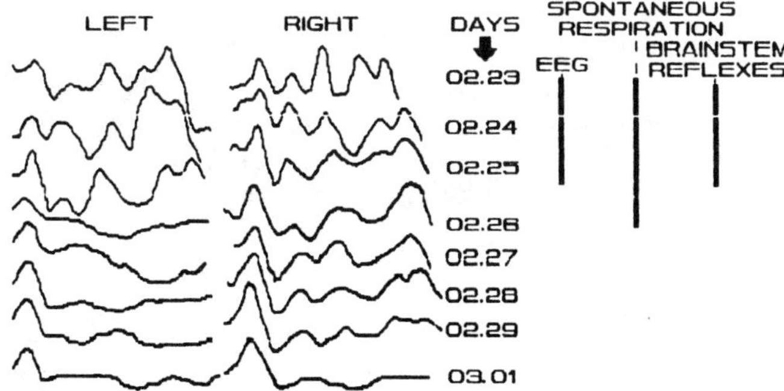

Fig 13–9.—The BAEP trend in patient 2 compared with ordinary brain death criteria. Right peaks persisted for approximately 3 days after cessation of cortical activity (electroencephalographic silence), spontaneous respiration, and brain stem reflexes. (Courtesy of Barelli A, Della Corte F, Calimici R, et al: *Crit Care Med* 18:322–323, 1990.)

studies) as an indication of irreversibility. When the usual precautions are taken (no depressant drugs on board, and so on), I've rarely, if ever, seen return to a functional level when these conditions prevailed. From any perspective, BAEPs are *not* essential in these circumstances.—R.R. Kirby, M.D.

Feasibility of Intracardiac Injection of Drugs During Cardiac Arrest

Jespersen HF, Granborg J, Hansen U, Torp-Pedersen C, Pedersen A (Copenhagen County Univ Hosp, Glostrup, Denmark)
Eur Heart J 11:269–274, 1990

13–37

The purpose of intracardiac injection (ICI) during cardiopulmonary resuscitation (CPR) is to introduce potentially life-saving drugs rapidly into the coronary circulation. Wider application of ICI has been hampered by repeated warnings of its dangers. On the other hand, practical experience with the systematic use of ICI in small series of patients has shown the risk to be quite acceptable for the circumstances. A 7-year experience with ICI in a large series of patients treated in a coronary care unit was reviewed.

Since 1967 ICI has been the routine method for administering inotropic drugs for cardiac arrest with ECG asystole or electromechanical dissociation occurring in the coronary care unit. Intracardiac injection is usually given by trained nurses who use the parasternal approach into the right ventricle, followed by continued external cardiac massage. During the 7-year study period, 543 ICIs were administered to 247 patients with cardiac arrest. Only 1 injection was given to 30% of the patients, 2 injections to 41%, 3 injections to 18%, and between 4 and 8 injections to 12%. Isoproterenol and epinephrine were the most commonly injected drugs.

Of the 247 patients treated with ICI, 122 could not be resuscitated; 45 died within 1 hour after CPR; 80 survived for more than 1 hour, 19 of whom were discharged alive. Autopsy was performed in 182 of the 228 fatal cases. A left-sided pneumothorax was demonstrated in 9 of the 80 patients who survived CPR for more than 1 hour and a right-sided pneumothorax in 2 patients. Eight of those 11 patients were treated with pleural drainage. Hemothorax was not demonstrated. A minor hemopericardium with no visible rupture of the myocardium or the aorta was found in another 3 patients who survived for more than 1 hour after ICI. Lesions of the coronary artery or myocardium attributable to the ICI were not seen. During cardiac arrest, drug treatment by ICI carried out by experienced staff with good technique presents a low risk that is quite acceptable for the circumstances.

▶ The 7.7% hospital discharge rate does not seem to be any better (and may be worse) than that reported in other studies in which ICI was not used as the standard approach to resuscitation. Why didn't the investigators have a comparable group of patients resuscitated by "conventional" measures? In my view, this study is potentially dangerous in advocating therapy based on poor scientific methodology.—R.R. Kirby, M.D.

14 Management of Pain

Postoperative

Reduction of Postoperative Morbidity Following Patient-Controlled Morphine

Wasylak TJ, Abbott FV, English MJM, Jeans M-E (McGill Univ; Montreal Gen Hosp)
Can J Anaesth 37:726–731, 1990   14–1

Patient-controlled analgesia (PCA) allows postsurgical pain management to be individualized, but its effects on morbidity remain uncertain. The influence of early PCA with morphine on functional recovery was examined in 38 women who had a hysterectomy. Patients either received morphine intravenously in the recovery room and intramuscularly on the ward on an as-needed basis, or they received a loading intravenous dose of 8 mg when pain began and then PCA for 48 hours. The amounts of morphine overall were similar in the 2 groups.

Pain control was better throughout with PCA and less variable over time. Minute ventilation recovered more rapidly in the PCA group. Oral temperature became normal a day earlier in this group and patients were ambulatory sooner and were discharged earlier. Patients who had PCA reported less discomfort 2 weeks after discharge; pain interfered less with daily activities and food intake.

Early self-titrated pain control enhances recovery from abdominal surgery. A more thorough understanding of how morphine, used in this way, promotes functional recovery may allow extension of these findings to more seriously ill patients.

▶ The use of PCA has been received enthusiastically by patients, physicians, and nursing personnel. Interestingly, there are few studies to demonstrate a decrease in the amount of medication administered or in postoperative morbidity. This is one of the few studies to demonstrate a decrease in postoperative morbidity. I wonder if this is because we are finally becoming sophisticated to the point of being able to assess postoperative progress in an intelligent manner.—G.W. Ostheimer, M.D.

Comparison of Two Methods of Intravenous Administration of Morphine for Postoperative Pain Relief

Zacharias M, Pfeifer MV, Herbison P (Southland Hosp, Invercargill, New Zealand)
Anaesth Intensive Care 18:205–209, 1990   14–2

Patient-controlled analgesia (PCA) was compared with continuous infusion of morphine in 60 patients in ASA class 1 and 2 who had major abdominal surgery. The PCA group received morphine, 1–3 mg/hr, in background infusion and demand bolus doses of .5 mg with a lockout interval of 10 minutes. Control patients received a dilute infusion of morphine solution at a rate of 1–4 mg/hr via a volume pump.

Most of the 60 patients underwent cholecystectomy via a midline incision. The total morphine requirement was significantly less in the PCA group. Pain scores were comparable in the 2 groups. One patient in the PCA group had significant respiratory depression in the immediate recovery period. Twice as many patients in the PCA group required an antiemetic.

Properly supervised continuous infusion of morphine is as effective as PCA for postoperative pain relief. The advantages of PCA have been exaggerated because it provides a better method of administering opiates than traditional intramuscular administration.

▶ I agree with the authors that intravenous infusion is preferable to intramuscular administration of opioids for pain relief. Going the next step to determine if continuous infusion is preferable to PCA may require consideration of factors as cost, nursing surveillance, and patient acceptance.—R.K. Stoelting, M.D.

Randomized Trial of Postoperative Patient-Controlled Analgesia vs Intramuscular Narcotics in Frail Elderly Men

Egbert AM, Parks LH, Short LM, Burnett ML (Univ of Kansas, Wichita; Wichita State Univ)
Arch Intern Med 150:1897–1903, 1990   14–3

The advantages of patient-controlled analgesia (PCA) theoretically would benefit the frail elderly patient, but most studies comparing it with intramuscular injections have involved younger, healthier individuals. In a prospective randomized study, 83 men older than 60 years who had major elective surgery were given PCA with morphine sulfate or intramuscular morphine injections as needed. More than half of the patients had chronic lung disease and more than 40% had coronary artery disease.

Analgesia was improved significantly by PCA, as judged from mean 3-day pain scores. No increase in sedation resulted from the use of PCA. Both postoperative confusion and severe pulmonary complications were significantly more frequent in patients given intramuscular injections than in those using PCA. Most patients rapidly mastered PCA, and those who previously received intramuscular injections reported that PCA was easier to use. Serum morphine levels on the first postoperative day were less variable with PCA.

Patient-controlled analgesia is a worthwhile approach to postoperative analgesia in high-risk elderly men of normal mental status. The technique has been used effectively in patients with liver or kidney disease, congestive heart failure, chronic obstructive lung disease, or psychiatric illness. Recovering alcoholics have also been managed successfully with PCA.

▶ This is a nice study that points out well the advantages of PCA. Even so, although PCA represents a major advance in postoperative pain relief, there are certainly problems with it not identified in this article.—R.D. Miller M.D.

Brachial Plexus Block With Opioids for Postoperative Pain Relief: Comparison Between Buprenorphine and Morphine

Viel EJ, Eledjam JJ, de la Coussaye JE, D'Athis F (Centre Hosp Univ, Nimes, France)
Reg Anesth 14:274–278, 1989   14–4

The efficacy and side effects of opioid injection into the brachial plexus for postoperative relief of pain were evaluated in 40 patients aged 18–90 years who underwent surgery on an upper extremity under brachial plexus block via the supraclavicular technique. In addition to 40 mL of .5% bupivacaine, 20 patients received morphine hydrochloride, 50 µg/ kg, and 20 received buprenorphine hydrochloride, 3 µg/kg. Using a 3-point pain scale, the quality of analgesia in the 2 groups was compared every hour for 6 hours, every 2 hours for the next 6 hours, and then at 12, 24, 36, and 48 hours.

Analgesia was consistently superior with buprenorphine, compared to morphine, and the duration of analgesia was nearly twice as long. The side effects were pruritus in 2 patients who received morphine and nausea (3 patients) and vomiting (1 patient) among those who were given buprenorphine. There were no differences in hemodynamic parameters between the 2 groups, and respiratory indices were not depressed in either group.

Buprenorphine injected into the brachial plexus sheath provides superior and longer lasting postoperative analgesia than morphine. There are no major side effects with buprenorphine.

▶ That pain relief can be provided by the introduction of opioids in a brachial plexus block is intriguing and controversial. I would caution the readers in concluding that this can clearly be accomplished. This study would have been strengthened by a group to which no narcotics were given.—R.D. Miller, M.D.

Using the McGill Pain Questionnaire to Study Common Postoperative Complications

Cohen MM, Tate RB (Univ of Manitoba, Winnipeg)
Pain 39:275–279, 1989   14–5

Many patients have postoperative adverse events that are considered to be "minor" but can compromise the quality of care. Overall patient satisfaction may well depend on the postoperative experience. The McGill

Pain and Nausea Questionnaires were used to quantify sore throat, muscle pain, headache, backache, and nausea in 253 patients, accounting for 8% of all surgical patients seen in a 3-month period. They had received inhalational or, for backache patients, spinal anesthesia.

The 25 most frequently chosen words were capable of distinguishing between the 4 pain-related problems. Five words (sore, tender, tiring, annoying, troublesome) were selected most frequently by all groups of patients. The only word uniquely chosen for backache was "miserable." Use of the 10 most common words correctly classified backache in 52% of patients, headache in 92%, muscle pain in 80%, and sore throat in 86%.

Except for backache, the Visual Present Pain Intensity scale correlated well with the standard-form word choices. They apparently measure the same dimension of intensity for these complaints.

▶ Cohen and Tate applied a series of methods to validate "words" used for pain. The "words" patients found most effective in analyzing pain were "sore," "tender," "tiring," "annoying," and "troublesome." One would question why the authors didn't just use a visual score for pain. Perhaps because they wanted to be able to continue to use the pain score during phone conversations and for phone follow-up. Anyone interested in doing pain research is commended to read this article; anyone doing clinical pain research almost certainly needs to read this article before starting that project; and anyone treating chronic pain should read this article to better understand what patients are saying when they talk to you.— M.F. Roizen, M.D.

Additional Reading

Strømskag KE, Minor B, Steen PA: Side effects and complications related to interpleural analgesia: An update. *Acta Anaesthesiol Scand* 34:473–477, 1990.

Chronic

A Controlled Trial of Transcutaneous Electrical Nerve Stimulation (TENS) and Exercise for Chronic Low Back Pain
Deyo RA, Walsh NE, Martin DC, Schoenfeld LS, Ramamurthy S (Univ of Washington; Univ of Texas, San Antonio)
N Engl J Med 322:1627–1634, 1990   14–6

The efficacy of transcutaneous electrical nerve stimulation (TENS), a program of stretching exercises, and a combination of both was studied in patients who had had low back pain for a median of 4.1 years. The patients were randomly assigned to treatment groups: 36 had daily treatment with TENS, 36 had sham TENS, 37 had TENS plus exercises, and 36 had sham TENS plus exercises.

After 1 month, there were no clinically or statistically significant treatment effects of TENS on any of 11 indicators of outcome. There was also no interactive effect between TENS and exercise. Overall, pain indicators improved by 47% with TENS and by 42% with sham TENS, which was not a significant difference. Patients in the exercise groups had significant improvements in self-rated pain scores, a decrease in the frequency of pain, and higher levels of activity compared with patients in the nonexercise groups. The mean reported improvement in the exercise groups' pain scores was 52%, compared with 37% in the nonexercise groups. After 2 months, however, most patients had stopped exercising and the initial improvements were gone.

Treatment with TENS is no more effective than treatment with a placebo in patients with chronic low back pain. Treatment with TENS adds no apparent benefit to that achieved with exercise alone.

▶ So much for TENS for chronic low back pain!—G.W. Ostheimer, M.D.

Quantification of Biomedical Findings of Chronic Pain Patients: Development of an Index of Pathology
Rudy TE, Turk DC, Brena SF, Stieg RL, Brody MC (Univ of Pittsburgh; Pain Control and Rehabilitation Inst of Georgia, Decatur)
Pain 42:167–182, 1990   14–7

Chronic pain is a complex phenomenon that includes psychosocial and behavioral aspects that interact with pathologic changes to produce an integrated perceptual experience and behavioral response. Problems in assessing and quantifying the biomedical signs and symptoms that may be related to reports of pain were addressed.

Twenty-three biomedical procedures commonly used to evaluate patients with chronic pain were subjected to reliability testing. An initial study showed that 17 of the 23 procedures can be applied in the clinical setting with an acceptable level of reliability. Fifty-five consecutively referred patients with chronic pain and 5 physicians participated. The procedures were combined into a standardized Medical Examination and Diagnostic Information Coding System, the MEDICS, a form designed to be simple, self-explanatory, and economical. Procedures demonstrating excellent clinical significance included a test for soft tissue trigger points, the plain radiograph, the thermogram, electromyography, CT, and contrast radiography.

A weighted scoring approach was developed, based on current medical consensus, to yield a general index of pathology that is independent of the number of procedures used to assess patients. The MEDICS approach may be used with a heterogeneous group of patients.

▶ This is an intriguing article. Wouldn't it be wonderful if we had some numerical way of objectively quantitating the intensity of pain, especially based on biochemical derived data?—R.D. Miller, M.D.

Celiac Plexus Neurolysis With the Modified Transaortic Approach
Lieberman RP, Waldman SD (Univ of Nebraska; Pain Consortium of Greater Kansas City, Leawood, Kan)
Radiology 175:274–276, 1990   14–8

Celiac plexus neurolysis frequently is used to treat pain from upper abdominal cancer that resists systemic narcotic analgesics. Errors in needle placement are common with the classic posterolateral approach. As an alternative, a transaortic technique was tried in 124 patients with pain resulting from intra-abdominal malignancy—most often pancreatic or colon cancer. Fifty-four blocks were performed on an outpatient basis; CT guidance was used in all cases.

Technique.—The skin entry site is below the 12th rib about 7 cm to the left of the midline. A 20-gauge Hinck needle is advanced through the anesthetized skin toward the aorta (Fig 14–1), and the course is confirmed by CT scanning (Fig 14–2). After aspiration of aortic blood, the needle is advanced slowly through the anterior wall of the vessel, and the aspiration test is repeated. If no blood is obtained, iothalamate meglumine 60% mixed with bupivacaine is injected, and a CT scan is obtained to confirm appropriate spread. Dehydrated alcohol is injected; the patient remains prone for 20 minutes and supine for another 20 minutes.

Marked relief of pain occurred in 91% of patients, and 43% required no narcotic analgesic. One patient reported worse pain after the procedure. Pain relief persisted at 6 weeks. Ten patients required intravenous fluids for hypotension and 4 of them received ephedrine as well. In no case did orthostatic hypotension last longer than 24 hours. The transaortic approach now is preferred for celiac plexus neurolysis.

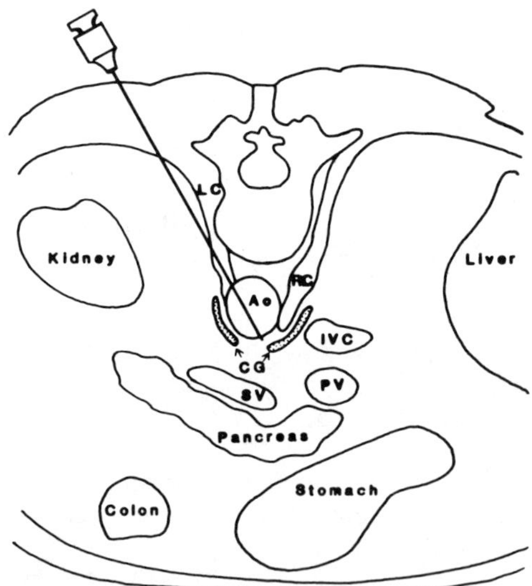

Fig 14–1.—Transaortic approach to celiac plexus neurolysis. Cross-sectional diagram at the L1 vertebral level. Patient lies prone, and the skin entry site is below the 12th rib. *Abbreviations:* CG, celiac ganglia; *Ao,* aorta; *LC,* left crus; *RC,* right crus; *SV,* splenic vein; *PV,* portal vein; *IVC,* inferior vena cava; *C,* colon; *K,* kidney; *S,* stomach; *P,* pancreas, *L,* liver. (Courtesy of Lieberman RP, Waldman SD: *Radiology* 175:274–276, 1990.)

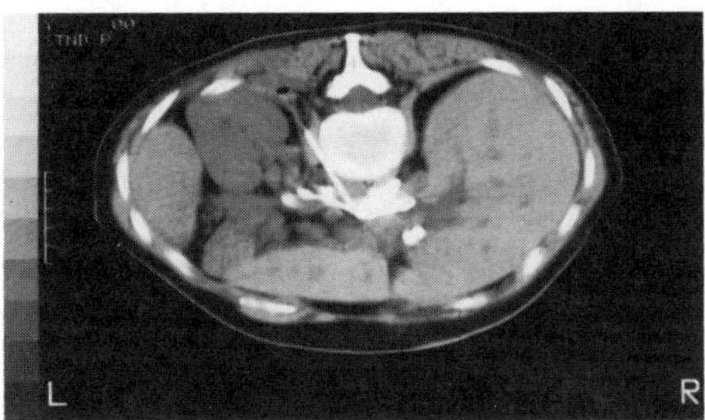

Fig 14–2.—Spread of contrast material anterior to crura indicates correct needle position for alcohol injection. *L,* left. (Courtesy of Lieberman RP, Waldman SD: *Radiology* 175:274–276, 1990.)

▶ Although this looks to be a very reasonable approach to the celiac plexus, the authors provide no objective data as to the superiority of this technique over others.—R.D. Miller, M.D.

Has the Analgesic Efficacy of Neurolytic Celiac Plexus Block Been Demonstrated in Pancreatic Cancer Pain?

Sharfman WH, Walsh TD (Cleveland Clinic Found; Cleveland Clinic Cancer Ctr)
Pain 41:267–271, 1990   14–9

Except for a small number of patients who have curative operations, there is no definite treatment for pancreatic cancer, and palliation of symptoms should be the prime concern in most cases. The optimal therapy for pancreatic cancer pain has not been established, but oral opiates remain the mainstay. Although neurolytic celiac plexus block (NCPB) is claimed by some to be the most effective, least hazardous treatment for pancreatic cancer pain, few patients undergo this procedure.

During the past 25 years 15 reports on the use of NCPB for pancreatic cancer pain have been published in the English literature. A review of these series yielded data on 480 patients with pancreatic cancer who underwent NCPB for pain. Of the 480, 418 were considered to have had at least a satisfactory response. The reported response rates were consistently high within individual series, and ranged from 70% to 95%.

However, a critical review of these studies revealed several major deficiencies in all 15. None of the studies was prospective or had a randomized controlled design. Quantitative pain assessment was carried out before performing NCPB in only 1 series. None of the series reported specifics on analgesics or dosages used before NCPB. Information on patients after NCPB was also limited because post-NCPB pain was quantitatively assessed in only 4 series. Only 8 studies provided information on whether the benefits of the block lasted until death. Data from the 6 largest series of patients having NCPB are shown in the table.

Although a review of the literature suggests that NCPB in the management of pancreatic cancer pain is safe when performed by an experienced anesthesiologist, the data do not confirm that NCPB is effective in pro-

Efficacy Data From 6 Largest Series of NCPB in PCP

Series (N = patients)

	Bridenbaugh et al.	Moore et al.	Thompson et al.	Hagedus	Orwitz and Sundararao	Brown et al.
Pre-NCPB						
Were all patients on opiates?	−	−	−	−	+	−
Were analgesic dosages specified?	−	−	−	−	−	−
Was there a quantitative assessment of pain?	−	−	−	−	−	−
Was there a qualitative assessment of pain?	−	−	+	−	−	−
Post-NCPB						
Were patients able to stop or decrease opiates?	+	+	+	+	+	−
Were analgesic dosages specified?	−	−	−	−	−	−
Was there a quantitative assessment of pain?	+ *	−	−	+ *	−	−
Was there a qualitative assessment of pain?	−	+ *	+ *	−	+ *	+ *
Was the duration of relief specified?	+	+	−	−	+	−

Note: +, data reported; −, data not reported.
*Time not specified.
(Courtesy of Sharfman WH, Walsh TD: *Pain* 41:267–271, 1990.)

viding acute or long-term analgesia, nor are the indications for its use clearly defined. Thus NCPB should be considered an option in the management of pancreatic cancer pain, but it cannot be recommended as the treatment of choice on the basis of available data.

▶ This group is challenging the widespread view that an NCPB is effective therapy for the treatment of pancreatic cancer pain. Based on a review of the literature, the authors question this conclusion. On a nonscientific basis, I have performed NCPBs for 14 years in such patients and believe it is quite effective. Do we need further studies? Does the choice of neurolytic agent matter (e.g., phenol vs. alcohol)?—R.D. Miller, M.D.

Additional Reading

Fernandez E: Headaches associated with low spinal fluid pressure. *Headache* 30:122–128, 1990.

Zatzick DF, Dimsdale JE: Cultural variations in response to painful stimuli. *Psychosom Med* 52:544–557, 1990.

G

Gaba DM, 97, 107
Gadalla F, 223
Galicich J, 149
Galimberti CA, 49
Gamsu HR, 56
Ganansia M-F, 205
Gandolfi AJ, 35
Garman JK, 124
Gatt S, 191
Gatti G, 49
Gaudreault P, 143
Gazmuri RJ, 347, 351
Gee MH, 336
Geurts JWM, 178
Gevaudan M-J, 347
Ghignone M, 177
Gholkar VR, 173
Giner JS, 324
Giudici MC, 218
Glosten B, 97
Glynn MFX, 283, 284
Gnanadev DA, 170
Goitein KJ, 188
Golan M, 304
Gold BS, 152
Goldberg ME, 208
Goldfarb G, 34
Goldman G, 176
Goldsmith CH, 11, 12
Goldstein DE, 168
Gomez GA, 90
Gomez-Arnau J, 236
Goodarzi S, 330
Goodman NW, 206
Goodnough LT, 306
Goor DA, 304
Gorbutt N, 295
Gottfried SB, 336
Gottlieb JE, 336
Gouin F, 104, 347
Gould SA, 317
Goulet B, 143
Granborg J, 354
Gravenstein JS, 96
Gravenstein N, 114
Graybeal JM, 248
Green S, 151
Green W, 112
Greenall F, 56
Greenough A, 56
Gregg RW, 342
Gregoire FM, 205
Grimbergen CA, 26
Grinand MR, 205
Grolleau D, 161
Gross D, 328
Gross JB, 126
Grossman JE, 110
Groth S, 275
Grounds RM, 323
Grunau RVE, 178
Guay J, 143

Gueller GE, 325
Guerraty AJ, 285
Guiblin H, 295
Guillen J-C, 104
Guinard J-P, 124
Guiney TE, 174
Gunther RA, 316
Gupta B, 258
Guzman RF, 307
Gwinnutt CL, 57

H

Haasio J, 120
Haberer JP, 264
Hackl W, 138
Haig MJ, 186
Haisch CE, 115
Hall J, 334
Hall RI, 160
Hamer-Hodges DW, 309
Hamilton WK, 11, 12
Hammond JS, 90
Hammond WG, 312
Hannallah RS, 145, 179
Hanning CD, 245, 291
Hansen DD, 181
Hansen TW, 36
Hansen U, 354
Hardin NJ, 115
Hardy A, 340
Hardy J-F, 106
Harken AH, 285
Harlow DJ, 322
Harmer M, 226
Harmey J-L, 225
Harper NJN, 43, 57
Harris CE, 323
Harrison GG, 7
Hart BB, 69
Haselby KA, 148
Hashimoto H, 156
Hatano Y, 54
Hatley RM, 183
Hauch MA, 47
Hawkey C, 295
Hawkins ML, 116
Head N, 101
Healy JMS, 134
Hechtman HB, 176
Hedderich GS, 285
Heffron JJA, 134
Heier T, 249
Heilbronn Y, 117
Hempelmann G, 167
Hendler JM, 344
Hendrickson M, 308
Henriksen E, 81, 85
Henthorn TK, 267
Henzel D, 72
Herbison P, 355
Herrick IA, 341
Hershenson MB, 180

Hibbard BM, 200
Hickey PR, 181
Hickey S, 114
Hill J, 60
Hinman DJ, 185
Hirakawa M, 270
Ho ET, 146
Höckerstedt KAV, 349
Hodge B, 95
Hoekje PL, 244
Høgskilde S, 42
Holcroft JW, 112
Holley FO, 263
Holley HS, 26
Hollingsworth-Fridlund P, 331
Hollmén AI, 222
Hompland SJ, 256
Hopeman A, 285
Horiguchi R, 156
Hornbein TF, 168
Horrow JC, 68
Horton JW, 324
Hosking MP, 162, 269, 289
Houghton PWJ, 5
Hovorka J, 292, 294
Howard RA, 211
Howard RJ, 89
Howell CG, 183
Howie MB, 61
Hoyt DB, 331
Huang SKS, 277
Hubbard AK, 35
Hull CJ, 268
Hultén JO, 133
Humphrey H, 334
Hunter DN, 63
Hurley RJ, 122
Hurst JM, 346
Huttunen P, 222
Hwang SS, 41
Hynson J, 97

I

Isern S, 36
Isert P, 191
Ivankovich AD, 256

J

Jacobi M, 167
Jacobs HK, 77
Jacobs S, 313
Jacquinot P, 225
Jardin F, 340
Järvinen A, 163
Jawan B, 121
Jeans M-E, 355
Jensen G, 275
Jensen TK, 91
Jespersen HF, 354
Joel S, 39

BUSINESS REPLY MAIL

FIRST CLASS   PERMIT No. 135   ST. LOUIS, MO.

POSTAGE WILL BE PAID BY ADDRESSEE

PAT NEWMAN
Mosby-Year Book, Inc.
11830 Westline Industrial Drive
P.O. Box 46908
St. Louis, Missouri 63146-9988

FREE Examination Privileges

Yes! I'd like to review a new Year Book. Please send me a FREE 30-day examination copy of the book(s) checked below:

[ ] Year Book of **Anesthesia**® (22137)	$57.95
[ ] Year Book of **Cardiology**® (22114)	$57.95
[ ] Year Book of **Critical Care Medicine**® (22091)	$54.95
[ ] Year Book of **Dermatology**® (22108)	$57.95
[ ] Year Book of **Diagnostic Radiology**® (22132)	$57.95
[ ] Year Book of **Digestive Diseases**® (22081)	$57.95
[ ] Year Book of **Drug Therapy**® (22139)	$57.95
[ ] Year Book of **Emergency Medicine**® (22085)	$57.95
[ ] Year Book of **Endocrinology**® (22107)	$57.95
[ ] Year Book of **Family Practice**® (20801)	$54.95
[ ] Year Book of **Geriatrics and Gerontology** (22121)	$54.95
[ ] Year Book of **Hand Surgery**® (22096)	$57.95
[ ] Year Book of **Hematology**® (20418)	$54.95
[ ] Year Book of **Health Care Management**® (21145)	$54.95
[ ] Year Book of **Infectious Diseases**® (20420)	$54.95
[ ] Year Book of **Infertility** (20414)	$54.95
[ ] Year Book of **Medicine**® (22087)	$57.95
[ ] Year Book of **Neonatal-Perinatal Medicine** (22117)	$54.95
[ ] Year Book of **Neurology and Neurosurgery**® (22120)	$57.95
[ ] Year Book of **Nuclear Medicine**® (22140)	$57.95
[ ] Year Book of **Obstetrics and Gynecology**® (22118)	$57.95
[ ] Year Book of **Occupational and Environmental Medicine** (22092)	$57.95
[ ] Year Book of **Oncology** (20415)	$54.95
[ ] Year Book of **Ophthalmology**® (22135)	$57.95
[ ] Year Book of **Orthopedics**® (20417)	$54.95
[ ] Year Book of **Otolaryngology – Head and Neck Surgery**® (22086)	$57.95
[ ] Year Book of **Pathology and Clinical Pathology**® (22104)	$57.95
[ ] Year Book of **Pediatrics**® (22088)	$54.95
[ ] Year Book of **Plastic and Reconstructive Surgery**® (22112)	$57.95
[ ] Year Book of **Psychiatry and Applied Mental Health**® (22110)	$57.95
[ ] Year Book of **Pulmonary Disease**® (22109)	$54.95
[ ] Year Book of **Speech Language and Hearing** (21144)	$59.95
[ ] Year Book of **Sports Medicine**® (20419)	$54.95
[ ] Year Book of **Surgery**® (22084)	$57.95
[ ] Year Book of **Ultrasound** (21170)	$75.00
[ ] Year Book of **Urology**® (20416)	$54.95
[ ] Year Book of **Vascular Surgery**® (22105)	$57.95

*All Year Books are published annually. For your convenience, we will add your name to our subscriber list and send you an announcement of each future volume about 2 months before publication. The new volume will be shipped to you unless you complete and return the cancellation notice enclosed with the announcement and we receive it within the time indicated. Don't forget, you may cancel your subscription at any time. The Year Book is yours FREE for 30 days, and may be returned for full credit. Return postage is guaranteed.

NAME/ACCT. NO.

ADDRESS

CITY/STATE/ZIP

Prepaid orders are shipped postage free; add $3.50 per order to cover handling. Other orders will be billed a shipping and handling charge. Please add applicable sales tax. Prices quoted in U.S. dollars. Canadian orders will be billed in U.S. funds. All prices subject to change without notice.

Mosby-Year Book, Inc. • 11830 Westline Industrial Drive • St. Louis, MO 63146

MC-0277